AFTER ANESTHESIA

A Guide for PACU, ICU, and Medical-Surgical Nurses

Kay E. Fraulini, M.S.N., R.N.
Staff Nurse Recovery Room Guy's Hospital
London, England
Formerly, Staff Nurse and Practitioner/Teacher
Post Anesthesia Care Unit
Rush-Presbyterian–St. Luke's Medical Center
Instructor, College of Nursing
Rush University
Chicago, Illinois

564748

**Appleton
&Lange**
Norwalk, Connecticut/ Los Altos, California

JACKSON LIBRARY
LANDER COLLEGE
GREENWOOD, S.C. 29646

0-8385-0078-1

87 88 89 90 91/ 10 9 8 7 6 5 4 3 2 1

Prentice-Hall of Australia, Pty. Ltd., Sydney
Prentice-Hall of Canada, Inc.
Prentice-Hall Hispanoamericana, S.A., Mexico
Prentice-Hall of India Private Limited, New Delhi
Prentice-Hall International (UK) Limited, London
Prentice-Hall of Japan, Inc., Tokyo
Prentice-Hall of Southeast Asia (Pte.) Ltd., Singapore
Whitehall Books Ltd., Wellington, New Zealand
Editora Prentice-Hall do Brasil Ltda., Rio de Janeiro

Library of Congress Cataloging-in-Publication Data

Fraulini, Kay E.
  After anesthesia.

  Includes index.
  1. Anesthesia. 2. Therapeutics, Surgical.
3. Surgical nursing. I. Title. [DNLM: 1. Anesthesia—
methods—nurses' instruction. 2. Anesthesia—nursing.
3. Postoperative Period—nurses' instruction.
4. Recovery Room—nurses' instruction.
WY 154 F845a]
RD82.F73   1987   617'.96   86-28712
ISBN 0-8385-0078-1

Design: Kathleen Peters

To my father, **Leno Fraulini,** *in loving memory.*

Contributors

Diane Randall Andrews, M.S., R.N.
Formerly, Unit Leader, Post Anesthesia Care Unit, Rush-Presbyterian–
St. Luke's Medical Center, Chicago, Illinois

Anne C. Borchardt, B.S.N., R.N.
Formerly, Staff Nurse-C, Post Anesthesia Care Unit, Rush-Presbyterian–
St. Luke's Medical Center, Chicago, Illinois

Nancy J. Brent, R.N., M.S., J.D.
Nurse-Attorney in Solo Law Practice, and Associate Professor of
Nursing, Graduate Program, St. Xavier College, Chicago, Illinois

Daniel W. Gorski, D.D.S., M.D.
Chairman, Department of Anesthesiology, Louis A. Weiss Memorial
Hospital, Assistant Professor, Loyola University School of Dentistry,
Maywood, Illinois

Franklin B. McKechnie, M.D.
Immediate past President, American Society of Anesthesiologists, Winter
Park Memorial Hospital, Winter Park, Florida

Kay Atkinson Wright, C.R.N.A.
Staff Anesthetist, Louis A. Weiss Memorial Hospital, Chicago, Illinois

Contents

Foreword

This book easily imparts the sense of the strong commitment that Kay Fraulini has to improve the quality of care for patients who are recovering from anesthesia. The theme of striving for excellence permeates the entire volume. The interesting way in which the contents are organized appears designed to invite all her peers in this specialty area to join with her in a search for excellence. The contents provide a strong baseline for this endeavor and have all the elements in place as the norms for high quality care.

The scholarly discussion of the literature ranges widely over each component of postanesthesia care. The review of clinical studies coupled with astute clinical observations enables the reader to gain insight into the demanding requirements of nursing care in this setting. The means of applying science to nursing care in a carefully reasoned way is highlighted. The effectiveness of this type of endeavor is portrayed through the use of many specific case examples. When the process of care is modeled by using the methods of science as a rigorous conceptual approach, understanding is facilitated and becomes feasible.

The nuances of the pharmacology and anesthesia and subtle variations of how each drug differs in effect on individual patients is one of the major strengths of this volume. While the present state of the art is thoroughly depicted, the promise of the future is greatly enhanced. From this base, significant adjustment to new knowledge can be managed more easily. Competence is inherent in the way data are presented. If every patient undergoing anesthesia received the quality of clinical nursing care portrayed in this volume, a highly desirable advancement in nursing practice will have taken place.

Luther P. Christman, Ph.D., R.N., F.A.A.N.
Chicago, Illinois

Preface

It is with a commitment to the professional practice of nursing—and beyond that, to the specialty of perianesthetic nursing—that I have written *After Anesthesia*. The need for nurses to explicate nursing practice in this highly specialized arena is beyond question. I have examined postanesthesia nursing within a conceptual frame of reference, which eliminates the need to address the various surgical specialties and specific postoperative care of postanesthetic patients. Instead, the commonalities of complications and nursing care, which transect surgical specialties, are grouped into concepts. Problems in oxygenation and tissue perfusion, immobility, pain and perception, for example, are described to show how they relate to the nursing process in any postanesthetic nursing situation.

I do not discuss whether or not the recovery room is a critical care unit. I believe that debate has been resolved and that postanesthesia recovery has assumed its unequivocal place in critical care. There is some confusion, however, over what to call the unit that has previously been known as the RR or PAR. I recognize and accept the American Society of Post Anesthesia Nurses recommendation that the area be known as the Post Anesthesia Care Unit (PACU).

Chapter 1 provides a look at the past. Knowledge of our roots is important as we define and redefine the rapidly changing profile of the perianesthetic nurse. Much attention is devoted in this book to the postanesthesia nurse. Theory and research surrounding the concept of that role is presented, divided into five components: practice, education, research, consultation, and administration. Greater knowledge of self and role is essential for the PACU nurse intent on furthering professional development and increasing effectiveness within the larger organizational structure.

Not to be forgotten, of course, is the PACU nurse's almost constant collaboration with the anesthesiologist. Because we interface with these medical specialists on a daily basis, consideration must be given in any PACU nursing text to the practice of anesthesiology. My colleagues and mentors in anesthesia have contributed the chapters on medical practice.

The concluding chapters attempt a look at the future. As you read this, however, the future may have become the present. One of the greatest challenges facing scientists is the processing and dissemination of information prior to its obsolescence. The knowledge explosion which has occurred over the past 25 years continues to escalate. Increased technology will continue to exert a profound influence on nursing. Nursing, and especially PACU nursing, must respond with increased efforts toward building a systematized body of knowledge based on research. To this end, a research thread has been woven throughout *After Anesthesia*. It is my intention to contribute to the science of PACU nursing.

This is an intermediate text on anesthetic care, neither a fundamental nor an exhaustive work on the subject. It is a clinical reference, to be used by nurses taking care of the preanesthetic and postanesthetic patient. I have attempted to answer most of the questions encountered in practice. The book is meant to stimulate the nurse to read further, to go to other sources, possibly to other disciplines. This text can be viewed as an important evolutional step in the professional development of PACU nurses.

I chose the title, *After Anesthesia: A Guide for PACU, ICU, and Medical/ Surgical Nurses*, so that the book could reach nurses who prepare the surgical patient for anesthesia and subsequently assume responsibility for the patient following his or her stay in the PACU. The nurse on the surgical floor is in desperate need of this information. Luther P. Christman says, "One cannot use knowledge one does not have." Most surgical nurses do not have knowledge of anesthesia as it relates to postoperative care. This book is targeted, therefore, to PACU nurses, nurses on the surgical units, student nurses, nurse managers with responsibility for ORs and PACUs, and possibly nurse-anesthetists.

I hope that both the content and organization of this book will meet the needs of nurses who care for the anesthetic patient.

Kay E. Fraulini

Acknowledgments

Deserving of recognition are the family, friends and co-workers who kept me from losing courage in this long and tedious enterprise.

I am grateful to my colleague/mentor, Dr. Shirley Fondiller, who fostered my expansion as a writer and enabled me to see and appreciate journalistic talent in others. I have known many excellent practitioners, educators, and researchers; only a small percentage, however, are also excellent writers. I am fortunate to have encountered some of these special people, and I am indebted to them for their efforts as contributing authors.

I appreciate the support and contribution of many PACU nurses. It is those team interactions over many years that shaped my own professional development and created an atmosphere in which the needs of PACU nurses could be identified. The following text represents a response to an overwhelming need for scientific information. A notable contribution to this endeavor was made by my colleagues Diane Cashen, R.N., and Sheila Duggan, R.N. Lynette Lane Gilbert, R.N., deserves recognition as the person who finally provided me with a title.

I have taken the liberty of speaking for all PACU nurses when I express appreciation to Drs. M. Sue and Robert Vaughan for their major contributions in the area of perioperative research. *After Anesthesia* would not have been possible without the work of such investigators.

I appreciate the considerable talent and effort of my typists, Vicki D. Carter and Katrina Greening.

Marion Kalstein-Welch's contribution as my acquisitions editor deserves acknowledgment. She was consistently supportive and encouraging and her efforts added new meaning to the word facilitator. The book reached its final stage of completion under the direction of Nancy Buckwalter. Added to the usual demands of production were the problems of working with an author living abroad. Her flexibility and efficiency assured the timely conclusion of this project.

A guiding force throughout my life has been my mother, Leona. In this, as in most other accomplishments, she offered those elements of a relationship which are almost essential to realizing one's goals.

PART I

Introduction

Chapter 1

Development of the Postanesthesia Care Unit

Franklin B. McKechnie
Kay E. Fraulini

MEDICAL PROGRESS AND THE NEED FOR PACUs

Until the early 1940s, the Postanesthesia Care Unit (PACU) simply did not exist. Occasionally a surgeon would keep a postoperative patient on the surgical floor for a time to monitor for complications, but the concept of a designated area for all postoperative patients, along with a concentration of personnel and equipment, had not been conceived. There are at least three reasons why this was so.

First, the types of anesthetic agents available were limited. Gas (nitrous oxide), oxygen, and ether (GOE) were the most common anesthetics, although thiopental was used extensively both for induction and, with nitrous oxide, for maintenance. Cyclopropane also was used, but not to the degree that it would be after 1947, when the relaxant agents were introduced.

Ether was considered the best anesthetic for major abdominal surgery because it produced excellent relaxation if given in adequate quantity, could be used with a high concentration of oxygen, particularly in a closed breathing system, and tended to support ventilation. Because of these three features of ether, many cases—thoracotomies in particular—

were maintained with an assisted respiratory technique rather than by the common controlled respiratory technique used today.

It was believed that by controlling respirations with ether one lost the best sign of the depth of anesthesia and, therefore, was in danger of overdosing the patient. In actuality, assisted respiration often became controlled as carbon dioxide was washed out. Usually near the end of the procedure it was fairly easy to reduce the ventilated volume and respirations would soon be reestablished. Thus in the routine type of case, respiratory insufficiency was less likely to be a postoperative complication.

A second reason that the concept of the PACU was not developed earlier was that the types of operative procedures commonly done did not involve open or even superficial heart procedures; a thoracotomy was considered a major undertaking. Presumably many cases handled now would have been considered too great a risk in the 1920s and 1930s, and even into the 1940s. Certainly the geriatric group of patients has increased greatly since that time, with all of their attendant respiratory and cardiovascular problems requiring good immediate postanesthetic care. Prior to the late 1940s the geriatric operative population was simply not large enough to require a separate recovery area. There is no question that the PACU would have been created eventually, particularly after curare was introduced, but before that there was little necessity for it.

A third factor in the late arrival of the PACU is that prior to World War II there was more than enough help in the hospital. Nurses were generally overworked and underpaid, but there always seemed to be plenty of them, both as students and as graduates. Many hospitals had their own schools, and patients who were to undergo surgery frequently brought their own private duty nurses to the hospital. Consequently, there was rarely a problem in assigning a nurse to stay with each patient during the recovery period.

In the absence of a PACU, operated patients were returned to their rooms for recovery. Depending on the severity of the surgery and the risk to the patient, a nurse or student nurse was assigned to sit and watch the patient and help to forestall complications. Pulse and blood pressure were duly recorded, and patients were assisted when they vomited. This was by no means an uncommon event and could last for some hours—if not days—following ether anesthesia. Suction apparatus was rare, although available. So, too, was oxygen, but the means to ventilate patients artificially were almost nonexistent. The pharmacokinetics of ether enabled many patients to survive surgery in spite of—not because of—the person who administered the anesthesia and also despite the inadequate postoperative care and facilities of the time.

The First PACUs

This is not to say that no one had addressed the matter of postanesthetic care facilities. Florence Nightingale suggested in her book *On Hospitals* that the patient be placed in a small room adjacent to the ward with clean sand on the floor, clean bed clothes, and windows to admit sunlight and fresh air. In 1904, G.C. Crandon, a Boston physician, designed a room specifically as an anesthesia recovery area to be part of a new addition to the Boston City Hospital's surgical suite. Crandon's idea was that all patients with abdominal surgery who might run the risks of vomiting, abdominal distention, or discomfort from ether anesthesia would go to this room, where a nurse would administer a warm water lavage to remove as much of the ether as possible. Crandon's book does not say whether such a room was ever built; correspondence with his son did reveal that Dr. Crandon was considered to have held rather radical ideas.

Warfield Firor, as a young neurosurgeon at Johns Hopkins Hospital, kept poor-risk patients following brain surgery in a separate room on the surgical floor, with himself and a nurse in attendance, until the patients could be safely returned to their own rooms. This was done largely because of surgical need rather than the anesthetic, and would compare more to an intensive care unit than to a PACU.

The literature contains a number of references to keeping patients in separate areas postoperatively not necessarily for their own care but to protect other patients in the hospital from witnessing vomiting, dying, and screams of pain as the patients recovered consciousness.

It was World War II and its demands on personnel that gave rise to the modern PACU as we know it. In January 1942, anesthesiologist Donald Stubbs had six pediatric patients in Washington (D.C.) Hospital who would be receiving avertin fluid for premedication. Because avertin is an exceptionally long-lasting agent as well as a profound respiratory depressant, Dr. Stubbs had trained a number of nurses to take care of these patients postoperatively. On the particular day in question, Dr. Stubbs had six patients and only two of his specially trained nurses. Realizing that there was a nonsurgical pediatric patient occupying a large room, Dr. Stubbs moved that patient out and put the six avertin patients and the two nurses together, and thus began the first PACU.

Several months later, John Lundy, a physician at the Mayo Clinic, arrived in Washington to give Dr. Stubbs the practical portion of the examination for the American Board for Certification. Dr. Lundy became interested in the PACU and, realizing its potential, went back to the Mayo Clinic and established such a room there. He also began to write articles about the concept and its requirements, calling the area a Post-Anesthetic Room.

As time passed and with the greater use of cyclopropane combined with relaxant agents, which often depress the respiratory exchange of the patient into the postanesthesia period, the need for a recovery area became widely recognized. By the end of the 1960s almost all hospitals had some sort of space close by the operating rooms where staffing and equipment were concentrated for the specific care of patients emerging from anesthesia.

Raising the Standards of PACU Care

Despite the recognition by the hospitals of the value of the PACU, the education of the nurses and other employees working there lagged behind. The same was true of the rules and regulations governing PACUs as well as Joint Commission on Accreditation of Hospitals (JCAH) standards. All too often the PACU was used for many purposes other than the recovery of the anesthetized patient. Joseph Civetta, MD, of the University of Miami has described the PACU as having rubber walls, always able to expand and accommodate more patients and more activities. If the hospital was full, new patients were sent to the PACU. If necessary, recovered patients were kept there overnight until space was found in the intensive care area or on the floors. Patients who needed a transfusion, a nerve block for treatment of pain or for diagnosis, dressing changes, or other routine procedures were sent for treatment to the PACU.

Most often, too, the PACU was considered by the hospital administration and the nursing administration as an area "down there somewhere," where the least experienced nurse or aide could learn to take blood pressures, count pulses, learn how to chart, and so on. The newly employed person often received no training in the care of the partially paralyzed, unconscious, anesthetized patient. The surprising fact is that more patients did not get into trouble.

Thus, the education of PACU nurses was for the most part left up to the hospitals in which they worked. Usually the responsibility for education fell to the anesthesiologist, and so it ranged from being excellent to being nonexistent. Unfortunately, the latter was more common than the former. There was no organization with a primary concern related to the education of PACU nurses. They either received their education from the hospital doctors or they learned how to do things themselves. The standard of care, therefore, varied widely, and as long as JCAH basic principles were satisfied, no one was greatly concerned.

A 1968 lawsuit acted as the impetus for change. The case was that of a healthy, active, 5-year-old boy who suffered from increasing visual problems because of congenital ptosis of both eyelids. Surgery was carried out with endotracheal nitrous oxide–halothane anesthesia without incident. The child was taken to the PACU still anesthetized but breathing adequately. At this time the PACU had five patients and two attendees—a registered nurse who was in charge and an aide who had been employed only a day or two earlier. The 5-year-old made a sixth patient, and since he seemed to be all right, he was left to the aide for care. She placed the child on his back and put splints on both arms to keep him from touching his eyes after he awakened. Shortly thereafter, she said that the child was not breathing and that she could not feel a pulse. A code was immediately called. Prompt response and therapy recovered a badly brain-damaged child, incontinent and with uncontrolled extremity movements, unable to walk or even to hold his head up without being strapped in a wheelchair.

It was determined that the boy now had the mentality of a 6-month-old infant.

Upon reviewing this case, the Board of Directors of The Florida Society of Anesthesiologists agreed that this catastrophic event was rare, but nevertheless it should not have occurred. The treatment of the child was well below generally accepted standards. The board also realized that although anesthesiologists depend regularly on the skills of PACU nurses to bring their patients successfully back to consciousness and full activity, no one was teaching them what to do or how to do it, nor was anyone assuming the responsibility for their training. The board agreed, therefore, to sponsor a seminar specifically aimed at teaching PACU nurses what they ought to know for better patient care. The first of these seminars took place in 1969.

Attendance at these seminars grew rapidly, reaching 800 to 900 a year, and many states followed Florida's lead and organized state recovery room organizations. The primary goal of all these organizations was and remains education of the PACU nurse.

In the late 1970s, a group of nurses got together to form a national organization. A board was selected, and after hard and often frustrating work the American Society of Post-Anesthesia Nurses (ASPAN) was born. Its first meeting was held in St. Louis in 1982. At about that time the American Society of Anesthesiologists offered to hold several seminars for PACU nurses. ASPAN has continued to grow, with the launching in 1986 of the *Journal of Post Anesthesia Nursing* and attendance at recent annual meetings exceeding 1000.

DEVELOPMENT OF PACU NURSING AS A SPECIALTY

Little has been written about the development of PACU nursing as a specialty. The two most influential factors were probably the advances in anesthesiology over the past 25 years (part of the knowledge explosion that has affected all disciplines) and, related to this, the societal pressures that brought about changes in the profession of nursing as a whole (for example, continuing education and university preparation). It was inevitable that nurses who found themselves working in PACUs would have to respond.

Van Dam (1984) provides a historical overview that spans the last several decades. It is interesting to note also that technological (apparatus) innovation has contributed to the forced specialization of nurses in the PACU. It is no longer considered adequate postanesthetic nursing care to take a pulse and provide an emesis basin.

The year 1960 may be viewed as a pivotal year; it was then that the journal *Anesthesiology* began to publish basic anesthesia research. This was preceded by such events as the formation of the American Board of

Anesthesiology in 1937 and the recognition of anesthesiology as a specialty by the American Medical Association.

Clinically, three new agents arrived between 1942 and 1946. This led to new anesthesia apparatus; previously there had been many deaths due to faulty apparatus. The 1940s also saw the introduction of syringes and hypodermic needles. It is interesting that ECG monitoring was available in 1915 and permitted the observation of hydrocarbon–epinephrine dysrhythmias. And yet as recently as 1950 no one knew anything about digitalis; there were no antiarrhythmic drugs and patients received cyclopropane. Twenty-five years ago the only heart drugs were procainamide and digitalis.

It was not until 1968 that oxygen was given with nitrous oxide. The 1970s witnessed the introduction of intravenous anesthesia.

During a lecture at Loyola University in 1984, Van Dam cited the following literature that chronicles recent advances and setbacks in clinical anesthesia:

- "Anesthetic, Circulatory, and Respiratory Effects of Fluothane."
- "Halothane Anesthesia as a Possible Cause of Massive Hepatic Necrosis."
- Summary of the National Halothane Study (one of the few times a national study was undertaken to solve a problem. Halothane had the best mortality record and cyclopropane the worst).
- "Nephrotoxicity Associated with Methoxyflurane Anesthesia" (four people at Peter Bent Brigham Hospital, Boston, with renal failure required transplants).
- "Massive Hepatic Necrosis after Fluroxene Anesthesia—A Case of Drug Interaction."
- In 1964, an article appeared in *Anesthesiology* entitled "Metabolism of Volatile Anesthetics." Further knowledge was gained regarding enzyme induction and pharmacokinetics. Information appeared on the hereditary aspects of malignant hyperthermia and biochemical changes in malignant hyperpyrexia. A major contribution came from the work of Eger, Saidman, and Brandstaters on "Minimum Alveolar Anesthetic Concentration: A Standard of Anesthetic Potency." Theories of narcosis continue to proliferate—for example, lipid solubility and reversal of narcosis by increases in atmospheric pressure.

Today the surgical patient is older, and we are learning that the patient's response to anesthesia is different. Patients are also younger than they have ever been: for example, procedures such as correction of hydrocephalus are being done in utero. Transplantation, microsurgery, and surgical treatment of dysrhythmias have appeared on the surgical scene.

There is no doubt that the complexity of today's patient and anesthetic management demands specially trained nurses in the PACU. Just as medical practitioners need a broad knowledge base, so also do PACU nurses. When one traces the development of anesthesia, it becomes apparent that the nurse's quest for knowledge and growth, coupled with the physician's demand for highly competent colleagues, has resulted in the specialty of postanesthesia nursing. Just as many new anesthesia residents are double-boarded, so will many nurses seek advanced preparation as specialists in perianesthetic care (see Chapter 16).

A brief look at the sociology of nursing in the recent past will add to our insights about the development of postanesthesia nursing as a specialty.

Continuing Education in Nursing

The post–World War II era intensified the need for in-service education. The population was increasingly mobile; no longer could administrators count on a staff that had grown up within the institution. Changes in nursing education ended the use of students as the primary source of labor. The rapid development of medical technology mandated staff who understood its uses and abuses. The concomitant proliferation of new and exotic drugs necessitated in-depth knowledge of pharmacology and drug management. Other examples abound; one of the primary examples, once the full potential in this area is realized, will be the use of computers as nursing tools.

Mandatory Continuing Education. With the recognition of the knowledge explosion of the 1960s, the need for systematic continuing education (CE) began to be documented. At that time the half-life of knowledge was estimated at 5 years; as of 1978 that estimate had been reduced to 2 to 2½ years! As the "expiration date" for knowledge has been pushed forward, mandatory CE as a valid remedy for keeping nurses current has been increasingly legislated. Two types of legislation have been utilized:

1. Enabling legislation. The state board of nursing of a given state is granted the authority to require CE for license "if" and "when" the board deems this necessary.
2. Directive legislation. The state board of nursing is directed to require evidence of CE from nurses seeking relicensure and is given the authority to set up the requisite rules and regulations for the process.

California was the first state (1974) to direct mandatory CE. Kansas, Florida, Minnesota, New Mexico, Iowa, Kentucky, and Massachusetts have followed suit.

Clearly, continuing education offerings have fostered the development of postanesthesia nursing as a specialty. The question, of course, remains as to why PACU nurses did not organize as a national group until 1980. For decades the varied settings in which nurses practice has influenced the development of professional organizations and groupings within organizations. This has been followed by a significant proliferation in the number and type of professional publications and journals. For professional organizations with specialized memberships, publications serve as a means of communication. We can speculate that in an ironically circuitous fashion it is the lack of communication from publications from a nationally organized group that has hindered the recognition of postanesthesia nursing as a specialty.

Examples of other groups include the American Association for Nurse Anesthetists (1931), the American Association of Industrial Nurses (1942), the Association of Operating Room Nurses (1957), and the American Association of Critical Care Nurses (1970).

One has to ponder the effects that changes in basic preparation programs have had on the field of postanesthesia nursing. The growing strength of baccalaureate programs in the late 1960s and early 1970s established significant changes in nursing curricula. Philosophically, these curricula specified that nursing students be oriented primarily to patients rather than tasks or routines, and the curricula established priorities in the care of a group of patients. Mandatory rotations through the operating room and the PACU disappeared from most programs. This left (and still leaves) a large number of potential nurse leaders unexposed to the PACU. Undoubtedly this accounts for the delayed development of this group as a specialty. Without creative, informed leadership, any group will flounder.

We must communicate our need for talented nurses to the university. Postanesthesia nursing must get its message to students, especially to undergraduate students, who can start planning to specialize at the graduate level in this field. This can provide the groundwork for doctoral study and a growing cadre of scholars who will generate a scientific knowledge base from which the practice of postanesthesia nursing will evolve. Until this happens, little more can be written about the development of PACU nursing as a specialty.

PHILOSOPHY OF POSTANESTHESIA NURSING

Within nursing, philosophies have sometimes been confused with theories. The PACU nurse needs to experience the process of philosophical thinking in its broadest sense. She or he needs to understand the pursuit of wisdom and to develop a personal philosophy of nursing.

Nursing, as an intensely human profession, requires of its practitioners the qualities of self-understanding, empathy, and understanding of people from all walks of life. In her classic article "The Nature of Nursing," Virginia Henderson called for the liberalizing effect of general education, noting that the "personality of the nurse is possibly the most important intangible in measuring the effect of nursing care."

Thoughts about nursing philosophies should really begin when nurses are in their basic educational program. This is probably best accomplished by a "marriage" of the sciences and the humanities through the undergraduate core curriculum. Students should be exposed to values. In nursing education, administrators and faculty are reexamining closely their philosophy and objectives as they move toward curriculum change. Philosophical statements may vary from school to school, but most institutions enunciate beliefs that require implementation through studies in the humanities as well as in the sciences. Philosophy is important because it searches for the ultimate explanations and causes of being.

A person becomes a person in the encounter with other persons and in no other way (Secord and Backman, 1964). To be human is to feel. All too often people allow themselves to think their thoughts but not to feel their feelings. The only way to develop sensitivity to one's self and to others is to recognize and feel feelings—painful ones as well as happy ones. A balanced sensitivity to one's feelings gives a foundation for empathy with others. Sensitivity to one's self and to others may determine the extent to which nurses are able to develop themselves and to fully utilize themselves with others. Honesty toward self promotes authenticity and sensitivity toward others, and it lays a foundation for primary prevention. A nurse attains and promotes health and higher level functioning to the degree that she or he forms person-to-person relationships as opposed to manipulative relationships.

Nursing, in its broadest sense, involves the whole patient—body, mind, and spirit; promotes health and health preservation by teaching and by example; ministers to the sick; and gives services to the family and community as well as to the individual.

In a sense, nursing recapitulates the evolution of man. A profession, as does mankind, has a growing edge on which the fittest survive; it is improved and refined and gradually, through succeeding generations, achieves a higher order of performance, public value, and prestige. Since original thinking and new knowledge largely constitute this growing edge for the profession, scholarly productivity is a natural, inescapable standard for survival for the individuals who make up the profession.

Nursing as a Science

While we work toward the development of a science of nursing and the validation of its concepts and theories, we can increase our knowledge and understanding of people—biologically, intrapersonally, interpersonally, and as members of society. We can use that knowledge to sharpen our observations of their requirements for nursing care. We can increase our skills in perception and our ability to think logically, soundly, and searchingly regarding cause and effect, to the end that the important factors pertinent to establishing realistic and appropriate objectives in nursing care are considered. We can seek to base our approaches to patients on firmer foundations by clarifying in our own minds what we are trying to do, why, and what scientific knowledge is involved (Johnson, 1959).

The practice of nursing rests on a scientific foundation supported by research. Nurses are committed to using theory as a foundation for practice, to the development of professional standards of competence, and to interdisciplinary efforts to improve the health care delivery system.

Socialization of nurses comprises the development of a professional "soul," the development of human wisdom and professional competence, and the opportunity to use scientific inquiry, interdisciplinary efforts, and social and natural sciences to acquire profound knowledge on a particular subject.

Believing in the dignity and worth of the individual, nurses help individuals and groups in society to attain, maintain, and restore health. And, in accordance with the holistic philosophy of man, the patient's needs determine the environment in which the patient is served.

Nursing care concerns primarily the recipient of nursing—the patient—rather than nursing itself. The imbalance may lead to confusion in establishing nursing goals or developing appropriate plans of nursing action. A knowledge of people and their responses to stress provides the foundation for any health service—for nursing care, medical care, or social casework—and it is knowledge that nurses share, with all professional health workers.

Nursing integrates personal, professional, and societal values. Values are broad, nonspecific qualities esteemed by the group. Values may include such ideas as truthfulness, honor, or the worth of human life. Norms, standards, or rules that guide and regulate behavior are set by the social system and are accepted by most of the members of the system.

Individuals should make the best use of what they have in order to do the most that they can. This is an individual phenomenon as each person has different resources and a different maximum potential from any other. If illness is considered a deviation from normal, it can also be considered a characteristic of health. The deviation may occur as a biological imbalance, an alteration in psychological makeup, or a social conflict.

Interpersonal relationships in nursing are based on perception, judgment, action, reaction, interaction, and transaction (King, 1971). It is nursing's function to recognize, view, interpret, verify, analyze, and synthesize. Johnson and Martin (1958), in a sociological analysis of the nurse role, discuss function as the consequence of activities rather than the activities themselves. They attempt to clarify nursing function by looking at "what the nurse is basically doing for the patient"—that is, the nurse's role and contribution with respect to the maintenance of the social system of doctor–nurse–patient. It is their contention that the primary role of the nurse within this system is to maintain its internal equilibrium through managing the tensions that arise among the system members. The nurse is aware of consumer expectations for health care services, and as a health care advocate is a guardian of patient rights.

Personal Versus Institutional Philosophy

The nurse in the PACU must adapt her or his personal philosophy of nursing and patient care to that of the institution. A clash of philosophies can be very frustrating both for the nurse and for the employing organization. It behooves the nurse to inspect carefully the institutional philosophy before signing an employment contract.

When one is thinking of creating an effective organization, such as a nursing care unit, a philosophy must be developed. This philosophy serves as the foundation for the goals and objectives on which the unit will function.

The PACU is a critical care unit. Dr. W. Leigh Thompson, president of the Society of Critical Care Medicine, has proposed that "only the nurse makes a critical care environment. The machines, the computers, the physicians are adjuncts to the nurse. We may afford more complex machines in the future but we cannot replace the nurse." The essence of postanesthesia care is nursing care. The patient's total dependency demands the skilled and intelligent vigilance of the nurse. Data exist to support the fact that patients are no less susceptible to physiologic crises in the PACU than in the operating room. Yet the number of people responsible for the patient in the operating room is five to ten times greater than in the PACU. Within minutes after the termination of a surgical procedure, the operating room team of several members transfers all responsibility to one person: the PACU nurse. Moreover, the PACU nurse may be accountable for more than one patient. The responsibility that this implies is awesome.

The PACU nurse must be a thinker. The complexity of the role and the needs of the patient demand this. Because of the nature of the specialization, the PACU nurse must have full appreciation and understanding of how specific anesthetics impact preexisting or complicating conditions within the context of the patient's medical or surgical intervention. The postanesthesia nurse's knowledge of anesthesia (both the pharmacodynamics and pharmacokinetics) and drug interactions should be second only to the anesthesiologist's. This is essential if astute patient assessments are to be made.

The nursing process (assessment, planning, implementation, and evaluation) is the basic framework for the provision of quality nursing care within a primary nursing model. The patient should receive care by nurses proficient in the practice of postanesthesia nursing. This includes skill in patient assessment, problem-solving, and emergency intervention. All of this must be accomplished in what is very often a frenetic environment with constant triaging of patients. Attempts must be made to treat the patient holistically. Although biological homeostasis may be a priority of care, behavioral concerns should focus on stress, adaptation, coping, time, space, anxiety, and so on. Although there may not be an opportunity to explore them in depth, cultural and spiritual needs should nevertheless be recognized. The nurse promotes individual human dignity and privacy.

The nurse acts to safeguard the physical environment. This is accomplished through a multidisciplinary approach. The PACU should be supplied with the equipment required to provide postanesthetic care and emergency intervention.

Communication within and between departments must be considered a priority for the PACU nurse. She or he must be skilled at negotiating care for postanesthetic patients. It is recognized that the PACU must be a highly collaborative area involving nurse and physician. The interdependency between these two disciplines is basic to patient survival. Possibly more than any other unit in the hospital, the potential for peer relationships exists here. Colleagueship should be a goal of the health professionals who have so much invested in this acute phase of the patient's hospitalization. Communication must also be supported between the PACU and the surgical floors, the other intensive care units, laboratory, radiology, respiratory therapy, biomedical engineering, internal medicine, transportation, and so on.

The postanesthesia nurse has professional responsibilities that include practice, education, research, administration, and consultation. Nursing education is a lifelong process. The nurse is obligated to update knowledge and clinical skills through continuing education. Staff development, orientation, and patient/family teaching are aspects of the education component.

PACU nurses should actively participate in clinical research and communicate research findings to their peers. Nurses are encouraged to contribute constructively through publications and lectures.

Qualified and talented leaders are essential to the effective management of the unit. Nurses in leadership positions must be adept in personnel administration.

Finally, the role for the postanesthesia nurse as a consultant will in all likelihood expand. The postanesthesia nurse's expertise in perianesthetic care—which includes respiratory management, pain management, and patient teaching—should be shared with other health care professionals as well as the consumer.

BIBLIOGRAPHY

Bullough V & Bullough B: The Care of the Sick: The Emergence of Modern Nursing. London: Croom Helm, 1979.

Deloughery G L: History and Trends of Professional Nursing (8th ed.). St. Louis: C.V. Mosby, 1977.

DeYoung L: Dynamics of Nursing (4th ed.). St. Louis: C.V. Mosby, 1981.

Ellis JR & Hartley CL: Nursing in Today's World: Challenges, Issues, and Trends (2nd ed.). Philadelphia: Lippincott, 1984.

Fondiller S: Nursing history in the undergraduate curriculum: Renewal and relevance. Deans List 4(4), 1983.

Henderson V: The nature of nursing. American Journal of Nursing 64(67), 1964.

Horvath N: Essentials of Philosophy. New York: Barron's Educational Series, 1974.

Johnson DE: A philosophy of nursing. Nursing Outlook 7(4):198–201, 1959.

Johnson M & Martin H: A sociological analysis of the nurse role. Americal Journal of Nursing 58:373–377, 1958.

King IM: Toward a Theory for Nursing. New York: Wiley, 1971.

Saunders L: Permanence and change. American Journal of Nursing 58:969, 1958.

Secord PF & Backman CW: Social Psychology. New York: McGraw-Hill, 1964.

Van Dam L: Changes in anesthesia over the last 25 years. Paper presented at Loyola University of Chicago, Anesthesiology Department, Maywood, Ill., July, 1984.

PART II

The Postanesthesia Nurse

Chapter 2

The Role of the Postanesthesia Care Unit Nurse

Kay E. Fraulini

Because the postanesthesia nurse functions within the larger organizational structure of the hospital, it is necessary to examine some sociological theories that are important for all health practitioners. Chapter 2 limits itself to role theory. Chapters 3 and 4 cover other organizational concerns.

The present chapter begins with a broad theoretical definition of role and continues with a brief description of its relevancy to nursing and the PACU. The chapter concludes with a look at four proposed components of the PACU nurse's role.

DEFINITION OF ROLE

"Role" means following not "merely a set of behaviors or expected behaviors, but a sentiment or goal which provides unity to a set of potential actions" (Turner, 1959, p. 26). Turner (1968) suggested that:

> In any interactive situation, behavior, sentiments, and motives tend to be differentiated into units, which can be called roles; once roles are differentiated, elements of behavior, sentiments, and motives which appear in the same situation tend to be assigned to the existing roles (p. 4).

Thus, role is used here in the symbolic interactionist concept developed by George Herbert Mead (1934) and elaborated in contemporary literature. Role in this sense is conceptualized as a way of coping with an imputed other role (Cottrell, 1942; Turner, 1962); it does not deny the importance of the situation but considers situation as an additional factor in defining roles.

Role is a useful concept in interpreting interactions with "significant others" and in understanding the context in which behavior takes place. Through this concept such interpretations can be made without losing sight of the standardized effects of society's demands on an individual. Role theory emphasizes the notion that human behavior is not a simple matter of stimulus–response reaction, but the result of a complex interaction between ego and society. It synthesizes the culture, the social structure, and the self by considering culture and social structure from the individual's level.

There are three major schools of thought in role theory. The first is the Lintonian approach, which views roles as culturally given prescriptions (Linton, 1936, 1945), while the second defines role in terms of the actions and expectations of individual members of a society (Parsons, 1951; Parsons & Fox, 1952; Sarbin, 1954, 1968).

The third school of thought conceives of role as stemming from interaction with actors in a social system. Following this view, role emerges in a designated reciprocity in which an interaction or a social exchange occurs, and is seen in terms of relevant other roles. The role that the actor elects to play is a derivative of his or her voluntary actions that are motivated by the returns expected and, indeed, received from others. In addition, the role assumed by an interactant in a given situation is validated when others indicate acceptance of that role allocation. Thus, roles chosen by the patient are validated by the acceptance of his significant others, such as the nurse and members of his family. Once a role evolves, the need to reciprocate in role behaviors becomes actually a need for benefits received in order to continue receiving them. As Gouldner pointed out (1960, p. 176), reciprocation acts as a starting mechanism in the interaction process. The exchange process, the rewards and losses, and the ratio between them continue to influence the development of the role played by the ego in the significant other's presence (Blau, 1964, pp. 145–146).

Through interaction and the role-taking processes with the significant other, each person's roles are discovered, created, modified, and defined. These roles are thus incorporated in the ego's self-conception. In general terms, then, self-conception is actually a conception of how one relates to major significant other roles.

RELEVANCY OF ROLE TO PACU NURSING

It is critical that nurses understand the concept of role. Many of our present and future challenges relate to role: role stress, role strain, role overload, and role transition. Role transition denotes a change in role relationships, expectations, or abilities. This requires people to incorporate new knowledge, alter their behavior, and thus change their definition of themselves in their social context.

The nurse must keep in mind that the PACU is a social system. For decades sociologists have attempted to conceptualize the culture of a typical hospital ward. What was observed many years ago, however, was that the operating room society was different from the rest of the hospital. Burling and associates (1956) pointed out the physical and psychological isolation of the operating room. To maintain asepsis and facilitate work flow, the operating suite is always separated from the hospital as a whole. It has its own floor or part of a floor, and patients are taken to surgery and brought back to their beds by orderlies. Other hospital personnel rarely visit it; casual visiting is prohibited.

This isolation of the operating room means that to other employees it is strange and forbidding. They are on the "outside" and apt to be both curious and in awe about what occurs in the sanctum.

Conversely, the surgical staff, from doctors to maids, develop a strong feeling of camaraderie. They recognize their status and role as a special group. Their world is the operating room, not the hospital. This results in great warmth and cohesion, and the sharing of many values (pp. 267–268). Some of these observations concerning the operating room may be applied to the PACU as well.

Another sociological perspective of nurse and patient roles in the PACU is provided by Minckley (1968) in an article about man's territoriality. She comments that Goffman (1963) describes certain types of people as being "open" and available for social contact at all times because of the uniform they wear. Examples are police officers, from whom the passerby seeks direction; or priests, who may be accosted by strangers for advice. There is a silent assumption that no excuse need be made by the approaching person in order to initiate social contact with these "open" persons. This is not so in ordinary social contacts. Nurses, being such open persons in the PACU, are continually asked for services and attentions.

Minckley observes that doctors who are present in the PACU do not receive much verbal recognition from patients. In general, patients remain quiet when a doctor leans over them to make observations, and some do not even respond to questions from doctors unless the doctors repeat the questions with greater volume and insistence. It is as though patients have nothing to give to the doctor, or perhaps that the doctor's questions force them to give answers at a time when they have no energy to give to anything. On the other hand, the nurse is viewed by the patient as a giver of comfort and services, and PACU patients demonstrated far more alertness and were more verbal in the presence of nurses.

The open person who is the nurse must supply services as well as treatments that the patient may not have requested but that are part of the doctor's plan of care; because of this, nurses become more and more accustomed to tactfully forcing their presence on the patient at those times that best suit nurses' own schedules. Perhaps because nurses are treated as open people by everyone from patients to hospital administrators, nurses treat patients as open people too, who need not necessarily be approached in the polite social manner. Or perhaps patients are viewed the way Goffman sees old people or the very young, as "being engaged at will" because the accoster has nothing to lose in the encounter. Patients do what they can to defend themselves within their limited territory which has no visible walls, by trying to become nonpersons, using the mechanism of "civil inattention." But then, nurses may accept patients at face value and treat them like nonpersons.

Because there is such a constant pressure on nurses in the PACU to perform nursing tasks for patients who are in semiconscious or nonperson states, nurses must seek outlets for their own aggression. In essence, their territory is overrun by patients whose needs may be so demanding as to be overwhelming. So when demands temporarily subside, or when there is a lull in pace, nurses seek escape into the heart of their own territory, which in Minckley's PACU was a small alcove at one end of the room. They used this area for their backstage socialization and for release of tension and aggressive feelings; having thus refueled their energies, they could return to the onstage territory again.

Backstage behavior for tension release could not always be confined to that area, however. Frequently it took place in the aisle between the rows of patients. Friendly exchanges between staff members, kidding or joking communications about situational difficulties, or other interpersonal exchanges not related to the patients or their care, were common. The patients seemed to show some resentment of these lighthearted comments made within their hearing. Especially laughter seemed to offend them, probably by intensifying their sense of confusion, nonbeing, and victimization. However, patients dutifully refrained from intruding on the encounters between staff members, remaining nonpersons for varying lengths of time. Occasionally, patients seemed to resort to other mechanisms when they felt they had been denied attention long enough: they would groan, call out, grasp a passing nurse, vomit, or ask for the bedpan.

FOUR COMPONENTS OF THE PROFESSIONAL NURSE ROLE

It is generally accepted today that the role of the professional nurse contains expectations in at least four areas—practice, education, administration, and research. This must be true of the PACU nurse as well. Rush-Presbyterian–St. Luke's Medical Center has proposed a role emphasis geared to the different educational levels (Fig. 2-1). A nursing "levels of practice" (LOP) system (see Appendix 2-1) was also developed at

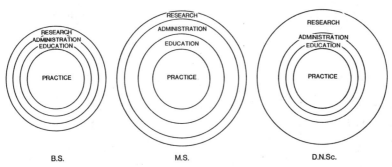

Figure 2–1. Role emphasis in the different educational levels. *(Courtesy of Rush University College of Nursing, Rush-Presbyterian–St. Luke's Medical Center, Chicago.)*

Rush, to provide professional advancement, increased status, and financial gains for achievement in clinical practice.

The LOP system, which in other settings is referred to as horizontal or lateral promotion, took several years to develop at Rush. During that process it became apparent that in addition to the evolution of the system itself, plans would be needed for accomplishing the meshing of the LOP with already existing policies such as those for job performance review (merit evaluations) and the salary compensation structure. Therefore, in addition to providing professional advancement, increased status, and financial gains for achievement in clinical practice, the system also was planned to provide behaviorally stated job descriptions to be used as a management tool for orientation, progress inventory, and staff development. Behaviors expected in each level are categorized into the four components of the professional nursing role: clinical practice, administration, education, and research. There are four classifications within the LOP—A through D, with A being the beginning practitioner and D requiring advanced skills. The system provides behavioral expectations for merit review within a classification as well as the "horizontal" promotion aspects from level to level within the staff nurse role. Placement within and progress through the levels are not tied to educational achievements or length of experience as such, but rather to the demonstration of achievement of the behaviors associated with each level (Ulsafer-Van Lanen, 1981).

It is not the intent of this chapter to discuss lateral promotion systems in depth but to illustrate how the four components of the professional nursing role can rationally be built into staff nurse positions at all levels. Even though the nurse may experience organizational or sociological differences in the PACU, she or he nevertheless must meet the role requirements set forth for all nurses in clinical practice. And, as illustrated in Figure 2-1, although the role emphasis changes as the nurse progresses through the educational process, the four basic components still comprise the role.

BIBLIOGRAPHY

Blau PM: Exchange and Power in Social Life. New York: Wiley, 1964.

Burling T, Lentz EM, & Wilson R: The Give and Take in Hospitals—A study of human organization in hospitals. New York: Putnam's, 1956.

Cottrell LS Jr.: The adjustment of the individual to his age and his roles. American Sociological Review 7:617–620, Oct., 1942.

Goffman E: Behavior in Public Places. New York: Free Press, 1963.

Gouldner AW: The norm of reciprocity: A preliminary statement. American Sociological Review 25:161–178, April, 1960.

Hardy ME & Conway ME: Role Theory—Perspectives for Health Professionals. New York: Appleton-Century-Crofts, 1978.

Linton R: The Study of Man. New York: Appleton-Century, 1936.

Linton R: Cultural Background of Personality. New York: Appleton-Century, 1945.

Mead GH: Mind, Self and Society, introduction by C W Morris. Chicago: University of Chicago Press, 1934.

Melels AI: Role insufficiency and role supplementation—A conceptual framework. Nursing Research 24(4): July–August, 1975.

Minckley B: Space and place in patient care. American Journal of Nursing 68:510–516, March, 1968.

Parsons T: The Social System. Glencoe, Ill.: Free Press, 1951.

Parsons T & Fox R: Illness, therapy, and the modern urban American family. Journal of Social Issues 8:31–44, 1952.

Sarbin T: Role Theory. In G Lindzey (Ed.), Handbook of Social Psychology (vol. 1). Cambridge, Mass.: Addison-Wesley, 1954, pp. 223–258.

Sarbin T: Role Theory. In G Lindzey & E Aronson (Eds.), Handbook of Social Psychology (2nd ed.), (vol. 1.) Cambridge, Mass.: Addison-Wesley, 1968, pp. 488–567.

Turner RH: Role taking as process. Los Angeles: University of California, 1959. Unpublished manuscript.

Turner RH: Role Taking: Process vs. Conformity. In A Rose (Ed.), Human Behavior and Social Process. Boston: Houghton-Mifflin, 1962, pp. 20–40.

Turner RH: The Self-Conception in Social Interaction. In C Gordone & KJ Greigen (Eds.), Self in Social Interaction. New York: Wiley, 1968.

Ulsafer-Van Lanen J: Lateral promotion helps skilled nurses in direct patient care. Hospitals 88–90, March 1, 1981.

Rush-Presbyterian–St. Luke's Medical Center Division of Nursing

Levels of Practice—Surgery

REGISTERED NURSE A

The registered nurse level A is a beginning nurse practitioner and has guidance and supervision from an experienced R.N. on the staff.

A. Clinical Practice

1. Interviews clients and their families to obtain the required nursing history, and records the data.
   a. Performs a nursing admission upon arrival to the unit. Includes data outlined on patient admission record: vital signs, allergies, medications, past hospitalizations, and gross physical symptoms.
   b. Involves the patient's family and significant others in obtaining the above data.
   c. Orients patient and family to physical surroundings and pertinent hospital routines.
   d. Records data on admission record, charts a pertinent note in the patient care record, and begins a skeletal care plan. Verbally communicates to other nursing staff any information that will promote continuity of care.
2. Develops nursing care plans and establishes priorities for patient care based on medical and nursing diagnoses.
   a. Uses observations and assessments to determine priorities in planning daily patient care.
   b. Assists preceptor or designate in the development of care plans by communicating observations, assessments, and priorities identified in day-to-day care.
3. Implements, utilizes, and begins to modify nursing care plans to provide care based on the behavioral and biological status.
   a. Applies written nursing care plans to daily patient care.

    b. Recognizes a diversity of patient's needs and begins to formulate a priority of needs for his/her patients.

4. Seeks guidance when performing nursing procedures which have not been mastered. Performs most activities on nursing skills check list and special unit procedures.
    a. Utilizes and updates nursing skills checklist.
    b. Seeks appropriate resource persons for guidance, i.e., unit leader or designate, preceptor, teacher-practitioner.
    c. Utilizes existing reference material, i.e., Policy and Procedure Manual, Standards of Care, rolodex, diet manual, library.

5. Attends conferences and seminars to gather information that will provide more comprehensive care planning.
    a. Attends unit conferences, R.N. meetings, nursing rounds, inservices and workshops.
    b. Shares information gathered from above sources with other members of the nursing team.

6. Takes direct, appropriate action in life-threatening emergencies.
    a. Knows where emergency equipment and emergency information are available (emergency cart, ECG, defibrillator, cardiac arrest policy and procedure, and fire code).
    b. Is functionally familiar with emergency measures to be taken in the case of a fire and of cardiac and respiratory arrests, including phoning per emergency code and performing cardiopulmonary resuscitation until help arrives.

7. Demonstrates beginning ability to communicate with the client, the client's family, and other health workers.
    a. Involves patient in planning care through preprocedural teaching, input into daily hospital routine, and providing information about special tests, etc., that will interrupt his/her routine. Documents such teaching in nursing notes and on care plan.
    b. Seeks information from family concerning approaches to patient's care and integrates this into care plan. Informs and instructs family of patient's activities.
    c. Coordinates patient's daily schedule with other health disciplines involved in care.

8. Communicates clearly and appropriately to co-workers both verbally and in writing.
    a. Begins to demonstrate the following communications skills:
        1. Gathers accurate information.
        2. Relays information clearly and concisely.
        3. Listens effectively and sorts out relevant information.
        4. Is discreet in the use of confidential information.
    b. Uses the above skills in giving and taking reports and verbal orders, in interaction with members of health care team and with patient and family, and in charting and care plans.

9. Observes symptoms and reactions of client.
   a. Recognizes significant symptomatic changes in client's condition, takes appropriate action involving recording incident and reporting to charge person and/or physician.
10. Anticipates and acts to maintain a safe environment for the client and others.
    a. Provides for patient's physical and psychological safety by such measures as bed in low position, side rails up as needed, aseptic technique, preoperative teaching.
11. Initiates appropriate intrainstitutional referrals.
    a. Makes nursing referrals to resource people available on the unit, i.e., dietician, teacher-practitioner, unit leader.
    b. Seeks assistance from preceptor or resource person in discovering and using avenues of referral beyond the unit level.
12. Accepts accountability for clinical care of his/her patients, and for others assisting in the nursing care of those patients.
    a. Held accountable for:
       1. Executing doctor's orders written for her/his patients.
       2. Administering treatments and medications.
       3. Being aware of procedures, tests, and appointments.
       4. Knowing patient's whereabouts.
       5. Practicing preventive nursing care measures.
    b. Follows up assignment given to another health care worker who is caring for his/her patients.
13. Assists in teaching patients and groups in established programs.
    a. Participates in teaching programs on patient care unit.
14. Identifies teaching needs of patients and families, and teaches health care principles based on nursing assessment.
    a. Identifies specific teaching needs.
    b. Identifies specific teaching plans.
    c. Assists in developing a teaching program.
15. Demonstrates awareness of the need to create a positive climate for interaction between the patient, family, health workers, and students.
16. Observes and preserves rights of patients.

B. Administration

1. Supports standards of nursing care for the department.
   a. Utilizes:
      1. Policy and Procedure manuals.
      2. Goals and objectives for department of surgical nursing and individual care units.
      3. Standards of care for surgical patients.
2. Supports existing policies and procedures.

3. Participates in formulating and evaluating standards of nursing care, and making recommendations for improvement of patient care.
   a. Participates in care conferences on the unit.
   b. Is aware of unit representation on various nursing committees, i.e., Standard of Care, R.N. Committee, Policy and Procedure Committee, Audit Committee, New Products Committee.
   c. Offers suggestions and feedback to committees through unit representative.
   d. Supports members of the health care team. Begins to participate in decision-making process and supports decisions of experienced members.
   e. Discusses and reviews his/her own values and expectations of patient care with preceptor or unit leader.
   f. Discusses observations of patient care given by others with an appropriate person, i.e., unit leader, preceptor or charge nurse.
4. Participates in interdepartmental activities as they relate to assigned patients.
   a. Takes into consideration interdisciplinary tests and therapies when planning patient's daily care.
5. Participates in self-evaluation and peer review as appropriate to the unit.
   a. Is involved in an on-going program of self evaluation both (a) formally with preceptor or unit leader at designated intervals and (b) informally within herself/himself and with peers.
   b. Initiates a promotional evaluation to level B at any time.
6. Participates in selection of assigned patients with unit leader, in consideration of needs of the area.
   a. Sets realistic goals of care.
   b. Mutually agrees upon a patient load to gain new experiences, with supervision.
   c. Begins to develop leadership skills in coordinating patient care by working with nurses experienced in the leadership role.

C. Education

1. Participates in development of self and other staff members.
   a. Participates in individual and group conferences.
   b. Participates in nursing care conferences.
      1. Attends and/or requests patient care conferences.
      2. Contributes to identification of patient care problems and needs.
      3. Contributes to the development of the plan of care for the patient being discussed.
      4. Brings current information and materials as input into conferences.

    c. Identifies own limitations in meeting educational needs of personnel and refers them to appropriate resources.

2. Assumes responsibility for own continuing education, utilizing both formal and informal resources.
    a. Requests opportunity to attend staff education and in-service programs available within the medical center.
    b. Requests and/or accepts supervision in performing new skills of assessment, practice, and documentation.
    c. Utilizes educational resources such as library, skills lab, teacher-practitioners, and more experienced nurses in the area.
    d. Participates with unit leader in selecting topic for inservice.
    e. Accumulates own continuing education credits as relevant to his/her practice.

3. Demonstrates the ability to apply basic teaching-learning concepts.
    a. Identifies content needed by the learner(s) and readiness to learn.
    b. Organizes and presents the content at a rate and in a manner which the learner can understand.
    c. Evaluates the learner's comprehension of the content via return demonstration, recall in the learner's own words, and questions and answers.
    d. Provides the learner with supervised practice sessions as appropriate.
    e. Provides the learner with appropriate resource materials.

D. Research

1. Assists with identifying patient care problems for investigation.
    a. Discusses possible areas for investigation with unit leader, teacher-practitioner, and/or research nurses.
2. Cooperates in collecting data for research projects.
    a. Records data relevant to tools and/or projects, i.e., workload sheet, quality of care study, and assessment of new equipment.
3. Cooperates in applying research findings to patient care.

REGISTERED NURSE B

The registered nurse level B performs all behaviors of the R.N. level A. In addition, the R.N. level B demonstrates appropriate independent judgments and decision-making skills.

A. Clinical Practice

1. Serves as primary nurse for his/her caseload.
    a. Assists unit leader or designate in choosing caseload according to skills and areas of interest.

b. Makes independent judgments based on acquired knowledge, skills and scientific principles.
2. Assesses and records the behavioral and biological status of patient and family by obtaining information pertinent to the health status (a) prior to admission, (b) during the period of care, and (c) anticipated after discharge.
   a. Obtains a beginning psychosocial history, including spiritual background, home environment, job, activities of daily living, economic background, education, effects of past illnesses and hospitalizations, expectations of this hospitalization.
   b. Obtains a physical history, including patient's knowledge of condition, physical assessment of nutritional status, skin condition, mental and emotional status, motor and sensory abilities, and elimination and sleep patterns.
   c. Formulates an individualized care plan within 24 hours of patient's admission based on initial interview, medical workup, clinical data, and laboratory data.
   d. Identifies needs and approaches specific to that patient.
   e. Identifies problems of a specific nursing nature and independently institutes nursing measures as indicated.
   f. Integrates both short- and long-term goals into his/her plan of care.
3. Maintains current care plans based on continuing assessment of the patient's status, evaluation of the effectiveness of nursing interventions, and consideration of alternatives for nursing care.
   a. Implements care plans by identifying specific approaches to patient's needs on nursing care cardex and communicates this information to nursing staff through report and conferences.
   b. Revises care plan according to patient's changing condition through periodic (every 3–5 days or postoperative) evaluation of needs and approaches.
   c. Involves other members of the health care team in the process of revision.
4. Anticipates emergencies based on nursing assessment, and takes appropriate action.
   a. Anticipates common postoperative complications and knows their prodromal symptoms.
   b. Correlates changing symptoms with scientific knowledge of system reactions.
   c. Makes observations, takes immediate action, reports to doctor and follows through with treatments and records.
   d. Insures emergency equipment is in order and accessible at all times.
   e. Can anticipate and obtain equipment and medications needed for care plan in an emergency situation, i.e., G.I. bleeding, shock, cardiac arrest, evisceration, respiratory arrest.

    f. Is able to delegate specific responsibilities to other staff members and auxilliary personnel during an emergency.

    g. Utilizes resources available for back-up in an emergency situation.

5. Initiates interaction with other members of the health care team for the purpose of coordinating direct patient care efforts and/or operating as the patient's advocate.

    a. Is aware of all the departments available as resources to the patient.

    b. Takes the necessary steps to make informal referrals (dietary, volunteer's office, teacher-practitioner).

    c. Suggest formal referrals to physicians when necessary and follows through making sure it goes through channels expediently.

    d. Maintains communication lines, written and verbal, with any and all departments involved in his/her patient's recovery (i.e., chest physical therapy, physical therapy, occupational therapy, extended care, respiratory therapy, etc.).

    e. Anticipates and prepares patient for any stressful situation.

    f. Knows and understands coping mechanisms and can identify specific mechanisms used by her/his patients.

    g. Allows a patient to act out within a safe environment.

    h. Utilizes resources available to patient for help: chaplain, volunteers, psychiatric nurses.

6. Plans and implements health teaching programs for patients and families, utilizing community resources as needed.

    a. Initiates a discharge plan, recognizing the patient and his family as a part of a community outside the hospital.

    b. Knows services to contact that can contribute to discharge planning by direct contact with the patient's community (extended care nursing, social services, family services).

B. Administration

1. Participates in committees, based on departmental needs and personal interests.

    a. Makes monthly reports to unit about committee activities.

    b. Involves other nurses in committee projects.

2. Participates in developing unit objectives.

    a. Works with other members of nursing team on the unit in establishing realistic yearly goals for the unit and reviewing progress toward past year's goals.

3. Demonstrates beginning leadership skills.

C. Education

1. Assists with clinical supervision of students.

    a. Facilitates the application of Rush College of Nursing core material.

    b. Knows the expected competencies of the student he/she is supervising.

    c. Reviews the objectives of the educational experience.

    d. Prepares client for experience by interpreting educational program and securing permission where indicated.

    e. Reviews with the student and/or faculty the outcomes of nursing intervention.

2. Assumes teaching roles within the health care team as appropriate.

    a. Initiates, organizes and conducts patient care conferences.

    b. Is a behavior model and/or preceptor for level A R.N. as well as other health care workers.

    c. Assumes teaching roles with staff in areas of clinical expertise.

    d. Demonstrates procedures and interprets policies to other members of the health care team.

    e. Participates in educational programs of professional and lay community agencies in accordance with expertise and interests.

3. Participates actively in in-service programs including orientation of new personnel.

    a. Assists in orienting personnel to any technical tasks.

    b. Discusses protocol and procedures with new personnel specific to area of practice.

    c. Participates in the in-service programs of other agencies as necessary.

4. Plans and conducts care conferences on the unit.

    a. Involves other disciplines in care conferences.

    b. Demonstrates the use of other resources in the preparation and presentation of conference materials.

D. Research

1. Applies concepts from current health reports to patient care.

2. Evaluates the effectiveness of new methods and communicates outcome.

    a. Discriminates between those new methods that were successful and those that were not.

    b. Identifies why new methods were successful or not.

3. Participates in critically evaluating existing nursing practice.

    a. Brings ideas to hospital committees and offers suggestions for improvement of nursing practice.

    b. Assists in establishing standards and levels of practice.

4. Identifies problems in the clinical practice of nursing which are suitable for investigation.

    a. Makes perceptive observations of nursing care and patient problems and reports findings to proper channels for possible research.

REGISTERED NURSE C

The registered nurse level C performs all behaviors of the R.N. level B. In addition, the R.N. level C demonstrates leadership skills in the delivery of nursing care.

A. Clinical Practice

1. Serves as a resource for other nursing personnel in assessing patient and family status and planning nursing care.
    a. Acts as a consultant for other staff members by using sophisticated interviewing techniques.
    b. Conducts interviews on a regularly scheduled basis with long-term patients and their families concerning areas of prognosis, progress, discharge planning, realistic goals for recovery, family coping mechanisms.
    c. Evaluates care plans developed by Level A and B nurses and works with them to identify more subtle patient needs.
    d. Encourages and directs nurses at other levels in regular revision of care plans to meet changing patient needs.
2. Provides direct nursing care to patients whose condition requires an intensive degree of nursing skill.
    a. Provides comprehensive care for complicated surgical patients who might also have underlying medical and emotional problems.
    b. Can easily assimilate a multitude of patient needs and establish priorities.
    c. Makes skilled nursing assessments and acts in a preventive manner to minimize complications.
3. Collaborates with health care team to assess patient progress, and to help direct and evaluate treatment approach.
    a. Makes daily rounds with physicians involved in the care of his/her caseload.
    b. Makes his/her own suggestions and brings suggestions from nursing staff to the physicians regarding progress, treatments and reactions to treatments, and unmet patient needs.
    c. Assumes responsibility for the quality of patient care not only self-administered but also administered by other levels of nursing and health care workers.
    d. Makes rounds to observe care given and the patient's response to care.
    e. Approaches other staff members and makes specific recommendations to improve patient care.
4. Initiates interdisciplinary and intradisciplinary patient care conferences.
    a. Identifies the patient who requires an intradisciplinary conference.

    b. Organizes intradisciplinary conferences and schedules them on a regular basis for identified patients.

    c. Involves Level A and B nurses in input for such conferences.

5. Teaches groups of patients with similar learning needs.

    a. Identifies groups of surgical patients with common problems and organizes teaching on a group level.

    b. Acts as a teaching consultant within her surgical specialty area, i.e., orthopedics, cardiovascular, general surgery, G.U. surgery.

6. Demonstrates an ability to utilize the resources of the medical center and other health care agencies.

    a. Supports and/or directs staff to utilize resources.

    b. Keeps staff informed of additional resources as they become available.

    c. Encourages staff to share information they have gained from resources.

    d. Supports and/or directs staff to report appropriate feedback to resources utilized.

B. Administration

1. Interprets and implements procedures, policies and nursing care objectives to patients, families, and health care workers.

    a. Is functionally familiar with policies, procedures and nursing care objectives and can clarify them to other levels of nursing.

    b. Insures application of policy and procedure and nursing care objectives on the patient care unit.

2. Guides in establishing and evaluating standards of clinical nursing practice.

    a. Participates on departmental and divisional committees concerned with standards of practice.

    b. Participates in the evaluation of Level A and B nurses and other health care workers on his/her unit at regularly scheduled intervals.

3. Demonstrates leadership skills in the practice setting, such as unit leader or unit leader-designate.

    a. Assumes leadership responsibilities of patient care unit as indicated.

    b. Makes realistic assignments based on anticipated workload and staff capabilities.

    c. Is able to delegate and direct other members of nursing team in a coordinated effort to ensure quality of patient care, and takes responsibility for such.

    d. As a charge person, maintains contact with administrative resource person above her/him.

4. Interprets patient-related administrative policies to all disciplines on the unit.

5. Initiates action toward attaining unit objectives.

    a. Familiarizes nursing team members with goals and objectives of unit and elicits their participation in attaining goals by setting up "specific action" programs and bimonthly progress meetings.

C. Education

1. Demonstrates the ability to direct clinical learning experiences of staff and students.
    a. Identifies learning needs of personnel and students.
    b. Collaborates with nursing faculty in the development of clinical learning experiences for personnel and students.
    c. Develops educational objectives for specified learning groups.
    d. Bases a teaching plan on subject's abilities and motivation to learn.
    e. Develops a means to evaluate effectiveness of teaching.
    f. Demonstrates ability to integrate core concepts with clinical practice.
        1. Selects patients manifesting core concepts or calling for nursing behaviors covered in core curriculum.
2. Assists with staff development by implementing planned in-service programs, teaching rounds, and team conferences, and utilizing available continuing education resources to initiate new programs.
    a. Uses experiential teaching to upgrade skills and competencies of staff.
    b. Utilizes continuing education resources in medical center and community to avoid duplication.
        1. Attends continuing education programs to meet own learning needs.
        2. Supports attendance of other staff to continuing education programs.
    c. Works effectively with staff and student groups.
        1. Seeks to evoke maximum participation of every member.
        2. Solicits opinions, evaluations, analysis, suggestions and expression of feelings.
        3. Clarifies and expands the ideas of others through examples, illustrations, and explanations.
        4. Integrates information.
        5. Keeps the group directed toward its goals.
        6. Gives feedback.
        7. Provides critiques when necessary.
    d. Evaluates the program outcomes.
    e. Modifies content or approach as indicated.

D. Research

1. Assists with the development and implementation of nursing and health related studies.
    a. Identifies methods of implementing conclusions of research.

2. Serves as a nursing resource for interdisciplinary research.
   a. Collaborates with nonnurses in the development and implementation of health related research.
3. Introduces concepts from health care research for application in the clinical setting.
   a. Analyzes published nursing research.
      1. Distinguishes between facts and opinions.
      2. Identifies cause–effect relations.
   b. Demonstrates concepts in practice and interprets to others.

REGISTERED NURSE D

The registered nurse level D has demonstrated the ability to perform the behaviors expected of the R.N. level C. In addition, the R.N. level D provides nursing leadership in management of the patient care system.

A. Clinical Practice

1. Provides guidance and direction in initiating and implementing change to improve the quality of care given.
   a. Involves all levels of nursing personnel in planning for change.
   b. Offers direction in setting realistic short- and long-term goals to improve patient care.
   c. Supports and/or directs staff in implementing change.
   d. Recognizes staff's contributions in planning and implementing change.
2. Serves as a consultant.

B. Administration

1. Assists in formulating and initiating unit or departmental policies, procedures and nursing care objectives.
   a. Identifies policies and objectives that need to be written or revised.
   b. Actively participates on committees that formulate policies and objectives.
   c. Brings back information from such committees to staff members and supports methods of implementation.
   d. Plans ways to involve staff in departmental and divisional decision making.
   e. Recognizes staff's involvement in formulating policies and objectives.
2. Participates in the evaluation of the effectiveness of care given on the unit.
   a. Supports planning for methods of evaluation.
   b. Supports consistent evaluation.

3. Interprets medical center policies and procedures.
   a. Reinforces follow through of policy and procedure.
   b. Offers staff ways to be involved in the change of policy and procedures.

C. Education

1. Develops, conducts, and evaluates in-service and continuing education programs utilizing internal and external educational resources.
   a. Contributes to curriculum development and program planning.
      1. Discusses with practitioner/teacher or core coordinator the appropriateness of curriculum in achieving student objectives.
      2. Offers suggestions based on background experience and literature for upgrading and/or enriching the curriculum.
   b. Serves as a resource to level C R.N. in planning in-service programs.
   c. Participates in group planning of continuing education programs.
      1. Rush Medical Center–sponsored endeavors.
      2. Community agency sponsored programs.
   d. Actively seeks out educational resources within the medical center and community.
      1. Investigates what resources are available in response to specific learning needs.
      2. Maintains a file, listing, or other compilation of resources.
   e. Uses learning theories and principles of effective communication in working with individuals and groups.
      1. Helps student think through a problem using knowledge gained rather than giving a direct answer or sending the learner to a printed source.
      2. Remains supportive and nonjudgmental.
2. Identifies for the unit issues in education and practice that have not been attended to and makes recommendations for correcting these.

D. Research

1. Proposes hypotheses for research.

Chapter 3

Tactics for the Postanesthesia Care Unit Nurse-Administrator

Diane Randall Andrews

The nurse-administrator in PACU is routinely faced with the need to adapt organizational plans to the unique characteristics of the PACU setting. This chapter is intended to assist in that process by providing examples of applicable administrative tactics tempered to meet the needs of the area.

Tactics, in a practical sense, are a combination of administrative concepts or theories used to attain the goals of the organization. Numerous factors, at all organizational levels, effect the choice of one tactic over another. The organizational philosophy and structure are primary influences. It is at this level that basic beliefs, such as the desire for growth of professional autonomy, find substance, as in the application of a decentralized management system.

Decisions regarding nursing practice follow the philosophical commitments of the organization, but they are structured in a way that addresses the character of the profession. Thus, the use of a primary nursing model may be a natural progression of decentralization efforts. New goals and corresponding tactics may be added as institutional goals are individualized to the nursing department. One result might be the decision to implement creative staffing tactics to increase job satisfaction.

Within the PACU a variety of influences contribute to the tactics employed by the nurse manager. External regulatory agencies such as the Joint Commission on Accreditation of Hospitals (JCAH) may impose standards against which acceptable performance is measured. The JCAH accreditation manual (1982) requires orientation, in-service training, policy and procedure, unit design, and equipment specifications for special care units which exceed those of general care areas. The nurse-administrator must incorporate the responsibilities implied by those expected outcomes into educational and standard-setting tactics.

The nurse-administrator must also identify and incorporate the tactics of nonnursing influences in the PACU. The medical director will bring one set of practices, the attending physicians another. Administrative and support service personnel will impose yet another set of variables. In many cases the nurse-administrator has a dual responsibility to report to both a nursing supervisor and a medical director. Negotiation between those groups may be necessary.

The nursing staff members themselves may affect the choice of management tactics. It is unlikely that self-directed, motivated staff members will reach their full potential with the use of highly structured tactics. In the same fashion, the nurse-administrator must identify her or his own leadership style. Only when all of these influences have been clarified can appropriate tactics for the PACU be selected and implemented.

A discussion follows of a number of common management tactics as they might be applied to the PACU. It is the responsibility of the nurse-administrator to develop each tactic to meet specific organizational and unit needs. The discussion has been divided into sections in order to provide examples related to four management functions: planning, organizing, directing, and controlling.

PLANNING

Philosophy

As was emphasized earlier, planning for the PACU must reflect institutional and departmental philosophy. From that beginning, a unit philosophy for management of patient care, education, research, and administrative practices can be identified. Incorporated into that philosophy are the principles against which nurses who specialize in postanesthetic care base their practice. Chapter 1 discusses the development of that base.

The leadership of the unit must then identify how its actions and those of the staff combine to support organizational, professional, and personal beliefs regarding the practice of nursing in the PACU. Example 1 demon-

EXAMPLE 1. PACU NURSING LEADERSHIP GROUP

The leadership of the Postanesthesia Care Unit recognize their responsibility to actualize the philosophical commitments of the Division of Nursing Affairs to clinical practice, educational endeavors, research and unit operations. Key to this is the ability of the professional nurse to effect decisions regarding the application of nursing practice standards. Therefore, the leadership holds that commensurate responsibility and accountability for clinical, educational and research activities must be delegated to the primary nurse. It is the role of the leadership group to coordinate and evaluate that process.

In keeping with this commitment, the leadership group supports the principles of primary nursing as defined in the PACU through the role of the total care nurse. Review of the collaborative efforts of the total care nurse within the Patient Care Committee and the Education/Research Committee is the responsibility of this body.

Nursing, as an applied science, collaborates with multiple interprofessional and intraprofessional groups in order to effect satisfactory patient outcomes. This process is essential to the delivery of high quality nursing care. In so much as the matrix structure and the unification model facilitate this end, they are implemented through the process of providing unit leadership.

Finally, it is acknowledged that the unit leader maintains responsibility to the Department of Operating Room and Surgical Nursing for all nursing activities that occur in the PACU. This includes accountability for unit management, teaching activities, clinical care and research. While some facets of these responsibilities may be delegated to others, those to whom the responsibility has been delegated maintain accountability to the unit leader in regard to those activities.

---

strates how one unit, operating within a matrix model, characterized its commitments.

The use of a leadership group itself is an example of a tactic used to support the organizational philosophy of decentralization. It facilitates movement of the responsibility for decision-making related to unit goal setting, quality assurance, review of patient care practices, education, and research systems to the individuals expected to implement the results of those decisions.

The PACU Nursing Patient Care Committee (Example 2) and the PACU Nursing Education/Research Committee (Example 3) were created to decentralize specific responsibility for those activities to staff. All unit activities then were placed under the review of one of those three committees. One outcome was the review of policies and procedures related to patient care by the Patient Care Committee prior to their submission to the nurse-administrator for formal approval. Similarly, the orientation

EXAMPLE 2. PACU NURSING PATIENT CARE COMMITTEE: PHILOSOPHY

The Postanesthesia Care Unit reflects the Division of Nursing Affairs' philosophy of nursing, which is based on the belief that the purpose of nursing is the provision of high quality, scientifically based nursing care.

The purpose of the PACU is to facilitate emergence from anesthetic agents, both regional and general, and to prevent complications from anesthesia, and medical or surgical interventions. Meeting the physical needs of the patient takes first priority upon patient entry into the recovery room. Once stabilized, the psychosocial, cultural and spiritual needs are integrated into the plan of care.

By utilizing the concept of total care nursing and the nursing process, (assessment, planning, implementation and evaluation), the PACU nurse demonstrates independent, interdependent, and dependent nursing actions that are based on clinical and theoretical knowledge in the perioperative and postoperative environment. Emphasis on the professional team approach not only allows channels of communication to remain open with all disciplines, but also maintains professional accountability to the PACU nurse.

EXAMPLE 3. PACU NURSING EDUCATION/RESEARCH COMMITTEE: PHILOSOPHY

In keeping with the Division of Nursing Affairs' philosophy, the PACU Education/Research Committee is committed to freedom of inquiry, excellence in practice, and the development of innovative thinking. The committee accepts nursing as an applied science and strives to develop the PACU nurse in the biological, behavioral and organizational sciences. Education is viewed as a lifelong process.

Research is a role component of every nurse in the PACU. Opportunities for clinical investigation are offered by the members trained in research methodology. Nurses are encouraged to contribute constructively through publication and lecture.

The Education/Research Committee recognizes the strong clinical focus of the university. Each nurse is responsible and accountable for his/her professional practice and is obligated to update knowledge and clinical skills through continuing education.

program and the in-service education program became the responsibility of the Education/Research Committee.

Nursing Care Delivery Models

Provided that the PACU nurse-administrator reports to the Department of Nursing, tactics to implement the department's philosophy regarding a particular nursing theory and/or nursing care delivery model must be considered. The nurse-administrator who works in an institution that applies either a functional or a team nursing model may find that little modification in the tactics employed on the general nursing units is necessary. However, the relatively short length of patient stay makes implementation of the primary model more difficult.

Key to the definition of primary nursing is the concept of 24-hour accountability. Modifications must be made to transfer the intent of the concept to the PACU. McConnell (1979) described the process used at Madison (Wisconsin) General Hospital. This process required review of all aspects of the PACU nursing care delivery system. Components of the system that required modification to elicit autonomy of the unit and each staff member were identified and changes were initiated. The result was a nursing care delivery system that held the unit accountable for all aspects of patient care delivery. Individual staff members were identified with individual patients, and they were held accountable for all aspects of the nursing care provided to those patients.

A similar modification took place at Rush-Presbyterian–St. Luke's Medical Center in Chicago. In order to identify the model that evolved from this process as an adaptation of the primary model used in the remainder of the medical center, it was labeled total care nursing (TCN). The standard of practice used to describe the model is demonstrated in Example 4. This standard was supported by numerous changes in existing standards, including policies related to the on-call system, admission and discharge, and record-keeping. The end result was reported by McConnell (1979).

Goals and Objectives

Once the philosophical components of the system have been identified and appropriate tactics for implementation stipulated, goals and objectives for the unit must be defined. As with the philosophy, these should follow the goals and objectives of the organization. The specific interests and needs of the PACU are then incorporated. Example 5 demonstrates the annual goals and objectives of the Patient Care Committee. Those statements that are measurable give substance to the philosophy and evolve annually to maintain the dynamic nature of the planning process.

EXAMPLE 4. PACU TOTAL CARE NURSING (TCN)

In keeping with the philosophy of primary nursing as implemented by the Division of Nursing Affairs, the Postanesthesia Care Unit has created a model which will support autonomous nursing care planning and delivery in a temporary care setting. This model has been designated as total care nursing (TCN) in order to differentiate it from the model which ascribes 24-hour accountability.

All patients admitted to the PACU will have an R.N. designated as the total care nurse assigned by the triage nurse. The TCN will be responsible for assessing, planning, implementing, coordinating, and evaluating all aspects of that patient's nursing care during his/her stay in the PACU. The TCN will be assisted in this process by an associate nurse.

POLICY
1. All patients admitted to the PACU will have an R.N. designated as TCN.
2. The TCN will take the initial patient report.
   a. The TCN will interview the anesthesiologist and anesthetist regarding the patient's history, physical status, surgical and anesthetic course and the plan for postanesthetic recovery.
   b. The associate nurse who assists the TCN will provide supplemental information regarding the admission assessment.
   c. The TCN will interview the members of the surgical team as necessary to determine the postoperative recovery plan.
3. The TCN and associate nurse will provide nursing care in accordance with the policies and procedures of the medical center and the PACU.
4. The recommended work load for the TCN is a maximum of two patients.
   a. A TCN will attend to one patient who is critically ill or unstable until the vital signs have been stabilized (i.e., patient requiring life support care).
   b. When the TCN has patient load as stated above, then she/he will admit patients as an associate nurse and assume full responsibility for the patient care until TCN is established.
   c. The TCN should attend to no more than three patients at a time.
5. When TCN leaves the work area, a specific nurse must be designated to take responsibility for the patients assigned to the TCN.
6. Approximately 15 minutes prior to a patient's discharge, the TCN should initiate preparations for discharge.
   a. Report is called by the TCN on all patients.
   b. When the TCN is to leave the work area and her/his total care patients are nearing discharge, every effort should be made to do the discharge assessment and call report to the nurse who will assume patient care responsibilities upon PACU discharge.

ORGANIZING

Organizational Structure
Organization of any activity requires knowledge of the structure of the system. Most medical centers use an organizational chart to clarify those

EXAMPLE 5. PACU NURSING PATIENT CARE COMMITTEE: GOALS

GOALS

1. Establish guidelines for the admission procedure to the PACU.
2. Develop standards for charting on the postanesthesia record.
3. Develop guidelines for respiratory management in the PACU.
4. Formulate criteria for pain assessment and management in the PACU.

OBJECTIVES

1. Investigate the recent literature regarding admission priorities (triage) in the PACU.
2. Evaluate the protocol and corresponding policy for admission to the PACU for this and other systems.
3. Redefine the admission protocol in the PACU as indicated.
4. Initiate a task force to examine the present record keeping systems in the PACU.
   a. Identify components of the current system
   b. Determine appropriateness of the current system
   c. Determine staff use of the current system through chart audits
   d. Redefine the system as indicated, including policy and procedure changes.
5. Formulate standards of care with the Department of Anesthesia and Department of Respiratory Therapy for postanesthesia respiratory management.
6. Incorporate respiratory management standards of care into the standardized plan.
7. Develop standards of care with the Department of Anesthesia for postanesthesia pain assessment and management.
8. Incorporate pain assessment and management standards of care into the standardized care plan.

relationships. However, charts usually stop just short of clearly defining relationships at the unit level.

In a centralized, hierarchical system, the job description may provide the necessary insight. Reporting relationships are stipulated. Job activities are specified functionally, and all interfaces are conducted in a vertical fashion through the hierarchy.

Decentralized systems with lateral interfaces may temporarily complicate a clear understanding of the communication system. Not only does the nurse-administrator report vertically but there may be a direct responsibility for horizontal communication to the medical director or hospital administrator. An organizational chart designed to reflect interactions at the unit level can identify the nature of those reporting and communicating relationships. In addition, specific statements in the unit's operational policy may further identify the scope of each individual's responsibility (Example 6).

Communication Systems

A clearly defined organizational structure promotes effective communication, but it does not assure it. A tactic significant to the success of any project is the organization of an adequate communication system. For staff members, this may mean monthly unit meetings, annual performance reviews, and individual goal-setting. These are techniques common to managers in all work settings. Extra unit communications are often not so routine.

Perioperative Role. One tactic that has been employed to improve communications between special care areas and the general care units is the use of preoperative assessment and teaching by personnel assigned to special care areas. This has been used predominately by operating room personnel, although some centers, for example, at the University of California at San Francisco, have involved PACU personnel.

Kneedler and Dodge (1983) define the perioperative role as "nursing activities performed by the professional nurse during the perioperative, intraoperative, and postoperative phases of the patient's surgical experience" (p. 24). Most programs initiate the perioperative role in the late afternoon, with preoperative rounds concerning patients scheduled for surgery the following day. This visit is intended to establish or validate nursing diagnosis through physical assessment, patient interview, and review of patient records. It is also used to supplement the preoperative teaching plan. An added benefit of involving the PACU nurse in the preoperative assessment and patient teaching programs is the opportunity for new avenues for interprofessional communications.

Implementation of this program does have some pitfalls. Martina (1981) identifies lack of educational preparation as a contributing factor in program failures. Bille (1979) acknowledges this element in patient education efforts, and recommends review of basic adult education principles to overcome the deficit. In addition, tactics must be implemented that provide both the time for the interviews and the motivation to conduct them.

Nurse-Consultant. PACU staff members have also been able to promote effective communications through use of the nurse-consultant role. Keithley and associates (1979) identify three capacities in which a nurse-consultant might be used: as a specialist, a resource person, and a process consultant. Although all roles are potential sources for consultation, PACU staff members would most likely be called upon to serve in the specialist's role. The "specialist's" contract is initiated to tap the special skills and knowledge of the PACU nurse as it relates to a patient management problem or the continuing education needs of the staff.

Some training for these nurse-specialists is usually necessary. As Oda (1982) suggests, possession of the specialized knowledge does not mean that an individual is prepared to function in a specialist's role. The functional process of nurse consultation must be learned. Lareau (1980, p. 81) has identified six steps in the process of nurse consultation:

1. Gaining entry into the system.
2. Negotiating or contracting.
3. Identifying the problem.
4. Developing interventions.
5. Intervening (either by the consultant or the consultee).
6. Evaluating (either by the consultant or consultee).

Steps three to six follow a familiar taxonomy, the nursing process, and will not be discussed further.

Step two, negotiation or contracting, requires mutual clarification of expectations and goals. Step one is key to the process, and requires special tactile planning. Several approaches may be used to gain entry into the system. The presentation of in-service programs increases the visibility of the consultant to staff as does the preoperative patient teaching program discussed earlier. Keithley and associates (1979) suggest the use of a consultant directory, formal consultation request forms, and professional business cards which can be easily distributed and posted on bulletin boards. Once initital contact has been made, efforts to demonstrate interest in serving the consultee and maintaining credibility are necessary.

MD/RN Interface. Possibly the greatest frustration for nurses is the quality of nurse–physician communication. This is magnified in the PACU due to the acuity of the patient's condition, the stress imposed by the need to "keep things moving," and the number of individuals involved in the patient's care. Systems must be organized to support effective nurse–physician communication. The reasons are multifaceted. Staff satisfaction, reduced patient injury, reduced malpractice claims, and staff productivity are suggested by Johnson (1983) as significant outcomes of improved communications.

EXAMPLE 6. SCOPE OF RESPONSIBILITY

OPERATIONAL RESPONSIBILITY

Medical director

The medical director is an anesthesiologist appointed by the chairperson of the Department of Anesthesiology. The medical director assumes Division of Medical Affairs and Medical College responsibility for the unit on a 24-hour basis. This includes, but is not limited to, the responsibility for the implementation of medical staff policies related to unit operations and for decision making in consultation with the responsible attending surgeon regarding the disposition of patients when the patient load exceeds optimal operational capacity. An alternate is designated by the medical director when he/she is unavailable.

Unit leader

The unit leader is a registered nurse appointed by the chairperson of the Department of Operating Room and Surgical Nursing. This individual assumes Division of Nursing Affairs and College of Nursing responsibility for the unit on a 24-hour basis. This includes, but is not limited to, the responsibility for the implementation of nursing staff policies related to unit operations and the management of patient care services. An alternate is designated by the unit leader when he/she is unavailable.

Director of operating room administration

The director of operating room administration is appointed by the associate administrator of surgical sciences and services. This individual assumes Division of Administrative Affairs responsibility for the unit on a 24-hour basis. This includes, but is not limited to, the responsibility for the implementation of administrative policies related to daily unit operations and the management of the unit's support services. An alternate is designated by the director of operating room administration when he/she is unavailable.

Support personnel

All support personnel functioning in the PACU are responsible to their line supervisors. Those supervisors are responsible to coordinate the activities of their personnel with the needs of the PACU as determined by the medical director, unit leader, and director of operating room administration.

PATIENT CARE RESPONSIBILITY

Medical director

In order to maintain a level of medical care commensurate with the needs of the patients and to maintain the channels of communication necessary to facilitate this function, the medical director is responsible for the coordination of the activities of the Division of Medical Affairs and Medical College personnel who practice in the PACU. The medical director shall ensure the quality, safety, and appropriateness of patient care services. The medical director acts as a medical and research consultant in the management of patients with respiratory and/or anesthetic related problems.

Unit leader

In order to maintain a level of nursing care commensurate with the needs of the patients and to maintain the channels of communication necessary to facilitate this function, the unit leader is responsible for the coordination of the Division of Nursing Affairs and College of Nursing personnel who practice in the PACU. The unit leader shall ensure the quality, safety, and appropriateness of nursing services. The unit leader acts as a nursing and research consultant in the management of patients with respiratory or anesthetic-related problems.

Anesthesiologist/Anesthesiology resident

The physicians assigned to the Department of Anesthesiology are responsible for the coordination of the medical care of the patient.

Surgeon/Surgical resident

The surgical attending staff and residents are responsible for the medical care of the patient as it relates to the surgical procedure and are kept informed of the patient's condition by the anesthesiologist and/or registered nurse.

Certified registered nurse anesthetist/Student nurse anesthetist

The CRNA/SNA is responsible to the attending anesthesiologist.

Staff nurse

The nurses assigned to the Department of Operating Room and Surgical Nursing, PACU, are responsible for the coordination of the nursing care of the patient.

PACU attendant

The PACU attendants are employed by the Department of Operating Room and Surgical Nursing. They are assigned directly to the PACU, and are responsible to the unit leader.

A framework used effectively to accomplish this goal includes the following tactics (Johnson, 1983, pp. 19–20).

1. Avoid charged words.
2. Build nurses' clinical competence and clinical credibility.
3. Create a problem-solving structure (solve problems at the lowest possible level).
4. Support the nurses.
5. Create a prospective problem-solving structure (collaborative practice committees).
6. Stop blaming the doctors—and start listening.

The first four tactics are established management precepts used in a variety of settings. Collaborative practice committees have already been used successfully in the operating room (Mailhot & Slezak, 1983) and in the intensive care unit (Bray, 1983). However, possibly the most significant aspect in establishing effective nurse–physician communications is the willingness to listen. Keelan and Stokoe (1983) emphasize the importance of understanding patterns used by individuals to communicate and the importance of being a good listener. Thus, if as much attention were paid to the process of communication as the product, stress would be decreased. The result would be a better nurse–physician relationship.

Committee Structure

The use of committees can be an effective management tactic. A committee has already been used by this author as a tool to facilitate decentralization and promote effective communications. It is important to organize committees in a manner that meets intended outcomes. This requires definition of purpose, membership, and responsibility. A document that describes these expectations helps to assure that all parties interpret the intent of the committee in a like fashion (Example 7).

DIRECTING

Standards of Practice

Much attention has been devoted in recent years to the tactic of establishing standards of practice for the PACU. Through the use of standards, nursing care is directed toward the patient-care goals established in the planning process. They are also an effective educational and evaluation tool.

The Association of Operating Room Nurses (AORN) first published standards in 1980. They evolved at the request of AORN members em-

EXAMPLE 7. COMMITTEE ORGANIZATION: PATIENT CARE COMMITTEE

The purpose of this committee is to coordinate all nursing activities, aside from education/research, intended to directly effect patient care in the Postanesthesia Care Unit. This responsibility includes:

1. An ongoing patient care needs assessment.
2. Development and revision of patient care protocols.
3. Planning for the implementation and evaluation of all PACU patient care programs.
4. Development of priorities, with unit leadership, for all committee activities and programs.
5. Coordination with department and divisional programs and committees which effect patient care in the PACU.

The chairperson of this committee attends unit administrative group meetings and is responsible for coordinating the committee's activities with unit's goals and objectives. The chairperson is responsible for committee leadership. This responsibility includes:

1. Establishment of a PACU patient care philosophy.
2. Development of committee goals and objectives.
3. Development and implementation of a plan by which to meet those goals and objectives.
4. Evaluation of patient care efforts.

The appointment of the PACU chairperson is made by the unit leader. To be qualified for this position the PACU staff member must meet the requirements of RNC as well as satisfactorily complete the interview process.

The work of the committee includes such current activities as standards of care, primary nursing, audits, new products, and infection control, as well as the creation of new programming as appropriate. In addition to reporting to the leadership group, it is the responsibility of this committee to interface with the Education/Research Committee for all projects which contain education or research components.

Projects for which this committee takes direct responsibility are:

Standards of Care (formerly Policy and Procedure)—to develop, review, and update a reference manual for nursing procedures specific to the PACU. This manual will support the standards of care established for both the Division of Nursing and specialty care areas.

Standardized Nursing Care Plans—to identify, develop, review and update PACU patient care protocols which serve as a minimum standard for patient care. This work will be compiled into a reference manual which will support the standards established within the Department of Operating Room and Surgical Nursing and by the Division of Nursing.

Total Care Nursing—to design, implement, evaluate, and modify as necessary a PACU nursing care delivery system which supports a philosophy of primary nursing as well as the aforementioned Standards of Care and Standardized Nursing Care Plans.

Nursing Audits—to systematically review nursing care delivery in the PACU, and to make recommendations for patient care based upon the outcome of those audits.

New Products—to establish a formal and continuing system for the evaluation and introduction into use of new or replacement patient care products used in the PACU. This process is intended to support established departmental, divisional, and organizational New Products Committees.

Non-PACU committees which articulate with the Patient Care Committee through their appointed PACU representative are:

Standards of Care—Department of Surgical and Operating Room Nursing.
Standards of Care—Special care areas.
Standardized Nursing Care Plan—Department of Surgical and Operating Room Nursing.

---

ployed in PACUs. The standards, based on the use of nursing process, are as follows (Standards of Nursing Practice, 1980, pp. 801–804).

1. The collection of data about the health status of the patient is systematic and continuous. The data are recorded, retrievable, and communicated to appropriate persons.
2. Nursing diagnosis is derived from health status data.
3. Goals for nursing care are formulated.
4. The plan of nursing care prescribes nursing actions to achieve the goals.
5. The plan for nursing care is implemented.
6. The plan for nursing care is evaluated.
7. Reassessment of the patient, reconsideration of nursing diagnosis, resetting of goals, and modification and implementation of the nursing care plan are a continuous process.

Each standard is accompanied by a set of assessment factors. For example, in the application of standard 1, the nurse is instructed to assess health data including current medical diagnosis, operative procedure, type of anesthesia, physical status, and physiological response.

The American Society of Post Anesthesia Nurses (ASPAN) has since produced its recommendations regarding PACU standards. Two documents were produced: the first outlines patient care standards (ASPAN, 1983a), and the second relates to management standards (ASPAN, 1983b). Together these two documents address the subjects of assessment, nursing diagnosis, care plan, implementation, evaluation, discharge, personnel, education, patient–staff ratio, and physical aspects of the PACU. As with the AORN standards, these statements are based upon the nursing process. However, they go beyond the patient care statements and provide recommendations regarding administrative support for those standards.

Recommendations regarding practice in the PACU have also been made by the American Society of Anesthesiologists. They are accompanied by a statement disclaiming the intent of the advisory to serve as either "a statement of medical opinion or as a standard of approved medical care" (ASA, 1978, p. 8). Nevertheless, these recommendations represent untested beliefs of the ASA regarding standards for the PACU.

The subjects addressed by this document are purpose, location, organization, nursing care, equipment, consultant physician role, isolation practices, control of radioactive substances, and policies. Particular care is taken to describe the nursing care component. Thus, reference to this document may assist in clarification of the functional role expectations of the anesthesia and surgical staff. An expanded but similar set of statements is provided by Brody and associates (1982).

Policy

Once nursing practice standards have been determined, continued application may be encouraged through the design or modification of written nursing policy and procedure, also referred to as standards of practice. The JCAH supports this written standard-setting process. Standard IV for Special Care Areas specifically states that written policies and procedures shall guide nursing care. At a minimum, policies and procedures are required to address the following (Chicago JCAH, 1982, p. 184):

- Admission and discharge of patients.
- A system for informing responsible physicians of changes in the patient condition.
- Explicit directions as to the location and storage of medications, supplies, and special equipment.
- The methods for procurement of equipment and drugs at all times.
- Responsibility for maintaining the integrity of the emergency drug system.
- Infection control.
- Procedures to be followed in the event of the breakdown of essential equipment.
- Pertinent safety practices.
- Regulations for traffic control, including visitors.
- The role of the unit in the hospital's external and internal disaster plans.
- Specifications as to who may perform special procedures, under what circumstances, and under what degree of supervision.

- The use of standing orders.
- The protocol for the handling of specific emergency conditions (p. 184).

Brody and associates (1982, pp. 96–99) add to this list, detailing the nature and scope of policies related to:

- Physician's orders.
- Nursing and administrative guidelines.
- Intravenous medication.
- Fluid and blood product administration.
- Environmental safety.
- Cardiopulmonary resuscitation.
- Infection control and epidemiological practices.
- Admission and discharge.
- Necessary equipment and supplies.
- Traffic control.
- Records and statistics.

The use of these guidelines in conjunction with the professional practice standards discussed previously can provide the foundation for a comprehensive policy and procedure manual. This manual then provides consistent direction for patient care practices.

Standardized Nursing Care Plan

Another means to encourage application of patient care standards is through use of a standardized nursing care plan. This plan should be individualized to each patient. Nichols and Barstow (1980) demonstrated that staff did use care plans even if they were considered imperfect; generation of a plan based upon accepted patient care standards could therefore serve as a conceptual tool for the organization of patient care activities.

The concepts addressed in such a plan may be based upon the outline provided by ASPAN for care plan development (ASPAN, 1983b). This document addresses priority setting, scientific knowledge base, communication of the plan, health status assessments, and specific nursing actions based upon previously formulated nursing diagnoses.

The AORN also recommends that the care plan be based upon nursing diagnosis (Standards of Nursing Practice, 1980). As postanesthetic complications commonly fall into several categories, specific nursing diagnosis statements could be anticipated. For example, the potential respiratory complication of airway obstruction secondary to soft tissue interference might be stated as the potential for ineffective airway clearance. Specific patient outcomes and suggested nursing interventions would follow the standards of practice statements adopted by the nursing unit. This would direct nursing actions toward behaviors compatible with the unit's standards.

Charge Nurse Role

An effective charge nurse is essential to efficient PACU operation. This individual's responsibilities include coordinating admission and discharge activity, supervising the maintenance of an appropriate nurse–patient ratio, and troubleshooting problem communications. The nurse- administrator may be expected to fulfill this function. However, recent trends appear to support the concept of 24-hour first-line accountability for unit management (Murphy, 1980). This has resulted in the decentralization of many new responsibilities to the nurse-administrator. The time spent in daily management must now be used for a full range of management functions. The PACU is particularly vulnerable to the effects of this change as the rapid patient turnover and high patient acuity create a very dynamic management environment, necessitating regular interventions.

In an attempt to reorganize their responsibilities, many nurse administrators have delegated the daily charge responsibilities to an experienced member of the nursing staff. In some centers the assignment is a permanent one, either to an assistant head nurse or to specified staff members. In others the responsibility is rotated among all eligible staff.

There are pros and cons to each tactic. Use of permanently assigned staff helps to assure management consistency and to ease communication. It does not promote understanding by all staff of decision-making and problem-solving processes. Thus, staff members may misinterpret the actions of the charge nurse, or be left helpless in a situation where the charge nurse is unavailable.

A rotating responsibility familiarizes all eligible staff members with the necessary management techniques. This helps assure cooperation between staff members and the charge nurse, as polarization between the two groups is less likely. Not only will staff members appreciate the responsibilities that fall to the charge nurse, but a "tomorrow it could be me" attitude will prevail.

An increase in individual autonomy is also possible. As staff members are prepared to make decisions and solve problems, they are less dependent upon the charge nurse. The charge nurse is now free to provide support to the nurse at the bedside rather than to intervene on her or his behalf unless requested to do so. Staff nurses receive satisfaction as a result of the opportunity to fully utilize their skills as professional nurses. The charge nurse is free to devote her or his attention to the overall organization of unit activities.

The difficulties that arise as a result of rotating charge responsibility are clarity of communication and consistency of technique. With so many staff members sharing daily operational responsibilities, confusion can occur. Non-PACU personnel have difficulty identifying the charge nurse. This is particularly true of long-term staff members who expect to identify the charge nurse without assistance and to then be about their business. Staff members also experience frustration because of the wide variety in decision-making and problem-solving techniques.

Once the delegation tactic is selected, it is necessary to develop tactics that support that model. One or two staff members who regularly assume the charge role may be easily oriented by the unit manager. Regular review and discussion of the role with this group and the staff group will most likely resolve any discrepancies in the interpretation of those responsibilities.

A large number of staff members functioning in the charge nurse role may require greater standardization of behaviors. Written guidelines to supplement the orientation and evaluation process can be an effective tool. In addition, consideration must be given to communication systems, both internal and external to the unit.

CONTROLLING

External Quality Review

Patient care controls for PACU may be internal or external. Examples of external controls include the accreditation process, review by state regulatory agencies, and the hospital quality assurance program. It is important that the nurse-administrator be familiar with the expectations of each of these bodies in order that tactics are implemented that ensure standard maintenance.

Outside agencies publish their standards, usually in the form of a manual made available to the hospital. The hospital quality assurance program may not provide its standards in so concise a format; it then falls to the nurse-administrator to characterize the process.

First the nurse-administrator must determine the nature of the review. Does it rely on documentation of appropriate structural elements (policy and procedure), process elements (observation), or outcome elements (retrospective chart audits)? Due to the limited length of PACU patient stay, this timing can significantly effect data accuracy. For example, a nursing process audit may not accurately demonstrate measurement of intake and output if the data is collected before the nursing assessment is complete. This would require that the nurse manager work with the quality assurance team to determine the most effective means to collect this data.

It may be necessary to eliminate or modify evaluative categories. Criteria related to health maintenance, home care planning, patient education, and family involvement are difficult to apply to all PACU patients. These statements must be eliminated or modified to reflect only the level of care realistic in the PACU.

Criteria must be defined clearly and provide reasonable measurement parameters. Unless that element is considered, the data produced may be meaningless. A statement regarding appropriate intervention for pain could produce a variety of responses on a retrospective chart audit without specific evaluative cues.

Finally, the nurse-administrator must determine the ability of the instrument to measure nursing care quality. An instrument designed to measure the quality of medical care does not necessarily reflect the quality of nursing interventions. This is not to say that such an instrument should not be used, only that the nurse-administrator should ensure that the data are correctly interpreted.

Internal Quality Review

In addition to compliance with the hospital quality assurance program, a unit audit of patient care practices is a valuable tool. Many nurse-administrators routinely perform this function via walking rounds. Another common and more objective tool is a retrospective chart audit by PACU staff. The data collection instrument should reflect the nursing standards of practice previously discussed. The resulting data should be systematically analyzed and formally reviewed with staff members. Finally, maintenance of acceptable patient care practices should be encouraged and modification of ineffective behaviors supported through individual staff evaluations.

Patient Care Conferences

Another means to review patient care practices is through the patient care conference. A traditional part of the team nursing model, this tool has been adapted to reflect the needs of primary nursing.

Kron (1966) originally described the patient care conference as a team planning tool. The objectives of the effort were the design of a patient care plan, coordination of team services in the implementation of that plan, and the promotion of team spirit and understanding.

With primary nursing it was necessary to shift the focus from the team effort to care plan communication. Mayer and Bailey (1979) outlined a "refocused" set of objectives to promote the patient care conference in a primary nursing model. The objectives are:

1. Description of the patient's care plan.
2. Explanation of patient care procedures and approaches.
3. Identification of rationale.
4. Solicitation of ideas for unsolved patient problems.

Use of these objectives shifted the intent of the conference from group planning to peer consultation.

The direct application of either set of objectives in the PACU is impractical due to the limited nature of the patient's stay. A feasible alternative is the patient care conference as a retrospective review. The set of objectives appropriate to the nursing care delivery model in use on the unit are applied to the case selected for presentation. Peer analysis and discussion stimulate both new learning and evaluation of patient care practices.

Morbidity and Mortality Review

Unlike the retrospective chart audit and patient care conference, which stimulate analysis of all nursing practices, the morbidity and mortality review concentrates on patients who have experienced complications. The activity is initiated by a staff member who determines the presence of significant events and records the findings in a morbidity and mortality log. These data are systematically correlated and the results are shared with staff for analysis of trends and review of contributing patient care practices.

At the same time, one or two case studies are selected for closer review using the format of the patient care conference. Nursing interventions that contributed to the incident or supported its resolution are targeted for discussion. Nursing practice standards are either reinforced or modified as a result.

REFERENCES

American Society of Post Anesthesia Nurses: Guidelines for management standards in the post anesthesia care unit. Breathline 83(3): 18, 1983a.

American Society of Post Anesthesia Nurses: Guidelines for standards of care in the post anesthesia care unit. Breathline 83(3): 17, 1983b.

American Society of Anesthesiologists: A practice advisory, 1978, p. 8.

Bille DA: Perioperative teaching: Rights and responsibilities. Critical Care Nurse 3(3): 19–20, 1983.

Bray K: Improving communication through an RN/MD advisory council. Critical Care Nurse 3(3): 19–20, 1983.

Brody DC, Shapiro AG, & Caine M: Criteria for Patient Care. In JS Israel & TJ Dekornfeld (Eds.), Recovery Room Care: Principles and Practice, Design and Equipment, and Staffing and Patient Care. Springfield, Ill.: Chas. C Thomas, 1982, pp. 86–115.

Chicago Joint Commission for the Accreditation of Hospitals: Accreditation of hospitals, 1982.

Johnson PF: Improving the nurse–physician relationship. Journal of Nursing Administration 13(3): 19–20, 1983.

Keelan JA & Stokoe SJ: Taking the stress out of O.R. communication. AORN Journal 37(5): 847–852, 1983.

Keithley JK, Shelley S, & Brenner JA: Help at hand: Using the nurse consultant. Nursing 79(11): 105–112, 1979.

Kneedler J & Dodge G: Perioperative Patient Care: The Nursing Perspective. Boston: Blackwell, 1983, p. 24.

Kron T: Nursing Team Leadership. Philadelphia: Saunders, 1966.

Lareau SC: The nurse as clinical consultant. Topics in Clinical Nursing 2:79–84, 1980.

Mailhot C & Slezak L: Nurse–physician committee eases tension in O.R. AORN Journal 38(3): 411–415, 1983.

Martina L: Opinions: How can we overcome barriers to preop interviews? AORN Journal 33(5): 1981.

Mayer GG & Bailey K: Adapting the patient care conference to primary nursing. Journal of Nursing Administration 9(6): 7–10, 1979.

McConnell EA: Primary nursing in the recovery room. AORN Journal 30(5): 1007–1010, 1979.

Murphy JS: Seventeen large hospitals surveyed: Trends revealed. Nursing and Health Care 1:34–37, 1980.

Nichols EG & Barstow RE: Do nurses really use standard care plans? Journal of Nursing Administration, 190, 10(5): 27–31, 1980.

Oda DS: Consultation: An expectation of leadership. Nursing Leadership, 5(1): 7–9, 1982.

Chapter 4

Strategies for the Postanesthesia Care Unit Nurse-Administrator

Diane Randall Andrews

Webster's *New Collegiate Dictionary* defines strategy as "a careful plan or method" and "the art of devising or employing plans or strategems toward a goal." The nurse-administrator uses a complex array of strategies to plan, organize, staff, direct, and control. The means by which these strategies are generated is often referred to as the management process. This process parallels the scientific method used by nurses in direct patient care: data collection and analysis, constitution of a plan, implementation of the plan, and evaluation. For the nurse-administrator, the process must be broadened to consider the impact of multiple impinging systems and the influence of numerous individuals. The strategic outcomes of the process may also affect sets of principles or procedures and those identified with them. Hence, the nurse-administrator must proceed with care through each of the management process steps.

Gilles (1982, pp. 1–6) suggests a systems approach to accomplish this task effectively. By this method, the input, processor, output, controls (evaluation mechanism), and feedback components of each strategic element are carefully identified.

The present chapter presents three strategic tasks common to the nurse-administrator in the PACU: staffing and scheduling, recording, and facilities planning. As was suggested, no strategy can be devised without adequate and accurate data. These data must then be interpreted and a plan unique to each setting must be designed, implemented, and evaluated.

This chapter is intended to guide the nurse-administrator in data collection and analysis through review of the variables which influence each topic.

STAFFING AND SCHEDULING

Probably no greater challenge faces a nurse-administrator than the design and implementation of an effective staffing and scheduling system. The system must ensure a work force able to meet organizational, departmental, and professional standards. It must be efficient to administer, cost-effective, and sensitive to nurse workload and patient acuity. It must employ an adequate number of staff members at the appropriate educational level, prepared to effect the goals of the system. Finally, a means of evaluation must be available.

Over the last few years, a number of scientific methodologies have been proposed to replace the more traditional approaches to nurse staffing. These were described by Stevens (1975, p. 132) as a mix of tradition, staff feedback, and staffing theory. The new designs quantify input and apply computer technology to process data and to calculate projected staffing. One example is the methodology developed by Medicus Systems Corporation (Norby & associates, 1977). This system applies data derived from patient classification, calculated direct and indirect nursing workload, and quality care monitoring to project staffing levels. Daily patient classification is used as an instrument to assist in short-term adjustment of these recommended staffing patterns. Nurse scheduling and management reporting capacity are additional features of this system (Byra & Pierce, 1974).

Nurse scheduling has also received much attention in the last few years. Staffing shortages and an increased emphasis on nurse satisfaction have contributed to more creative nurse scheduling schemes. In addition to trial and error or fixed, cyclic scheduling modes, a variety of nontraditional approaches have been used. Most of these offer an alternative to the traditional 5 day, 40 hour work week. Included in those schemes are plans that increase the use of part-time staff members and an extensive array of flexible shift schedules (American Journal of Nursing, 1981; Rasmussen, 1982).

Staffing

The design of a PACU staffing system relies on principles common to general unit staffing. However, these principles are applied in a setting with a highly dynamic patient census. This results in variable facility utilization. Determination of the effect of this variability requires collection and analysis of patient census, patient acuity, and nursing workload data.

Patient Census. The PACU census is dependent upon operating room caseload, and this may fluctuate dramatically—hourly, daily, weekly, and monthly. PACU staffing plans must meet peak patient census levels to permit efficient use of operating room suites and personnel. At the same time, however, the staffing plan must reflect low census periods to minimize overstaffing. In addition, the PACU may be used as a special procedures unit (for example, for electroconvulsive therapy treatments or placement of anesthetic nerve blocks), an overflow area for intensive care, and an outpatient recovery and discharge area. Staffing plans must predict as close as possible these additional requirements, and must also be flexible enough to permit short-term adjustments in staffing. Finally, emergency surgery requires emergency recovery. Staffing of the PACU must include a contingency plan for such events.

In order to determine the nature and frequency of census trends, data need to be collected and analyzed. The most readily available source of this data is a PACU census record that keeps track of admission and discharge times (Fig. 4-1). Unfortunately, analysis of this data can be

PRESBYTERIAN-ST. LUKE'S HOSPITAL
PACU CENSUS

Patient Name	Room No.	Procedure	Surgeon	Anesthesiologist	Time In	Time Out	Total Time

Figure 4–1. PACU census record. *(Courtesy of Rush-Presbyterian–St. Luke's Medical Center, Chicago.)*

cumbersome and time-consuming. A more convenient method uses case-by-case entry of census data into a computerized statistical program that summarizes the data according to specified parameters.

One such system is in use at Rush-Presbyterian–St. Luke's Medical Center in Chicago. Admission, acuity, and discharge information is recorded for each patient on a workload data collection tool (Fig. 4-2).

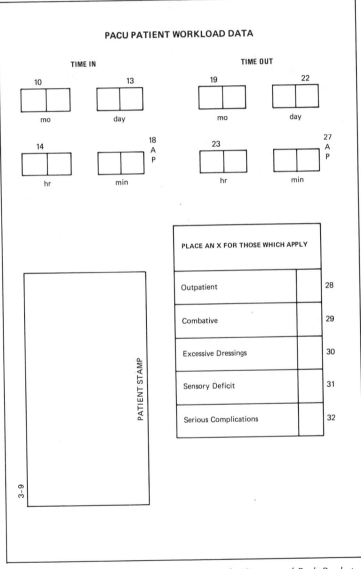

Figure 4–2. PACU workload data collection tool. *(Courtesy of Rush-Presbyterian–St. Luke's Medical Center, Chicago.)*

These data are processed according to a prescribed format, and a four-week printout is available to the unit manager (Fig. 4-3). This printout demonstrates yearly, weekly, and bihourly census trends. The data is combined with patient acuity data to suggest nurse staffing levels.

Patient Acuity. Just as census is unpredictable, so is acuity. All patients admitted to the PACU are expected to have baseline nursing care requirements as a result of surgery and anesthesia. In addition to these requirements, underlying disease or nonsurgically related health problems may increase the patient's acuity.

Patients may also require a variable amount of staff time due to rapid changes in acuity. At the time of admission, the patient may require the attention of several staff members. Once stabilized, the patient's nursing care needs may decrease dramatically. On the other hand, a sudden deterioration in the patient's condition may require an even greater number of staff members to render effective nursing care. Finally, unexpected surgical and anesthetic complications may result in significant shifts in patient acuity.

Patient classification offers the nurse-administrator a means to quantify patient acuity. A number of instruments are currently available. Some are designed to classify the needs of patients in critical care settings; these are directly applicable to the PACU setting (Cullen and associates, 1974; Duraiswamy and associates, 1981; Evans and associates, 1980). Others require adaptation.

In 1974 (Byra & Pierce), Rush-Presbyterian–St. Luke's Medical Center and Medicus Systems Corporation created a patient classification system that defined acuity in progressive categories of nursing time requirements. Unfortunately, this system did not discriminate adequately for PACU patients, who all tended to fall into the highest classification category. Therefore, in 1978 (Kronman & Burke) an adaptation of this model was completed for PACU use. Five additional discriminating factors were identified. Using modified classification categories, nursing staff members classify each patient (Fig. 4-2). Specified cues (Table 4-1) were provided to standardize interpretation. The acuity data were collected with census data, and these two measures were used to calculate actual nursing workload. Via weighted indices in hours per hour of nursing time (Table 4-2), this workload then forms the base for suggested nurse staffing determinations (Fig. 4-3). Trends in suggested staffing data can then be used to predict future staffing needs.

Nursing Workload. Perhaps the most difficult aspect of nurse staffing either to qualify or quantify is nursing workload. To do so requires a detailed analysis of all the direct and indirect components of nursing care. Norby and associates (1977) have devised a methodology for this purpose that relies on determination of the total workload for each staff group

UNIT STATISTICS	AVERAGE	06-07 TO 07-04	07-05 TO 08-01	08-02 TO 08-29	08-30 TO 09-26	09-27 TO 10-24	10-25 TO 11-21	11-22 TO 12-19	12-20 TO 01-16	01-17 TO 02-13	02-14 TO 03-13	03-14 TO 04-10	04-11 TO 05-08	05-09 TO 06-05
	TOTAL	TOTAL	TOTAL	TOTAL	TOTAL	TOTAL	TOTAL	TOTAL	TOTAL	TOTAL	TOTAL	TOTAL	TOTAL	TOTAL
CENSUS (FROM LOG)	833	903	816	860	813	883	837	804	694	809	870	863	812	870
CENSUS (REPORTED)	832	904	815	859	816	879	835	795	693	809	867	863	812	872
OUTPATIENT	29	26	27	33	32	27	30	30	17	27	25	32	37	43
% OF REPORTED CENSUS	3.5	2.8	3.3	3.8	3.9	3.0	3.5	3.7	2.4	3.3	2.8	3.7	4.5	4.9
COMBATIVE	59	97	58	67	45	59	50	49	37	71	63	74	71	73
% OF REPORTED CENSUS	7.1	6.3	7.1	7.7	5.5	6.7	5.9	6.1	5.3	8.7	7.2	8.5	8.7	8.3
EXCESSIVE DRESSINGS	81	115	88	83	85	62	52	63	63	109	93	93	87	63
% OF REPORTED CENSUS	9.7	12.7	10.7	9.6	10.4	7.0	6.2	7.9	9.0	13.4	10.7	10.7	10.7	7.2
SENSORY DEFICITS	369	380	343	400	353	365	363	385	313	363	413	395	369	359
% OF REPORTED CENSUS	44.3	42.0	42.0	46.5	43.2	41.5	43.4	48.4	45.1	44.8	47.6	45.7	45.4	41.1
SERIOUS COMPLICATIONS	98	123	113	86	79	76	76	60	75	104	115	128	143	112
% OF REPORTED CENSUS	11.8	13.6	13.8	10.0	9.6	8.6	9.1	7.5	10.1	12.8	13.2	14.8	17.6	12.8
AVE. STAY (HOURS)	2.17	2.26	2.25	2.33	2.08	2.24	2.14	2.28	2.20	2.32	2.12	2.03	2.00	1.97
PERSONNEL STATISTICS														
WEEKDAY 8A-8P *														
SUGGEST STAFFING	7.5	8.2	8.0	8.0	7.3	7.2	6.9	7.1	7.0	8.2	7.8	7.6	7.2	7.2
ACTUAL STAFFING	8.9	7.7	8.0	7.7	7.5	9.2	9.1	9.9	9.8	9.6	9.7	8.8	9.4	9.7
ACT-SUG STAFFING	1.4	-0.5	0.0	-0.2	0.2	1.9	2.1	2.8	2.8	1.4	1.9	1.1	2.1	2.4
WEEKDAY 8P-8A **														
SUGGEST STAFFING	1.2	1.5	1.0	1.1	0.9	1.4	1.2	1.5	1.3	1.4	1.1	1.1	0.9	1.0
ACTUAL STAFFING	1.4	1.2	0.9	1.4	1.1	1.5	1.6	1.5	1.7	1.5	1.4	1.4	1.5	1.3
ACT-SUG STAFFING	0.1	-0.3	-0.1	0.2	0.2	0.0	0.4	0.0	0.3	0.0	0.3	0.3	0.6	0.2
WEEKEND AND HOLIDAY 8A-8A **														
SUGGEST STAFFING	0.3	0.2	0.2	0.1	0.4	0.4	0.2	0.4	0.3	0.2	0.3	0.2	0.2	0.3
ACTUAL STAFFING	0.3	0.5	0.4	0.2	0.3	0.4	0.5	0.4	0.4	0.1	0.4	0.3	0.2	0.3
ACT-SUG STAFFING	0.0	0.2	0.1	0.0	0.3	0.0	0.3	0.0	0.1	0.0	0.1	0.1	0.0	0.0
SICK & ABSENT HRS	148.8	83.7	115.3	151.7	174.2	174.6	114.6	209.4	106.2	303.5	89.2	150.6	88.2	173.7
HLDAY & VACATN HRS	286.4	222.0	256.0	328.0	416.0	240.0	134.0	380.0	570.0	116.0	194.0	256.0	282.0	330.0
OVERTIME HRS	78.6	130.0	128.0	105.5	69.3	109.8	31.9	61.0	65.8	78.0	46.6	41.1	59.0	96.5
ON CALL HRS	117.8	76.5	54.2	597.0	660.0	40.8	26.4	20.6	19.4	17.9	2.4	6.5	3.9	5.6

*SUGGEST AND ACTUAL HOURS ARE AVERAGED OVER THE 12 HOUR TIME PERIOD FOR NON-HOLIDAY WEEKDAYS AND INCLUDE OVERTIME HRS. FOR REQUIREMENTS WITHIN THE PERIOD SEE PAGE 2.

**SUGGEST HOURS DURING NON-PEAK PERIODS DO NOT INCLUDE THE INDIRECT ACTIVITY CONSTANT.

Figure 4-3. PACU management report—nursing quality assurance. (Courtesy of Rush-Presbyterian–St. Luke's Medical Center, Chicago.)

WORKLOAD STATISTICS

WEEKDAY	WORKLOAD	TIME:	8A – 10A	10A – 12P	12P – 2P	2P – 4P	4P – 6P	6P – 8P	8P – 8A	AVERAGE DAILY ADMISSIONS
MONDAY		(03) ###								50.0
SUGGEST	STAFF		5.2	11.6	12.1	11.1	6.0	3.4	0.7	
ACTUAL	STAFF		10.0	12.3	12.8	13.2	10.5	3.9	1.2	
ACT-SUG	STAFF		4.8	0.6	0.7	2.1	4.5	0.5	0.5	
PATIENT CENSUS			4.8	11.6	12.6	10.4	4.2	1.5	0.3	
TUESDAY		(04) ###								43.5
SUGGEST	STAFF		4.6	7.2	8.1	8.7	6.2	3.1	1.4	
ACTUAL	STAFF		8.0	12.3	12.7	13.1	10.8	4.1	1.5	
ACT-SUG	STAFF		3.4	5.1	4.6	4.4	4.5	1.0	0.0	
PATIENT CENSUS			4.5	8.4	8.6	8.9	4.9	1.2	0.9	
WEDNESDAY		(04) ###								48.5
SUGGEST	STAFF		6.4	11.4	11.5	9.1	6.3	4.1	1.1	
ACTUAL	STAFF		7.5	11.4	11.7	12.0	10.1	3.6	1.5	
ACT-SUG	STAFF		1.0	0.0	0.1	2.9	3.7	-0.5	0.4	
PATIENT CENSUS			6.7	11.5	11.5	8.6	5.0	2.0	0.3	
THURSDAY		(04) ###								37.0
SUGGEST	STAFF		3.1	7.7	10.3	10.5	6.2	3.5	1.3	
ACTUAL	STAFF		8.2	10.3	11.0	11.3	9.4	3.9	1.3	
ACT-SUG	STAFF		5.1	2.6	0.7	0.8	3.1	0.4	0.0	
PATIENT CENSUS			1.7	7.9	10.5	10.2	5.2	1.7	0.7	
FRIDAY		(04) ###								46.0
SUGGEST	STAFF		5.4	8.2	10.0	7.6	5.4	3.6	0.6	
ACTUAL	STAFF		7.6	11.6	11.8	12.3	9.6	3.8	0.9	
ACT-SUG	STAFF		2.2	3.4	1.7	4.7	4.2	0.2	0.2	
PATIENT CENSUS			5.2	9.3	10.7	7.3	4.5	2.4	0.5	
WEEKDAY AVERAGE		(19) ###								45.0
SUGGEST	STAFF		4.9	9.2	10.4	9.4	6.0	3.5	1.0	
ACTUAL	STAFF		8.3	11.6	12.0	12.4	10.1	3.9	1.3	
ACT-SUG	STAFF		3.3	2.3	1.6	3.0	4.0	0.3	0.2	
PATIENT CENSUS			4.6	9.7	10.8	9.1	4.8	1.8	0.6	

Figure 4–3. (Continued)

TABLE 4–1. WORKLOAD MONITORING—PATIENT CLASSIFICATION CUES

Outpatient	Patients who undergo surgery as outpatients and are discharged to home from PACU.
Combative	Patients who become aggressive or agitated while waking up after their surgery. These patients need constant supervision to prevent them from injuring themselves.
Excessive dressings	Patients with extensive burns, complex dressings, excoriations, or dermatological problems requiring extensive care.
Sensory deficit	Patients who are blind, deaf, unable to speak or who speak only a foreign language.
Serious complications	Patients who require immediate nursing attention beyond that effort strictly required by other indicators to either avert or cope with a threatening situation. Examples include hemorrhaging, shock, drop in vital signs, arrhythmias, cardiac or respiratory arrest, anesthesia-related problems, and other drug reactions.

(Courtesy of Rush-Presbyterian–St. Luke's Medical Center, Chicago.)

(e.g., RNs) divided by the average workload capacity of each staff member, to quantify direct patient care requirements. Research based data collection instruments and calculations were generated for this task. Factors related to the indirect patient care requirements then were identified, and an average time requirement was calculated. Budgetary considerations such as time allowance for days off, vacation, and illness were quantified. From these determinations, average staffing needs for each category of employee on a shift-by-shift basis were projected. To this is added patient classification, census, and quality monitoring data to adjust suggested staff levels over time.

Even if a sophisticated methodology such as the one provided by Norby and associates is not accessible, the variables that affect nursing workload (aside from census and acuity) should be qualified as specifically as possible. These variables include:

- Organizational, departmental, and unit philosophy, goals, and objectives.
- Policies and procedures.
- Standards of practice (institutional and professional).
- Availability of support personnel, equipment, and supplies.
- Model of nursing care delivery (primary, team, and functional).
- Staff mix (RN, LPN, NA).
- Environmental constraints (patient cubicles).
- Indirect patient care requirements (role of charge nurse, in-service, orientation, and research).

TABLE 4–2. MODEL OF NURSING REQUIREMENTS

Indicator	Unweighted Value (Hours)	Weighted Value* (Hours)
Census	0.356	0.403
Outpatient	0.305	0.346
Combative	0.465	0.527
Excessive Dressings	0.458	0.519
Sensory Deficit	0.322	0.365
Serious Complications	0.355	0.402
Constants		
Direct	0.702	0.795
Average Indirect	1.156	1.310

Notes

1. All indicator values are stated in required nursing hours per day of patient length of stay.
2. Constant values are stated in terms of required nursing hours per day shift hour.
3. Average indirect hours are applied during day shift only in the reporting model.

*Weighted values include 13.3 percent allowance for personal and meal time. In the development report this allowance was limited to 6.7 percent for personal activities. For the purposes of the management report, 6.6 percent was added for meals because it was impossible to reasonably account for lunch in actual hours. *(Courtesy of Rush-Presbyterian-St. Luke's Medical Center, Chicago.)*

Recommendations by external agencies for nurse-to-patient ratio should also be considered. The American Society of Anesthesiologists (1978) recommends a maximum nursing workload of three patients. The Northwest Recovery Room Nurses Association (1980) and the American Society of Post Anesthesia Nurses (1983) have qualified nurse-to-patient ratios even more. They recommend that a 1:1 nurse-to-patient ratio be employed on admission and for the care of the unstable patients, with a second nurse available if necessary. A one nurse to two patient ratio should be applied to stable patients who have undergone complicated surgery or anesthesia, unconscious patients, and pediatric patients. A ratio of one nurse to three patients should be used only for uncomplicated adult patients.

Once these variables have been evaluated and qualified, they are analyzed in terms of census data and acuity data to predict the average nurse-to-patient workload for each institution.

Once average nurse-to-patient ratios are determined, these figures can be combined with census and acuity trends to predict nurse staffing. With allowances for vacation, holiday and sick time, days off, meals, breaks, and other time-related employee benefits, budgeted staff positions can be determined.

Scheduling

After staffing has been predicted and provided, attention can be turned to nurse scheduling. As was true of staffing methodology, the traditional methods of nurse scheduling often prove ineffective for the PACU. A scheduling system based entirely upon a division of available staff into standard day, evening, and night shifts according to projected workload may result in periods of under- and over-staffing.

The system in use at Rush-Presbyterian–St. Luke's Medical Center projects bihourly census and nurse workload as the basis for nurse scheduling. Staff hours are adjusted to provide appropriate levels of coverage by staggering personnel starting times (e.g., 7 A.M., 8:30 A.M., 9 A.M., 12 P.M., 3 P.M., and 11 P.M.). Ten-hour shifts and the use of part-time personnel offer increased flexibility.

In addition to provision of coverage for peak census periods and predictable periods of low census, the scheduling system must offer enough flexibility to provide nurse coverage for events with low predictability. Some institutions maintain a skeleton staff in PACU at all times. Others modify this approach through the use of an on-call system. Finally, some PACUs rely on the operating room staff, the intensive care unit, or general nursing units to provide postanesthetic care after a specified time of day. Whichever approach is selected, policies, procedures, and continuing education programs should be established to ensure equivalent standards of care for all postanesthetic patients.

RECORD KEEPING

Record keeping in any organization is a complex task. Large quantities of data must be recorded, collected, analyzed, stored, and made available for retrieval. This is a costly and time-consuming process on which present and future operations depend.

The health care industry is no exception in its need for efficient, effective record-keeping systems. In addition to the large amount of data that must be managed in the delivery and review of patient care, organizational records must be maintained for internal and external purposes.

The nurse-administrator faced with the challenge of monitoring patient care and organizational record keeping is well aware of the enormity of the task. Data are constantly circulated through the patient care area and within the organization. Unless the data are properly recorded, analyzed, and stored they are lost for future use.

Increased Data Collection Needs

The need for accurate records has become even more critical in recent years. The projected use of diagnostic related groups (DRGs) for reimbursement of medical costs provides a timely example. The reimbursable costs for each institution are calculated according to a two-stage process (Grimaldi & Micheletti, 1983b). First, the direct care costs are calculated using the actual cost of hospital-based physician's services, nonphysician hospital services, and the average cost of nonphysician services in the hospital's locale. Second, approved costs of hospital operation recovered in the direct care fee, such as overhead and capital expenses, are calculated. A reimbursement rate is then set for each rate year for each DRG within each hospital. Obviously, such determinations require a large amount of data. Inadequate or inaccurate records can have a significant influence on the ability of a hospital to recover its expenses.

Lest the failure to include nursing costs in the calculation of DRGs should lead some to believe that the record of nursing activities is less significant, a short discussion of activities proposed to qualify those costs is indicated. The architects of the prototype DRG plan have turned their attention to the calculation of the cost of nursing services. The relative intensity measures (RIMs) method has been presented as a valid and reliable indicator of prospective nursing reimbursement costs for incorporation into the DRG methodology (Caterinecchio, 1983). However, critics of the RIMs method point out statistical, methodological, and interpretive inaccuracies (Grimaldi & Micheletti, 1983a). Only with the data obtained through effective record keeping will nursing be able to substantiate or refute claims regarding the cost of nursing services.

Legal Necessity. The current legal climate also has emphasized the need for accurate, reliable medical records. The patient record bears a great deal of weight in legal proceedings. Not only does it serve as substantive documentation of the patient's medical course, it is scrutinized for errors of omission and commission, tampering, and the care with which the record was maintained (McCaman & Hirsh, 1979).

Conservation of the medical record thus becomes crucial to physician and hospital alike. Chapman (1980) points out the value of patient record retention in accordance with the malpractice statute of limitations. Enactment of the statute and application of the law to minors can vary widely in each state. Therefore, it is recommended that state malpractice acts be reviewed to determine minimal retention time.

The American Hospital Association has prepared a statement entitled Preservation of Medical Records in Health Care Institutions (Record Retention, 1977) which was intended to prompt uniformity in state laws in regards to the statute of limitations for the retention of medical records. In this document a minimum of 10 years is recommended for the retention of complete patient medical records.

In addition to the patient care record, guidelines should be available regarding the retention of other medically related and organizational records. These records are not only required for internal review but may be necessary as substantive documentation in legal and regulatory matters.

The American Hospital Association guidelines have been expanded upon by the Illinois Hospital Association. *A Record Retention Guide for Illinois Hospitals* (Illinois Hospital Association, 1977) provides retention guidelines for a broad range of patient care and organizational records. Both of these documents emphasize the fact that the recommendations are to serve only as guidelines.

The medical records department of each hospital usually has policies related to record storage. Familiarity with these policies will ensure that documents that relate to the patient care record are maintained in a similar fashion. Each health care institution is responsible for internal practice related to record retention until legal statutes are established.

Maintenance of Patient's Rights

Attention must also be paid to a patient's rights when one considers hospital record maintenance. The data maintained in the patient record are needed for insurance, research, audit, statistical, and occasionally legal purposes. At the same time the patient has the right to privacy and the physician has the responsibility of confidentiality.

It is well established that the right to ownership of the patient's record is that of the physician and the hospital (McCaman & Hirsh, 1979). However, the patient's rights regarding access to and disclosure of that information have been upheld (Hiller, 1981). A balance must be established in each institution to ensure that the data maintained in the patient record are not used in a fashion that would breach the rights of the patient.

Recording in the PACU

How does record keeping relate to the role of the nurse-administrator in postanesthesia recovery? Obviously, the preceding information can be applied to the PACU setting. Data must be collected and recorded both efficiently and accurately. Caution must be taken to ensure that record retention meets legal and regulatory needs. Data must be maintained in the record in accordance with the rights of the patient.

It is equally obvious that much of the responsibility for the maintenance of these records falls to the nurse-administrator and the PACU staff. The special challenge that recording offers the PACU is the constraint imposed by time. With most nursing units, the bulk of nursing records can be completed after immediate patient care needs have been met. This is not the case for PACUs. Comprehensive data collection must be handled in a timely fashion throughout the patient's relatively short stay. The primary instrument is the patient care record. Therefore, this record must be organized in such a manner that it supports rapid notations regarding the patient's surgical and anesthetic course, admission status, ongoing assessments, laboratory data, medication administration, and discharge status. This record must not be so bulky that its use is cumbersome, and should facilitate later use by non-PACU personnel and researchers. Finally, the record can provide primary data in collection of patient charges and can function as a postdischarge reference to the PACU nurse.

Figure 4-4 gives an example of a record designed to satisfy these requirements. Note that this is a one-page form that relies heavily on checklists and short notations. The data on the front of the record are recorded in triplicate to facilitate direct collection of patient medication and solution charges. The second copy is kept in the PACU for postdischarge reference, morbidity and mortality review, quality assurance audit, and research. The REACT scoring system, a new postanesthesia recovery score designed by Fraulini and Murphy (1984), has been incorporated into the record.

Although the use of this record should adequately reflect a patient's postanesthetic care, it is not intended to take the place of a cardiopulmonary resuscitation (CPR) record. A CPR record is designed to ensure concise, chronological recording of the events during cardiopulmonary resuscitation. Most hospitals have adopted a standard record for use at such times (Fig. 4-5). An alternative approach is the electronic clipboard, which has been demonstrated to increase the quantity of documentation during the first 20 minutes of CPR (Ornato & associates, 1981). In the event of complications during a patient's PACU stay, records that document those episodes in a systematic fashion may then be used to facilitate review of patient care practices (Fig. 4-6).

The PACU is experiencing an increase in the use of the facility for special procedures. One such use is for delivery of electroconvulsive therapy treatments. This usually requires eight to ten repeated sessions; the use of separate PACU and anesthesia records for each session may cause needless repetition of medical findings, may make retrieval of data across a number of records difficult, and may add unnecessary bulk to the patient record. Therefore, it may prove useful to develop a separate record for use by both nursing and anesthesia (Fig. 4-7).

FACILITIES PLANNING

PACUs as we know them are a relatively new invention (their history is summarized in the beginning of Chapter 1). By 1960 they became a common hospital feature. In the period following 1960, the PACU became the prototype for further consolidation of equipment and personnel into highly specialized areas. These included medical and surgical intensive care, emergency care, cardiac catheterization, and special procedure radiologic units.

Unfortunately for the PACU the status of leadership in special care was lost as newer, more modern intensive care facilities became available. Only now, with advances in anesthetic management, has the concept of the PACU experienced a rebirth.

This rebirth has often necessitated modernization of existing facilities. In some centers the relocation of the surgical suite into new facilities

Allergies: _____

ANESTHESIA SUMMARY

GENERAL Agents ☐ N₂O ☐ Halothane ☐ Isoflurane
☐ Enflurane

Muscle Relaxant _____
Antagonist(s) _____

INTRA-OP MEDS

REGIONAL ☐ Spinal ☐ Axillary ☐
☐ Epidural ☐

Agent(s) _____
Sedative _____
Sensory Level _____

FLUIDS (Intra-operative)
Loss: EBL ___ Urine ___ Other ___
Replace: IV ___ Blood ___ Other ___

MEDICATION

DRUGS | Dose | Route | Time | RN

IV ADDITIVES
DRUG | BOTTLE NO. AND SITE | RN

DISCHARGE SUMMARY

Airway ☐ None ☐ Oral ☐ Nasal ☐ Endotracheal
Support ☐

Resp. Quality

Br. R ☐ Clear
Sounds ☐ Clear
L ☐ Clear

☐ HHO₂ ___ % ☐ Room Air ☐ Ventilator
EKG: ☐ NSR ☐ Dry
Surgical Drsg./Site ☐

L.O.C. ☐ Alert ☐ Delirious ☐ Comatose
☐ Lethargic ☐ Stuporous
Neuro. ☐ Moves all extremities
Skin ☐ See P.A.R. Progress Notes
Condition

LINES/CATHETERS/TUBES
☐ As on admission
☐

Describe Change

Fluids (P.A.R.)
In: IV ___ Blood ___ Other ___
Out: Urinary ___ Discharge ___
☐ Report R.N. ___
☐ Called

Date ___ Admit Time ___ Disch. Time ___

OPERATION

SURGICAL TEAM

ANESTHESIA TEAM

ADMISSION SUMMARY

History/Comments:

Graphic Key
V Systolic
Λ Diastolic
Pulse ●
Pre-Op
B/P
H·R
Resp.
Temp.
REACT ∘

210	
190	
170	
150	
130	
110	
90	
70	
50	
30	
10	
0	

Airway ☐ None ☐ Oral ☐ Nasal ☐ Endotracheal
Support ☐

Resp. Quality

Br. R ☐ Clear
Sounds ☐ Clear
L ☐ Clear

☐ HHO₂ ___ % ☐ Room Air ☐ Ventilator
EKG: ☐ NSR ☐ Dry
Surgical Drsg./Site ☐

L.O.C. ☐ Alert ☐ Delirious ☐ Comatose
☐ Lethargic ☐ Stuporous
Neuro. ☐ Moves all extremities
Skin ☐ See P.A.R. Progress Notes
Condition

LINES/CATHETERS/TUBES
IV: Peripheal ☐ U.E. ☐ R ☐ L
☐ L.E. ☐ R ☐ L
Central ___
Type ___
Other ___

Arterial ☐ R ☐ L I.V. Site Check ☐
☐ Epidural ☐ NG ☐ Gastrostomy
☐ Urinary with Irrigation ☐ Urinary ☐ Jackson/Pratt
☐ Drains ___

I N T A K E
O U T P U T

Hemovac ___
Chest ___
Other ___

Admit By ___ Orders Checked By ___

Figure 4—4A. Postanesthesia recovery record (front). (Courtesy of Rush-Presbyterian–St. Luke's Medical Center, Chicago.)

P.A.R. PROGRESS NOTES

_____

_____

_____

_____

_____

_____

_____

_____

_____

_____

_____

_____

_____

_____

_____

_____

_____

_____

_____

_____

_____

_____

_____

ARTERIAL BLOOD GASES						LABORATOR/X-RAY			INITIAL	SIGNATURE & TITLE
						Procedure	Time	COMMENTS		
TIME						EKG				
pH						CXR				
pCO₂						SMA 6				
pO₂						CBC				
BE										
										REACTe SCORING
K+										(SEE POLICY FOR COMPLETE EXPLANATION)

REACTe SCORING
(SEE POLICY FOR COMPLETE EXPLANATION)

(R)espiration
0 - Ventilator
1 - Resp < 10 c̄ airway
2 - Resp < 10 s̄ airway
(E)nergy
0 - ō move legs
1 - moves legs,
  ō sustained head lift
2 - head lift, legs move
(A)lertness
0 - rousable c stimulation
1 - alert but dozes
2 - alert

(C)irculation Adults
(see policy for infants)
0 - B.P. < 80 syst. or
  weak pulse
1 - B.P. 80 syst. to WFL
  full pulse
2 - B.P. WFL, pre-op level,
  full pulse
(T)emperature
0 - Ax. T. < 95°F
1 - Ax. T. 95-96°F
2 - Ax. T. > 96°F

Figure 4–4B. Postanesthesia recovery record (back). _(Courtesy of Rush-Presbyterian–St. Luke's Medical Center, Chicago.)_

has prompted a total redesign of the PACU. This has placed many unprepared nurse-administrators in the role of facilities planner. And few nurse-administrators know where to start. Therefore, Figure 4-8, which diagrams a suggested PACU layout, and the following are intended as a guide for facilities modernization.

Getting Started

The job of unit modernization does not fall to one person alone. The nurse-administrator is a member of a planning group that also includes representatives from the medical staff and administration, the architec-

MEDICATION		Time	Amt.	Time	Amt.	Time	Amt.	Time	Amt.	Time	B.P.	Pulse
ADRENALIN	IV											
ATROPINE	IV											
SODIUM BICARBONATE	IV											
CALCIUM CHLORIDE	IV											
XYLOCAINE	IV											
ISUPREL	IV											

IV DRIP MEDICATION	Conc. Amt.	Infusion Time	Total cc's	Conc. Amt.	Infusion Time	Total cc's	Conc. Amt.	Infusion Time	Total cc's	Conc.	Time	Amt.
DOPAMINE												
ISUPREL												
XYLOCAINE												
LEVOPHED												

PACEMAKER:
TIME INSERTED: _____
TIME ON: _____
TYPE: _____ Transthoracic _____ Transvenous
Rate _____ MV _____

DEFIBRILLATION

Time	Amt. Watt/Sec.	Effect

ARTERIAL BLOOD GASES

Time				
PH				
PO$_2$				
PCO$_2$				
BE				
K$^+$				
Ca				

TYPE ARREST
RESP. ☐
CARDIAC ☐

EXTERNAL MASSAGE
TIME STARTED _____
TIME STOPPED _____

INTUBATION TIME _____
Nasal ☐ Oral ☐
Tubes _____

Figure 4–5. Resuscitation record. (Courtesy of Rush-Presbyterian–St. Luke's Medical Center, Chicago.)

PACU MORBIDITY and MORTALITY RECORD

Day of Surgery: _____

Patient's Name: _____

Patient's Age: _____

Patient's Hospital Number: _____

Surgical Procedure: _____

Surgeon/Team: _____

Anesthetic Agents Used:_____

Anesthesiologist/Team: _____

Nature of Incident:

_____

_____

_____

_____

_____

_____

Length of Stay: _____

Post-op Room: _____

Follow up: _____

_____

_____

Signature of RN: _____

Figure 4–6. PACU morbidity and mortality record. *(Courtesy of Rush-Presbyterian–St. Luke's Medical Center, Chicago.)*

tural firm, and other disciplines active in the unit (e.g., respiratory therapy). It is with this group that the planning process is organized, major issues are negotiated, and the final plan is approved.

The means of accomplishing modernization will vary with the complexity of the project and the institution. Zilm (1979) identifies careful organization of the planning process as key to project effectiveness, breaking it into three phases: (1) definition of milestones, (2) estimation of time requirements, and (3) projection of a timeline. This framework then serves as a guide against which task force efforts are measured. The central planning committee may also meet intermittently during the con-

PRESBYTERIAN-ST. LUKE'S HOSPITAL
1753 West Congress Parkway
Chicago, Illinois 60612

ANESTHESIA PRE ECT EVALUATION
AND
TREATMENT SHEET

Diagnosis:

Tests / Dates											Date	Pertinent Hx & Physical, B/P, P Consent, P.S., Teeths, Glasses, Etc.
CXR												
ECG												
Hgb, Hct												
WBC												
U/A												
COAG												
SMA 18												
Meds												

Rx 1	DATE		Rx 2	DATE		Rx 3	DATE		Rx 4	DATE		Rx 5	DATE	
Time	V.S.	Meds & Amts	Time	V.S.	Meds & Amts	Time	V.S.	Meds & Amts	Time	V.S.	Meds & Amts	Time	V.S.	Meds & Amts
COMMENTS			COMMENTS			COMMENTS			COMMENTS			COMMENTS		
Anes MD/CRNA			Anes MD/CRNA			Anes MD/CRNA			Anes MD/CRNA			Anes MD/CRNA		

Rx 6	DATE		Rx 7	DATE		Rx 8	DATE		Rx 9	DATE		Rx 10	DATE	
Time	V.S.	Meds & Amts	Time	V.S.	Meds & Amts	Time	V.S.	Meds & Amts	Time	V.S.	Meds & Amts	Time	V.S.	Meds & Amts
COMMENTS			COMMENTS			COMMENTS			COMMENTS			COMMENTS		
Anes MD/CRNA			Anes MD/CRNA			Anes MD/CRNA			Anes MD/CRNA			Anes MD/CRNA		

M/R FORM NO. 7822 3-79

Figure 4–7. Anesthesia pre-ECT evaluation and treatment sheet. *(Courtesy of Rush-Presbyterian–St. Luke's Medical Center, Chicago.)*

struction phase to review progress and resolve issues that arise after construction has begun.

Each of the representatives from the central committee are responsible for the direction of planning within his or her particular area. Ideally, a task force in each area addresses the project. A study by Becker (1980) indicates that employee involvement improves morale, offers creative and effective use of space and equipment, provides greater patient satisfaction, and elicits cooperation among hospital staff members. Unfortunately, subordinates often have only limited involvement in early plan-

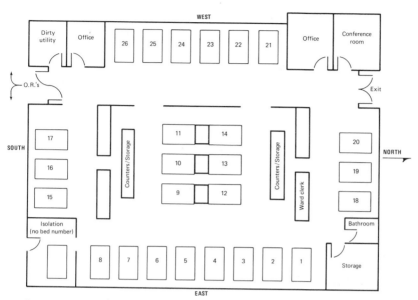

Figure 4–8. PACU layout and bed designations. *(Courtesy of Rush-Presbyterian–St. Luke's Medical Center, Chicago.)*

ning. Then, after the plan has been approved and is presented to the staff, valuable insights are made. By this time, significant changes may prove costly. Staff members may perceive that the project fails to meet their needs and may develop distrust of the system; enthusiasm is lost. To prevent this, a unit-based task force is strongly recommended.

Task force communications also have a significant influence on the project's success. As basic as it may seem, many problems might never have occurred if effective communication systems were established from the start. Robbins (1980, p. 358) points out that perfect communications are impossible due to barriers that interfere with the transference of meaning. To minimize the effect of these barriers, mutual understanding and interpretation must be promoted.

To begin, the unit manager should clearly define the charge to the task force, and all group meetings should be recorded via written minutes. Progress toward the stated objectives results from shared understanding of intended outcomes. The group is also able to monitor its communication system via the minutes and provide feedback as necessary when discrepancies occur.

Consultation with other individuals or departments is another reason to keep a written record of meetings, noting the content discussed and the agreements reached. Distribution of this record to all individuals involved in task force meetings allows perceptual differences that may distort or ignore the intended message to be detected (Gilles, 1982, p. 113).

Stevens (1975, p. 65) indicates that committee feedback to and from nonmembers is important to ensure project effectiveness. Any individual or department working with the unit and not meeting regularly with the planning committee should be kept abreast of planning. In addition, any decisions that affect operations in other areas, such as dress code, must be communicated.

The Plan

Whether the problem presented to the planning task force is modernization of the present facilities or the design and relocation of the unit to new facilities, the following broad areas must be considered:

- Physical layout
- Equipment
- Electrical/mechanical systems
- Communication systems
- Supply systems
- Unit operations
- Staff education

Each of these areas will now be explored in greater detail.

Physical Layout

The PACU should be located within or adjacent to the operating suite, as this will allow rapid patient transfer and ready access by surgical and anesthesia personnel. Access to a nonsurgical corridor permits entry by other personnel (respiratory therapists, laboratory technicians, and clinical consultants). This dual accessibility can result, however, in an overlap between street and operating room attire. Therefore, one of the first decisions to be made is that of dress code. If only operating room attire is permitted, a plan must support access of equipment and personnel into the area from nonsurgical corridors. If a mix of surgical and nonsurgical attire is permitted, the plan must seek to minimize the potential contamination of the surgical suite. Because nonrefutable infection control data are not available, it is recommended that a joint decision be made by a multidisciplinary committee representing the medical, surgical, and anesthesia staff, operating room and postanesthesia nursing, administration, and infectious disease/epidemiology. With this approach, the impact of the dress code restrictions on all of these groups will be known. It will also result in a mutual agreement regarding infection control practices.

Size. Badner and Laufman (1981) recommend 1.5 PACU beds per operating room. To evaluate if this figure is appropriate for a specific institution, each institution must consider acuity, length of stay, peak patient census, outpatient surgery needs, and use of the unit for special procedures and/or as an intensive care unit. Each of these variables will influence unit occupancy. The number of PACU beds should be planned to meet maximum expected occupancy.

Floor Plan. The space allowed for each patient should be sufficient to accommodate the hospital's largest stretcher, bed, or frame. Workspace must be adequate on either side and at the base of the bed to permit ready access of equipment and personnel. If cubicles are used to provide additional privacy or isolation, a minimum of 10 by 12 feet must be allowed for each (Badner & Laufman, 1981). Ceiling height must be sufficient to allow personnel movement under retractable ceiling IV extensions, or permit the extension of floor or bed IV poles to a sufficient height. Door width and height should accommodate all forms of traction.

Nurse-to-patient ratio is an important consideration in the design of a floor plan, since decisions on the number of bedspaces in each geographic area reflect those ratios. For example, if the recommended nurse-to-patient ratio is 1:2, a group of three bedspaces in a patient care area will result in either over- or under-staffing. Staffing is a particularly important consideration if cubicles or critical care areas are used. Creation of special care areas isolated from other patient care areas or the communication center ensures that the staff assigned to work in those areas are isolated as well. This requires design and modifications that support effective utilization of personnel.

The nursing station and communication center is key to the organization of patient care activities and traffic patterns. The station should be clearly visible to all patient care areas, located in such a fashion that patient movement into and out of the recovery room may be easily monitored, and large enough to support clerical and nursing activities. Present and future use of computers should be forecast, and appropriate space for terminals provided. In addition, a work station for medical staff that supports communication with clerical and nursing personnel is necessary. Isolation of the physician in a private conference room interferes with vital information-sharing at a critical point in the patient's postanesthetic or operative course. Finally, as the staff nurse is stationed at the bedside, provision for adequate counterspace and communications in that area is vital.

Utility rooms, supply rooms, offices, and conference rooms should be easily accessible but sufficiently isolated from the patient care area. If outpatient recovery is located within the PACU, an effort should be made to isolate the outpatient from the sights and sounds of the inpatient PACU. Dressing areas large enough to accommodate a wheelchair, sink, and toilet must be available. If a discharge area is not located elsewhere in the facility, a nourishment area and family waiting area are necessary.

The design of a floor plan must take into account all traffic patterns. The movement of the patient from the operating room into the PACU must be efficient to ensure rapid initiation of the recovery plan. Physical and visual barricades interrupt this process. As an example, visual obstacles that block a clear view of the operating room entrance may result in a "lost" patient and transport team as they seek direction to their PACU space. Ventilators, stretchers, narrow corridors, and short turning radii can impede the admission process. Carefully designed floor plans and the use of appropriate signs (Hospitals, 1979) promote the efficient movement of patients and personnel.

Equipment

Planning for equipment is a costly and time-consuming process. Numerous manufacturers offer merchandise with similar applications. The only way to determine the most appropriate equipment is to fully investigate each option. Care must be exercised to ensure that only equipment that meets the current and projected needs of the facility is considered. For example, a cardiac/pulmonary artery pressure monitoring device for each PACU bed is not necessary if only occasional or intermittent use is predicted. Rapid advances in clinical practice and technology may outdate equipment before it is installed. It is therefore necessary to forecast as closely as possible the present and future needs of the PACU by all users.

Consider the present clinical policies. Do they need to be updated or revised? Do not forget to consider the recommendations of state and national regulatory and accreditation bodies. Once these considerations have been evaluated, determine which equipment will most effectively support these patient care standards.

The head wall consolidates much of the standard patient support equipment. Kinney (1981) recommends a minimum of two oxygen and two suction, one compressed air, and eight three-pronged electrical outlets per bedspace. Additional suction outlets with high/low intermittent vacuum regulators may be necessary for centers with a case mix that includes a significant number of abdominal and thoracic procedures. Jacks for monitors, x-ray equipment, and ECG machines should be available. Equipment and outlets located at eye-level facilitate access and observation.

Early decisions regarding equipment storage in the PACU permit allocation of space appropriate to the size and anticipated use of the equipment. For example, undercounter storage for ventilators, an ECG machine, the emergency cart, and defibrillators in the patient care area keeps necessary equipment within easy reach of staff members yet eliminates clutter.

Electrical and Mechanical Systems

The electrical and mechanical systems for the PACU are intended to eliminate potential hazards and discomfort for patients and staff members. All electrical systems require grounding and connection to the hospital's emergency power source. Ventilation systems should promote air exchange patterns that minimize infection and anesthetic waste hazards. Heating, air conditioning, and humidification systems must promote maximum safety and comfort. Finally, lighting should not irritate the patient's eyes, should allow for accurate physical assessment, and should be flexible enough to permit high-intensity lighting in the event of an emergency.

Communication Systems

In any special care area, communication is vital. The hub of the communication network is traditionally the central nursing or clerical station. It is through this area that most incoming information is collected, processed, and disseminated. However, it should not be forgotten that the nurse at the bedside needs to communicate with many individuals inside and outside the PACU. The use of only a central communication center removes the nurse from the bedside and may compromise patient care. A mechanism to support routine and emergency communication at the bedside is vital to efficient unit operations. Hence, telephones and intercoms should be easily accessible to staff at the bedside.

The noise produced by communication and patient care activity must also be considered and reconciled. Special care areas, with their need to rapidly share a large volume of information, by their very nature are noisy. As a communication system is planned, every effort should be made to minimize excessive noise levels.

Supply Systems

Hospital supply, processing, and distribution systems will dictate the means by which the PACU is serviced. Whether shelves are hand-stocked or an exchange cart system is used, a 24-hour supply of all necessary items should be stored in the area at all times. Dumbwaiters, pneumatic tube systems, and other means of supply distribution should be available for "stat" delivery.

Supply storage must be accessible to PACU personnel. A small quantity of routinely used supplies should be stocked at each bedside. Other necessary items, such as pharmacueticals, should be available in the PACU. Provision for the storage of supplies in the patient care area facilitates their distribution. Open-rack shelving, movable exchange carts, and the elimination of excessive stock helps to prevent the collection of dust and debris.

Unit Operations

Whether you are modifying current facilities or planning for relocation to a new facility, these activities will have a profound effect on all aspects of unit operations. The need for modifications in unit policies and procedures must be determined. Systems that will be interrupted by construction require identification and temporary alteration. In the event of relocation, extensive analysis of unit operations facilitates the implementation of comparable or new systems (e.g., fire, safety, and admission and discharge procedures).

During construction, regular review of the new facility ensures that expectations will be met and unanticipated problems are discovered and rectified. Daily unit operations can also be monitored to ensure the effectiveness of altered systems. Staff members may modify their work patterns due to environmental changes and the responsibilities of facilities planning. A regular opportunity by staff members to review systems, express frustrations, and problem-solve can be effective in easing stress.

Staff Education

The final phase of facilities planning is the education of staff members in the use of the new or modified unit. Personnel must receive information regarding all new equipment and systems. An opportunity for all staff members to familiarize themselves with the new environment and equipment prior to opening the facility should be available. A mock admission, emergency, and discharge may assist with staff orientation.

Follow-Up

Once the new unit has been opened, an expected period of confusion and disorganization is likely to result despite all planning efforts. Coping with a new environment and new systems is frustrating to even the best-prepared staff. No matter how many complaints may have been made about the old facility, people may refer repeatedly to the "good old days."

This can be a very difficult time for staff members and those involved in the planning for the new unit. The evaluations made by those working in the new unit are affected by the stresses associated with the need to make multiple changes in work patterns. This may result in nonobjective statements. At the same time those who were closely identified with various phases of development for the new facility have a vested interest in the success of their alterations. Their response to staff evaluations may also be nonobjective.

Thus, recommendations may be accepted and systems changed before they have had a chance to prove effective, or recommendations may be ignored and true problems left to compromise the patient care process. The goal for the nurse-administrator during this period is to remain as objective as possible and to act on only those matters that appear to truly compromise the efficiency of unit operations. When the rash of complaints has subsided and the systems begin to function efficiently, a formal evaluation of the new facility can be made by both the unit and organizational task forces. These evaluation results can then be used to make necessary adjustments in unit operations.

REFERENCES

American Hospital Association: Preservation of medical records in health care institutions. Record Retention, 1977.

American Journal of Nursing: The demise of the traditional 5-40 work week? American Journal of Nursing 81:1138–1143, 1981.

American Society of Anesthesiology: A practice advisory for the recovery room. American Society of Anesthesiologists Newsletter 2:7–8, 1978.

American Society of Post Anesthesia Nurses: Guidelines for management standards in the post anesthesia care unit. Breathline 3(18), 1983.

Badner B & Laufman HE: Preoperative holding and postanesthesia recovery areas. In HE Laufman (Ed.), Hospital Special Care Facilities: Planning for User Need. New York: Academic Press, 1981.

Becker FD: Employees need a role in designing of work space. Hospitals 97–101, 1980.

Byra JR & Pierce FA: A personnel allocation and scheduling system for patient care units. Proceedings NCSC/HME 23, 1974.

Caterinecchio RP: A defense of the RIMs study. Nursing Management 14:36–39, 1983.

Chapman S: How long should you keep your patient's medical records? Journal of the American Medical Records Association 51:37–47, 1980.

Cullen DJ, Civetta JM, et al: Therapeutic intervention scoring system: A method for quantitative comparison of patient care. Critical Care Medicine 2:57–60, 1974.

Duraiswamy N, Welton R, & Reisman A: Using computer simulation to predict ICU staffing needs. Journal of Nursing Administration 11:39–44, 1981.

Evans SK, Laundon T, & Yamamoto W G: Projecting staffing requirement for intensive care units. Journal of Nursing Administration 10:34–42, 1980.

Fraulini KE & Murphy P: REACT: A new postanesthetic recovery score. Nursing, 14(4):101–102, 1984.

Gilles D: Nursing Management: A Systems Approach. Philadelphia: Saunders, 1982.

Grimaldi PL & Micheletti JA: A defense of the RIMS critique. Nursing Management 14:40–41, 1983a.

Grimaldi PL & Micheletti JA: Diagnosis Related Groups: A Practitioner's Guide. Chicago: Pluribus, 1983b.

Hiller MD: Computers, medical records, and right to privacy. Journal of Health Politics, Policy, and Law 6:463–497, 1981.

Hospitals: Sinage aids smart moves in medical center. Hospitals 53:27, 1979.

Illinois Hospital Association: A record retention guide for Illinois hospitals. Chicago: Illinois Hospital Association, 1977.

Kinney JM: The design of an intensive care unit. In E Laufman (Ed.), Hospital Special Care Facilities: Planning for User Need. New York: Academic Press, 1981.

Kronman B & Burke M: A staffing study report for post anesthesia recovery. Unpublished manuscript. Medicus Systems and Rush-Presbyterian–St. Luke's Medical Center, 1978.

McCaman B & Hirsh HL: Medical records—legal perspectives. Primary Care 6:682–92, 1979.

Norby RB, Freund LE, & Wagner B: A nurse staffing system based upon assignment difficulty. Journal of Nursing Administration 7:2–24, 1977.

Northwest Recovery Room Nurses Association: Off the cuff. Northwest Recovery Room Nurses Association Newsletter, 1980.

Ornato, JP, Fennigkoh L, & Jaeger C: The electronic clipboard: An automated system for accurately recording events during a cardiac arrest. Annals of Emergency Medicine 10:138–141, 1981.

Rasmussen SR: Staffing and scheduling options. Critical Care Quarterly 4:35–41, 1982.

Robbins SP: The Administrative Process (2nd ed.). Englewood Cliffs, N.J.: Prentice-Hall, 1980.

Stevens BJ: The Nurse as Executive. Mass.: Contemporary, 1975.

Zilm F: The planning process and development of a time line. Journal of Nursing Administration 9:40–44, 1979.

PART III

Perianesthetic Care

Chapter 5

Preoperative Involvement of the PACU Nurse

Kay E. Fraulini

WHO SHOULD VISIT THE PATIENT

This chapter was developed on the assumption that the majority of PACU nurses do not visit patients preoperatively. Although this may be true now, I believe that within the next decade we must make major efforts to expand the scope of the PACU nurse beyond the PACU. As our patients get sicker and our technology more complex, we must build our care on a well-developed nursing data base.

I therefore believe that the PACU nurse is one of the people who should visit the patient preoperatively. The concern here, of course, is that patients are not taxed with large numbers of personnel visiting them before surgery. We must try to avoid pure duplication of questioning and collecting information. Whenever possible, pooling of information should be the rule.

PREANESTHETIC ASSESSMENT

A major rationale for preoperative medical and nursing assessment is reduction in perioperative morbidity by optimizing preoperative status and planning the perioperative management. Other reasons for preoperative assessment include evaluation of risk for anesthesia and surgery and establishment of baseline function with which intraoperative and postoperative abnormalities can be compared. Perioperative mortality and morbidity increase with severity of preexisting disease. Therefore, preoperative evaluation and treatment should reduce perioperative morbidity and mortality.

PACU nurses should start thinking about the kind of information they want to include on their preanesthetic assessment. Anesthesia departments have been evaluating preoperative patients for decades, yet the rules are still fairly arbitrary. For example, Grogono (1977) collected preanesthetic assessment forms from 10 hospitals. Table 5-1 summarizes the information most commonly requested. Roizen (1981) further notes that most hospitals and many anesthesia departments have rather arbitrary rules for recommendations as to which tests should be performed on a patient prior to elective surgery.

Since the ordering of laboratory tests is not usually a nursing function, this will not be discussed in detail. The nurse should be able to evaluate whatever laboratory results appear in the patient's chart. This information can be used in developing the nurse's data base and plan of care. Table 5-2 gives an overview of laboratory tests that the nurse can expect to find in the chart of a "healthy" patient.

Vaughan and associates (1983) have identified certain risk factors that should be included in the nurse's preanesthetic assessment (Table 5-3).

TABLE 5–1. INFORMATION REQUESTED ON PREANESTHETIC ASSESSMENT FORMS FROM 10 HOSPITALS

In at Least Half the Forms	In Less than Half the Forms
Patient identification data (name, age, number, race, sex)	Room number
	Social security number
Date	Urinalysis
Diagnosis	Hematocrit
Proposed surgery	White cell count
Height	Other blood chemistry
Weight	Units blood ordered
Previous anesthetic details	Respiratory assessment
Hemoglobin	Central nervous system assessment
Pulse	Head, neck, mouth, eyes assessment
Blood pressure	Intubation assessment
Premedication	Gastrointestinal assessment
	ECG
	Smoking and drinking habits
	Estimate of blood volume
	Dental condition

(From Grogono AW & Kane PB. A PSRO record-keeping system for anesthesiologists. Anesthesia and Analgesia 56(1): 1977, with permission.)

TABLE 5–2. INDICATED SCREENING STUDIES ON ASYMPTOMATIC, HEALTHY PATIENTS SCHEDULED TO UNDERGO NONBLOOD-LOSS "PERIPHERAL" PROCEDURES

Age	Males	Females
Under 40	?SGOT/?BUN/?Glucose	Hemoglobin or Hematocrit ?SGOT/?BUN/?Glucose
40 to 59	Electrocardiogram BUN/Glucose ?SGOT	Hemoglobin or Hematocrit Electrocardiogram BUN/Glucose ?SGOT
Over 60	Hemoglobin or Hematocrit Electrocardiogram Chest x-ray BUN/Glucose ?SGOT	Hemoglobin or Hematocrit Electrocardiogram Chest x-ray BUN/Glucose ?SGOT

(From Roizen MF. Routine preoperative evaluation. In RD Miller (Ed.), Anesthesia (vol. 1), 1981. Courtesy of Churchill Livingstone.)

This study was designed to determine those risk factors associated with unfavorable outcome—*worse* or *serious cardiac* anesthesia related conse- quences (ARCs) in the operating room and PACU—and to predict the relative odds for occurrence of an adverse outcome. Vaughan and asso- ciates conclude that clinical factors strongly predictive of adverse outcome include age; ASA classification III; major organ system disease; preopera- tive intravenous antibiotic therapy (it was an unanticipated finding that multiple antibiotic therapy was as good a prognostic factor as some more obvious clinical indicators for *worse* or *serious cardiac* ARCs in the operat- ing room); abdominal incision; and prolonged operative procedure. More- over, if any ARCs occur in the operating room, and especially if *serious cardiac* ARCs occur intraoperatively, one can predict that *serious cardiac* or *worse* ARCs will result in the PACU.

ARCs were defined as pivotal occurrences requiring physician or nurse intervention that could lead, if not discovered or corrected in time, to an undesirable outcome. ARCs were categorized as follows:

- *Worse*—cardiac arrest or mortality.
- *Serious cardiac*—hypertension or hypotension (change > or < 35 percent of admission systolic pressure), dysrhythmias (from con- tinuous ECG monitoring), ventricular tachycardia, myocardial in- farction, or angina.
- *Serious pulmonary*—prolonged airway management, pneumothorax, aspiration pneumonia, pulmonary embolism, emesis with unpro- tected airway, pulmonary edema, hypoxemia, and hypercarbia (acutely).
- *Less serious*—unstable blood pressure, airway management problems, emergence delirium, electrolyte abnormalities, nausea and vomiting

requiring treatment, severe shivering, hypothermia ($< 34°C$ on PACU admission), or metabolic aberrations.

It is recommended that the data generated by Vaughan and associates be used in the nurse's preanesthetic assessment. For example, space should be provided on the record for information about patient age, ASA classification, major organ system disease, preoperative intravenous antibiotic therapy, incisional site, and length of time in the operating room. These factors should be sufficiently weighted to reflect the prospective risk that they represent. The information should be disseminated to the relevant personnel and should be utilized to make triage decisions.

What other patient data could assist the nurse? ASPAN Guidelines for Standards of Care in the Post Anesthesia Care Unit (see Chapter 9) recommend collecting the following preoperative data: electrocardiogram, vital signs, radiology findings, laboratory values, allergies, disabili-

TABLE 5–3. RISK FACTORS IN THE NURSE'S PREANESTHETIC ASSESSMENT

Risk Factors	Perioperative Location	
Patient Variables	*OR*	*PACU*
Age≥50 years	1.7 (1.1–2.5)[1]	NS[2]
ASA (PS) III	2.0 (1.1–3.4)	1.8 (1.0–3.2)
Hx major organ system disease	1.8 (1.2–2.6)	1.9 (1.3–2.9)
Preop antibiotic (IV) [multiple]	2.8 (1.1–7.0)	NS
Surgery Variables		
Incision:		
Abdominal	4.0 (1.9–8.9)	3.0 (1.4–6.3)
Peripheral	2.7 (1.5–4.9)	2.2 (1.2–3.9)
Length of surgery [≥120 minutes]	3.2 (2.0–5.0)	2.6 (1.6–4.1)
Packed RBC given [≥2 units]	3.4 (1.5–7.7)	3.2 (1.5–7.2)
OR crystalloid [≥3500 ml]	3.5 (1.8–6.7)	3.9 (2.0–7.6)
Anesthesia Variables		
Length of anesthesia [≥150 minutes]	3.4 (2.2–5.3)	2.7 (1.7–4.2)
PGY3 resident	2.7 (1.1–4.0)	NS
Agent: N$_2$O:Fent:Musc. Relaxant	2.0 (1.2–2.7)	2.1 (1.4–3.2)
Forane	NS	2.5 (1.1–5.8)
Controlled vent. (OR)	1.9 (1.3–2.9)	2.2 (1.5–3.4)

[1]Odds ratio presenting relative risk with number in ( ) denoting 95% confidence interval.
[2]NS = not significant.
(From Vaughan RW, Vaughan MS, Hagman RM, et al: Predicting adverse outcomes during anesthesia and surgery by prospective risk assessment. Abstract of scientific papers. 1983 annual meeting. Anesthesiology 59(3A), Sept., 1983.)

ties, drug use, physical or mental impairments, mobility limitations, and prostheses (including hearing aids).

There is growing awareness of the importance of the mental and emotional assessment. We know that despite similarities in medical conditions, patients often differ greatly in their recovery from surgery. The impact of a stressful event such as surgery is affected by how individuals interpret a situation and their emotional and behavioral reactions—in other words, how they cope. Coping is defined as the thoughts and actions taken to manage external and internal demands and conflicts among them that tax or exceed a person's resources (Lazarus & Launier, 1978).

Attending to patient's emotional needs is not only a desirable aspect of perioperative nursing but it may also be cost-effective by, for example, shortening postsurgical hospitalization. Patients benefit by receiving more than technically adequate nursing care. The PACU nurse, in planning care, could be expected to identify a patient's coping mechanisms and their effectiveness. As nurses look at individual coping patterns, they will become more expert in knowing when to intervene (Fraulini, 1983).

Cohen and Lazarus (1973) developed a classification system for coping styles. Preoperative patients were interviewed and classified into three groups based on whether they showed avoidance, vigilance, or both.

Patients in the avoidance category deny the emotional or threatening aspects of the upcoming surgery. They seem unaware of the medical conditions necessitating surgery, the nature of the surgery, and the postsurgical outlook. Also, these patients are unwilling to discuss their thoughts about the operation. At the other extreme is the vigilant patient. Such patients are too alert to emotional or threatening aspects of the upcoming surgery. They tend to seek out extensive knowledge about the medical condition, the nature of the surgery, and the postsurgical outlook. These patients are eager to discuss their thoughts about the operation.

Avoidance and vigilance, as judged from interview data, were rated on a scale from 1 to 10, with ratings from 8 to 10 implying vigilance and ratings of 1 to 3 implying avoidance. The middle group (ratings of 4 to 7) was designed for patients emphasizing neither vigilance nor avoidance behavior (Fraulini, 1983, pp. 1200–1204). Lazarus' sample of 61 patients showed that the vigilant group had the most complicated postoperative recovery, although only number of days in the hospital and incidence of minor complications were statistically significant.

After proper training in analyzing interview data, the nurse making a preanesthetic assessment could be expected to assign a coping rating to the patient. This information could possibly help the PACU nurse understand some of the patients' postanesthesia behavior—such as restlessness or delirium—and intervene appropriately. Further, this data could be used in making triage decisions. For example, the patient who is expected to have negative psychological reactions to surgery and anesthesia may be placed in a more supportive location in the PACU (see case studies presented in Chapter 10).

Table 5-4 is a proposed tool for the PACU nurse to use when making the preanesthetic visit. When this checklist is completed, it can be brought back to the PACU and filed in a preop box. The next day, when the patient arrives in the PACU, the primary nurse can pull this sheet and add the information to whatever is reported by the anesthetist or anesthesiologist. Also, the triage nurse can refer to these documents when making various triage decisions.

PATIENT TEACHING

Controversy continues to surround what, where, how, and when to teach preoperative patients. The question of whether preoperative instruction makes a physiological difference in postoperative recovery from surgery has yet to be consistently answered. Further research in the area is indi-

TABLE 5–4. PREANESTHETIC ASSESSMENT CHECKLIST

Patient name	Age[1]	
Identification band on and correct		
Nutritional status	Height	Weight
Elimination habits		
Allergies (drugs, foods, dye, tape, others)		
Emotional status		
Coping rating: avoidant 1–3		
middle 4–7		
vigilant 8–10		
Physical limitations (obesity, paralysis, others)		
Signs of infections		
Antibiotic therapy[1,2]		
Medications taken at home		
Medications taken in the hospital		
Past medical and surgical history (respiratory, cardiac, pulmonary emboli, thrombophlebitis, malignant hyperpyrexia, family history of anesthetic reaction)[1,2]		
Present medical and surgical history		
Respiratory	Cardiac	
Diabetic	Glaucoma	
Sickle cell	Others	
Incision[1,2]		
B/P	P	R
ECG	CXR	
Lab data		
ASA classification[1]		

[1]Prognostic risk factors.
[2]ASA classification

cated if definitive conclusions are to be reached. Preoperative teaching involves activities directed toward physically and emotionally preparing patients and their families for all facets of the operative experience. Preoperative teaching is done with the intent of enhancing the surgical patient's welfare and recovery.

Research in effectiveness of teaching formats has been done on healthy subjects, but there is belief that illness changes one's perspectives and abilities to learn (see "State-Dependent Learning" that begins on p. 97). Thus, research done on healthy subjects may not apply to ill subjects.

Preoperative Instruction

One of the most important and confounding questions the nurse must ask is what are the effects of preoperative teaching on physiological postoperative patient outcomes? Specifically, many investigators have studied preoperative teaching of coughing and deep breathing exercises. For example, Mezzanotte (1970) gave instruction in the techniques of bed exercises, coughing, and deep breathing, combined with information about what to expect postoperatively, to 24 patients in groups of four on the evening prior to the day of surgery. The patients were interviewed postoperatively and asked to evaluate the effectiveness of the preoperative instruction. All but one patient felt that the instruction had helped them learn to perform the exercises correctly after surgery. It should be noted that the value of this study is limited by the small sample size, possible investigator bias since she did the teaching and conducted the interviews, and failure to use an experimental design.

Lindeman and VanAernam (1971) studied the effects of preoperative teaching with the presurgical patient. The research was a comparative investigation of the effects of structured and unstructured preoperative teaching of deep breathing, coughing, and bed exercises upon postoperative ventilatory function, length of hospital stay, and postoperative need for analgesics. Preoperative teaching was done by registered nurses assigned to the surgical and pediatric units. Two different procedures were followed: teaching, which allowed nurses to teach what, when, and how they intuitively felt was adequate and correct; and structured preoperative teaching, which involved the implementation of an approach standardized for content and method. This method was implemented after a descriptive effective stir-up regime procedure was written, and an intensive and extensive staff development program was conducted for all nursing personnel.

Tests of ventilatory function were administered preoperatively and 24 hours postoperatively. The data showed that (1) the ability of subjects to deep breathe and cough postoperatively was significantly ($p < 0.05$) improved by the structured preoperative teaching method, (2) the mean length of hospital stay was significantly ($p < 0.05$) reduced by the implementation of the structured preoperative teaching method, and (3) there was no differential effect (p > 0.05) upon postoperative need for analgesia.

Lindeman (1972), utilizing the same teaching program developed for the previous study, compared the effects of group and individual preoperative instruction on postoperative ventilatory function, length of hospital stay, number of analgesics administered, and length of learning time in two groups of patients. Patients entering the hospital for elective surgery were randomly assigned on a weekly basis to either the group or individual teaching programs. The content presented and teaching methods used were the same in both groups. No statistically significant difference was found between the two groups in terms of the postoperative ventilatory function, length of hospital stay, or use of analgesic medication. A statistically significant difference was found between groups for the length of learning time, which was found to be less for those patients who received the group instruction.

Initial studies by Lindeman and VanAernam (1971) and Lindeman (1972) found structured teaching associated with improved pulmonary function. More recent studies evaluating the effectiveness of preoperative intensive teaching have been discouraging and somewhat contradictory. They have addressed the question of whether teaching programs make a difference in postoperative pulmonary status and whether group teaching is as effective as individualized instruction (Risser, 1980).

Carrieri (1975), in a study of 22 patients, set out to determine if there were differences in postoperative ventilatory capacity (measured by lung volume, flow rate, gas exchange, and pulmonary shunting) between upper abdominal surgical patients who experienced a teaching program that emphasized deep breathing and coughing and those who received the unstructured nursing approach then in use. No significant (p > 0.05) differences were found between the two groups when the data for each day were analyzed. However, the change in the forced midexpiratory flow rate from the preoperative day to the third postoperative day significantly (p < 0.05) decreased in the control group compared to the group receiving the teaching program. Thus, these data indicate that the teaching program may have decreased the incidence of small airway (2 mm or less) obstruction. The finding of lower mean forced maximum midexpiratory flow rate in the control group, in the presence of a mean forced expiratory volume for one second that was within normal range, suggests obstruction limited to the smaller airways.

The purpose of a study conducted by Felton and associates (1976) was to determine the effect of three nursing approaches to preoperative care of the surgical patient on the frequency of postoperative complications, ventilatory function, manifested anxiety level, and the patient's perception of psychological well-being. The sample was comprised of patients who were having "first time major surgery" requiring general anesthesia that did not represent "a realistic threat to life." Types of surgical procedures experienced were not reported. The findings supported the hypotheses that (1) patients who had experimental preoperative preparation would have a significantly greater decrease in preoperative to postoperative level of anxiety than those who did not, and (2) patients who received experimental preoperative preparation would have significantly higher scores on scales that measured psychological well-being. The second hypothesis was supported by data obtained from only one of the three psychological scales employed in this study. The investigators concluded that "Obviously, the experimental approach used in this study had no effect on the magnitude of decrease in postoperative vital capacity nor on the incidence of postoperative atelectasis or pneumonia" (p. 92).

Using the same teaching program developed and utilized in the Lindeman study (1972), Crabtree (1977) examined the effect of preoperative teaching of coughing and deep breathing exercises on postoperative ventilatory function, length of stay, and incidence of postoperative respiratory complications. Analysis of variance revealed no significant differences between research and control groups. These results contradict those of Lindeman and VanAernam (1971), but cannot be considered conclusive due to the small sample size (45 patients).

Archuleta and associates (1977) used a staff development model designed around a training model with a consultation role delineated by project staff members. The approach was designed through content developed for the retaining component. The content covered four areas: (1) principles of teaching and learning, (2) patient education, (3) cultural implications, and (4) respiratory care. The 265 patients in the unstructured teaching experimental group were from 11 participating hospitals. There was no statistically significant difference between the unstructured and structured groups on any of the five dependent variables. These included three postoperative ventilatory function test scores—forced vital capacity, maximum midexpiratory flow rate, and forced expiratory volume per second—and the length of hospital stay and number of postoperative analgesics.

A study conducted by King and Tarsitano (1981) replicated the Lindeman and VanAernam (1971) study with the exception of examining the amount of analgesic medication required. In contrast to the original study, no significant differences between groups was found for length of hospital stay.

In summary, there are no consistent answers to the question of whether preoperative instruction results in improved postoperative ventilatory status. Postoperative ventilatory changes are discussed in later chapters.

State-Dependent Learning. There is some question as to whether this is a variable in preoperative teaching. Generally the surgical patient receives a myriad of drugs in the perioperative period. The question arises whether it is best to attempt patient teaching the night before surgery, before preoperative drugs are given, or following surgery in the holding area or PACU. If a patient learns something while in a particular drug-defined state, later attempts to utilize the information while in a different state will prove more difficult than if the state had not been changed. (Ho and associates, 1978).

The Patient's Right to Know. The courts have not yet held specifically that a physician or a nurse has a duty to educate patients. To the extent that patient instruction is necessary to advise patients of the nature of proposed treatment or how to care for themselves, physicians and nurses have a duty to provide it; but extensive, general patient teaching is not required by law. Nevertheless, patient education is widely recognized as an important part of health care and may be provided by a variety of professional health personnel working in coordination with their patients' physicians (Bille, 1981).

There is no ideal method, time, or content for preoperative teaching. With this in mind, a proposed preoperative teaching program is presented in the appendix to this chapter.

Interestingly, studies show that patients receiving sensory information report less anxiety, and their expectations are more congruent with their actual experiences, than patients receiving only procedural information. Information given to a patient may lessen anxiety before or during a threatening procedure.

Hartfield and associates (1982), based on previous work by Johnson (1975), studied the effects of patient information about an impending threatening event—a barium enema. They found that patients who were told what most patients feel during the procedures had a less emotional response than patients who were told only about the procedure. Giving patients sensory information allows the patients to have expectations congruent with their actual experience.

Procedural information does not seem to affect patients' expectations, feelings, or anxiety. Because appropriate expectations are not based on procedural information, patients often have difficulty coping with the threat. When a patient's expectations are changed by the sensory information given, often changes are made in his or her coping mechanism. The changed coping method is more appropriate for the situation.

How coping, sensory information, and emotional response are related is not clear. More study is needed to determine how sensory information changes emotional response to a threatening situation.

DISSEMINATION OF INFORMATION

Once information about the patient is collected, it must be passed on to the appropriate personnel. Information which the nurse gathers should be shared with the physician as well as vice versa. There are many mechanisms for doing this (discussed elsewhere in the text).

REFERENCES

Archuleta V, Plummer OB, & Hopkins KD: A Demonstration Model for Patient Education: A Model for the Project "Training Nurses to Improve Patient Education." Boulder, Co.: Western Interstate Commission for Higher Education, 1977.

Bille DA: Practical Approaches to Patient Teaching. Boston: Little, Brown, 1981.

Carrieri V: Effect of an experimental teaching program on postoperative ventilatory capacity. In M Batey (Ed.), Communicating Nursing Research: Critical Issues in Access to Data. Boulder: Western Interstate Commission for Higher Education, 1975.

Cohen F & Lazarus R: Active coping processes and recovery from surgery. Psychosomatic Medicine 35:378–379, 1973.

Crabtree M: A cost benefit analysis of individual and group preoperative teaching. Unpublished master's thesis, University of Illinois, College of Nursing, 1977.

Felton G, Huss K, et al: Preoperative nursing intervention with a patient for surgery: Outcomes of three alternate approaches. International Journal of Nursing Studies 13:83–96, 1976.

Fraulini KE: Coping mechanisms and recovery from surgery. AORN Journal. 37:1198–1208, May, 1983.

Grogono AW & Kane PB: A PSRO record-keeping system for anesthesiologists. Anesthesia and Analgesia. 56(1):1977.

Hartfield MT, Cason CL & Cason GJ: Effects of information about a threatening procedure on patients' expectations and emotional distress. Nursing Research 205 (31) July/August, 1982.

Ho BT, Richards DW, & Chute DL: Drug Discrimination and State Dependent Learning. New York: Academic Press, 1978.

Johnson JE: Stress reduction through sensation information. In IG Sarason & CD Sprelberger (Eds.), Stress and Anxiety. New York: Wiley, 1975.

King I & Tarsitano B: The effect of structured and unstructured preoperative teaching: A replication. Nursing Research 31:324–329, 1981.

Lazarus RS & Launier R: Stress related transactions between person and environment. In LA Pevim & M Levis (Eds.), Perspectives in Interactional Psychology. New York: Plenum, 1978.

Lindeman CA: Nursing intervention with the presurgical patient: The effectiveness and efficiency of group and individual preoperative teaching. Phase two. Nursing Research 21:169–209, May/June, 1972.

Lindeman CA & VanAernam BV: Nursing intervention with the presurgical patient: The effects of structured and unstructured preoperative teaching. Nursing Research 20:319–322, July/August 1971.

Mezzanotte EJ: Group instruction in preparation for surgery. American Journal of Nursing 70(89):1970.

Owen PK: Excerpts from guidelines to patient teaching. In DA Bille (Ed.), Practical Approaches to Patient Teaching. Boston: Little, Brown, 1981.

Risser NL: Preoperative and postoperative care to prevent pulmonary complications. Heart and Lung. 9:57–67, Jan./Feb., 1980.

Roizen MF: Routine preoperative evaluation. In RD Miller (Ed.), Anesthesia (vol. 1). New York: Churchill Livingstone, 1981.

Vaughan RW, Vaughan MS, Hagaman RM, et al: Predicting adverse outcomes during anesthesia and surgery by prospective risk assessment. Abstract of scientific paper. 1983 Annual Meeting. Anesthesiology 59(3A), Sept., 1983.

APPENDIX 5–1

Health Teaching Program: Preoperative Preparation

PRINCIPLES

It is the goal of preoperative teaching to instruct all surgery patients before surgery; to decrease apprehension and promote recovery. Routine preoperative, preparation and recovery room procedures are explained to the patient; including coughing and deep breathing, postoperative exercises and relaxation skills, IVs, suction tubes, pain, medications, and other postoperative expectations; according to the type of surgery and the physician's requests and procedures.

GOALS

1. Have group presentations available for preoperative general education, followed with individual instruction.
2. Give preoperative instruction to allay fears, apprehension, and anxiety, and to promote comfort postoperatively and to hasten recovery.
3. Present the patient with information on what to expect.
4. Assist the patient to cooperate effectively in his own recovery.
5. Promote increase in patient turnover for more efficient utilization of hospital facilities.

OBJECTIVES

1. To facilitate recovery after surgery.
2. To supply information to improve patient's understanding of his part in recovery.

3. To alleviate fears that hinder recovery.
4. To describe in general, simplified terms what the patient can expect to see and do postoperatively.
5. To answer questions and to clarify misconceptions.
6. To demonstrate and practice any postoperative exercises and treatments for recovery.
7. To familiarize the patient with postoperative environment and equipment.
8. To allow time for and encourage verbalization of concerns. _____

PREOPERATIVE TEACHING WORKSHEET

Diagnosis:
Surgery:
Discharge:
Background Data:
Home Call:
Address:
Phone:

Knowledge	1		2		3		Comments
	P	F	P	F	P	F	
Preoperative Preparation							
Enema							
Skin prep							
Belongings							
Special tests							
Jewelry							
NPO							
Undergarments							
Gown							
Void							
Preop med (stay in bed)							
Surgery							
Define							
Time scheduled							
Family waiting room							
OR environment							
IV							
Anesthesia							
Suture line							
Dressing							
Drains/Tubes							
Foley							
Recovery							
PACU environment							
ET tube							
Oxygen mask/mist							

Frequent V/S	_____	_____	_____
ICU	_____	_____	_____
TC and DB exercises	_____	_____	_____
Relaxation skills	_____	_____	_____
Pain and medication	_____	_____	_____
Activity/ambulation	_____	_____	_____
Sore throat	_____	_____	_____
Equipment and Treatments			
Wound care, stitches	_____	_____	_____
Peri care	_____	_____	_____
Sitz bath	_____	_____	_____
IPPB	_____	_____	_____
Other	_____	_____	_____

P = patient; F = family; I = needs instruction on; 2 = needs reinforcement on; 3 = comprehends instruction/appropriate behavior; NA = not applicable (does not need instruction on).

(From Owen PK: Excerpts from guidelines to patient teaching. In DA Bille (Ed.), Practical Approaches to Patient Teaching. Copyright 1981 by Little, Brown and Company. Reprinted with permission.)

Chapter 6

Anesthetic Techniques

Daniel W. Gorski
Kay Atkinson Wright

The goals of anesthesia—analgesia, sedation, or muscle relaxation appropriate for the type of operative procedure and control of the autonomic nervous system—may be accomplished by a variety of drugs and techniques. Because of advances in the fields of medicine, pharmacology, and anesthesiology, pain control has become more of an exact science and less of an art, although the art aspect is still important. Given that pain control (analgesia) is of major importance to the anesthesiologist, he or she must consider the drugs and anesthetic techniques currently available to provide an adequate level of pain control for the individual patient. One axiom must not be forgotten: each person's pain experience is an individual experience. To assure a successful outcome during and after surgery, the drugs and techniques chosen to alleviate pain must be chosen carefully. This choice usually begins during the anesthesiologist's preoperative visit. At that time, the anesthesiologist considers the following points to arrive at a plan of anesthesia:

1. The needs and wants of the patient:
    "I want to be awake and see my baby."
    "I don't want to see or hear anything."
    "I'm afraid that if I go to sleep, I'll never wake up."
2. The needs and wants of the surgeon:
    "I'll need good muscle relaxation to resect that tumor."
    "I want to question the patient during the procedure."
3. The ability and skill of the anesthesiologist:
    "I can do a continuous lumbar epidural for both intraoperative and postoperative pain control."

Recent developments have led to the availability of an entire spectrum of pain control, as shown in Figure 6-1 (Malamed, 1985). Of prime importance is the division between the conscious and the unconscious state when considering which anesthetic technique to use. For example, if the goals of anesthesia can be met by regional anesthesia and conscious sedation (e.g., with the addition of intravenous valium), the benefits to the patient of remaining in the conscious state are well known (Table 6-1). However, if this patient had a full stomach and was sedated to a point of unconsciousness without airway protection, the risks to the patient (aspiration, partial or complete airway obstruction) are also well known. Such a patient should have his or her anesthetic plan revised to either avoid the state of unconsciousness or to protect the airway from possible aspiration by the induction and maintenance of general anesthesia utilizing a rapid sequence induction technique with appropriately applied cricoid pressure.

Anesthetic techniques and drugs utilized to achieve the appropriate level of anesthesia will now be considered. Table 6-2 lists the definition and a brief description of each anesthetic technique commonly used today (Office of Medical Applications of Research, 1985). Tables 6-3 and 6-4 list anesthetic drugs or agents commonly used to achieve the techniques outlined in Table 6-2 (Attia & Grogono, 1978). Charts 6-1 and 6-2 further amplify properties of the anesthetic drugs and agents identified in Table 6-4. The physiology of the patient, the pharmacology of the drugs or agents, and the physics of the various anesthetic techniques should interact in a beneficial way, achieving the goals of anesthesia and avoiding unwanted side effects or complications. Only an individual well trained in the above areas can make the administration of an anesthetic look easy and achieve a successful outcome.

Each technique outlined in Table 6-2 and each drug or agent used to produce an appropriate level of anesthesia can be associated with side effects or complications. The postanesthesia nurse needs to be watchful for the occurrence of those signs that foretell of impending problems and initiate prompt action to treat the problems. Problems associated with the various anesthetic techniques (Table 6-5) and anesthetic drugs or agents (Table 6-6) should be familiar to PACU nurses. Well-trained PACU nurses should be able to recognize as well as either prevent or treat many of them. In most cases, the treatment necessary to solve a problem is both obvious and easy, provided the problem is caught before any irreversible changes occur.

Patients who arrive in the PACU after receiving anesthesia require the watchful eye (and ear) of the PACU nurse. Recovering from the effects of general anesthesia, a patient may complain of pain and may appropriately receive an analgesic, such as morphine sulfate or demerol. The dose of drug administered requires careful titration to achieve the desired goal of pain relief without the unwanted complications of respira-

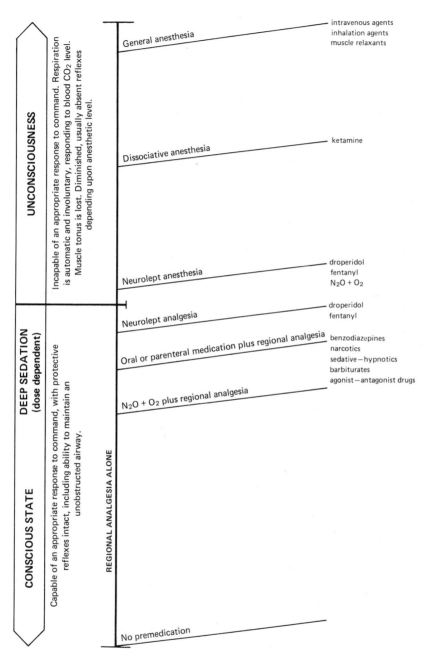

Figure 6–1. Spectrum of pain control, ranging from analgesia to general anesthesia.

TABLE 6–1. BENEFITS OF REMAINING CONSCIOUS

1. Patient capable of appropriate response to command
2. Protective reflexes (cough, gag) remain intact
3. Able to cooperate, if needed, with surgeon or anesthesiologist
4. Vital signs remain stable (as opposed to changing as the spectrum of pain control proceeds from conscious sedation to unconsciousness or general anesthesia)

tory depression, possibly leading to a respiratory arrest. Patients in the PACU have varying degrees of apprehension, anxiety, fear, and levels of awareness. The choice of appropriate measures that might be taken in the PACU to allay the triad of apprehension, anxiety, and fear, and to relieve pain, must consider the maintenance of an acceptable level of consciousness during a changing period of time: the emergence from anesthesia. For example, consider a patient who is semiconscious in the PACU after receiving general anesthesia. The patient complains of pain and yet intermittently falls asleep between pain complaints. Additionally, this patient's blood pressure is elevated and his respiratory rate varies from 6 to 18 breaths per minute. Would analgesics, antihypertensive agents, or sedative drugs be appropriate? This situation, not uncommon in the PACU setting, requires careful consideration.

In general the goal is to keep the patient as pain-free as possible. The alteration in mental status from sleep to full arousal is probably secondary to drugs given either preoperatively or intraoperatively (other reasons should also be considered—changes in electrolytes, hypoxemia, and so on). In this case, the anesthesiologist could control the excessive elevation of blood pressure with apresoline 5 to 10 mg intravenously, and carefully review the anesthesia record, noting what drugs were given preoperatively and intraoperatively. Knowing the drugs' duration of clinical action and their time of administration, the anesthesiologist may be able to determine which drug(s) could be causing the changing mental status. If a drug administered has an antidote, the anesthesiologist will consider its use. However, noting that the patient complains of pain when awake, it would be best not to administer naloxone to this patient even if the pupils were constricted and a narcotic were recently administered. The anesthesiologist will allow "tincture of time" (10 to 15 minutes) to pass, and be ready to administer additional narcotics, carefully titrating the doses and noting the patient's pain complaints and pattern of respiration. Many anesthesiologists utilize multiple drugs both preoperatively and intraoperatively which—due to their action and duration of clinical action—might have been responsible for this type of reaction in the PACU.

If this pattern occurs in multiple patients for prolonged periods (greater than 30 minutes), the PACU nurse should inform the anesthesiologist or anesthetist of the problem. Perhaps the next patient, with careful drug choice and manipulation, may have a smoother emergence from

TABLE 6–2. COMMON ANESTHETIC TECHNIQUES

Technique	Definition	Remarks
Conscious Sedation	State of anesthesia during which the patient remains conscious with some alteration of mood, relief of anxiety, drowsiness, and sometimes analgesia, but protective reflexes remain intact.	Drugs that depress the CNS produce a continuum of effects. Small doses (for example, Valium 2.5 to 10 mg IV) can produce this state.
Deep Sedation	Patient may sleep but can be aroused without difficulty. Minimal depression of protective reflexes occurs.	An increase in dosage of Valium given IV (from 10 to 20 mg) can produce this state.
General Anesthesia	A controlled state of unconsciousness—loss of consciousness from which the patient cannot be aroused. A reversible state providing analgesia, sedation, appropriate muscle relaxation, and appropriate control of the autonomic nervous system. Produced by either intravenous drugs or inhalation agents. There is a partial or (more common) a complete loss of protective reflexes.	Valium at a dose of 1 mg/kg can produce this state. Most commonly, general anesthesia is induced by a barbiturate (sodium thiopental) and maintained with N_2O, O_2 and narcotics or N_2O, O_2 and inhalation agents. Muscle relaxant drugs are added as needed.
Regional Anesthesia	The production of analgesia in a part of the body. Accomplished by either injecting local anesthetic into a vein (a Bier block or IV regional) or, most commonly, by placing local anesthetics in close contact with appropriate nerves to achieve a conduction block.	Successful regional anesthesia requires a thorough knowledge of anatomy, pharmacology of local anesthetic agents, and of alterations to the patient's physiology. These alterations can either be predictable changes (such as decreases in blood pressure secondary to the level of sympathetic blockage produced by spinal or epidural anesthesia) or unexpected (allergic reactions).
Spinal Anesthesia	Produced by administration of a local anesthetic into the lumbar intrathecal space. The local anesthetic blocks conduction in the spinal nerve roots, dorsal root ganglia, and probably the periphery of the spinal cord.	
Epidural Anesthesia	Accomplished by injecting the local anesthetic into the extradural space. The epidural space is usually identified by using a lumbar approach to reach that compartment between the dura mater and the walls of the spinal cord.	
Peripheral Nerve Blocks	Accomplished by injecting local anesthetic at a specific site(s) to block conduction of impulses and render a defined area anesthetic.	

TABLE 6–3. DRUGS USED TO ACCOMPLISH COMMON ANESTHETIC TECHNIQUES

Technique	Drug and Agent
Conscious Sedation	N_2O (nitrous oxide), O_2 (oxygen), and inhalation agents which require an appropriate anesthesia machine for administration. Barbiturates, narcotics, benzodiazepines, or antihistamines administered by the oral, rectal, intramuscular, or intravenous route. Intraoperatively, administration via the intravenous route of an agent like diazepam (Valium) allows titration to achieve anxiety control while the patient remains conscious. Drugs available for IV sedation are listed in Table 6–4.
Deep Sedation	In general, increasing the dose of any of the agents listed in Table 6–4 can produce an increase in the depth of sedation and can produce drowsiness and sleep. If the patient cannot be aroused easily, the state of unconsciousness has been reached.
General Anesthesia	A state of pain control that may be achieved by either inhalation agents (halothane, enflurane, or isoflurane—the fluorinated hydrocarbons) and/or intravenous agents (barbiturates, narcotics, narcotic agonist/antagonists, and benzodiazepines). The mechanisms for the production of this state are still unknown, although considerable emphasis is placed on depression of synaptic transmission as a probable mechanism. Potency of inhalation agents is measured using the minimum alveolar concentration (MAC) of an anesthetic at 1 atmosphere that produces immobility in 50% of those patients or animals exposed to a noxious stimulus. MAC is the most readily measured index of partial pressure of the inhalation agent at the anesthetic site of action—the brain. Breathing the anesthetic vapors causes a rise in anesthetic partial pressure in the alveoli. Diffusing from an area of high partial pressure to one of lower pressure, the anesthetic agent makes its way to the bloodstream where, depending upon the agent's solubility partition coefficient, the anesthetic agent will be "taken up" by the blood. Once the agent has saturated the blood, it is carried by the bloodstream to the vessel-rich organs (heart, brain, lungs, splanchnic organs, and liver). Again, by the process of diffusion, the anesthetic agent leaves the bloodstream and achieves a partial pressure in all the vessel-rich organs. The brain, at equilibrium, experiences the same partial pressure of the anesthetic as the alveoli, and as the partial pressure of the agent is increased (by increasing the inspired concentration of the anesthetic agent delivered through the vaporizer), the depth of anesthesia is increased. Patients in the PACU undergo a process opposite to that experienced during the induction of anesthesia. During emergence from anesthesia, the partial pressure of the agent in the alveoli is less and the agent travels from the brain to the blood and from the bloodstream to the alveoli, finally being exhaled from the body. Even though the agent has been discontinued, any circumstance that would keep the agent in the bloodstream (for example, depressed respirations) would maintain or slow emergence from the anesthetic state. Since the agent is transmitted not only to the brain but also to other organ systems (the vessel-rich group, skeletal muscle, and fat), the agent must leave all of those organ systems via the blood route. It is this continual exit of anesthetic agent from the various organ systems that maintains a

TABLE 6–3. (*Continued*)

Technique	Drug and Agent

blood level of anesthetic agent (and therefore a brain partial pressure of the agent). PACU nurses should be aware of this fact and observe the patient for a continual decline in anesthetic activity due to a continual decline in the agent's partial pressure which will be manifested by a return to consciousness.

Intravenous agents, by combination with receptor sites, achieve their anesthetic action by transmission to various sites in the brain and spinal cord. Blood levels of the intravenous agents are dependent upon protein binding, available storage sites for the drugs, and tissue levels. Blood levels are important in maintaining the clinical duration of drug activity. The tissue levels are dependent upon pH, pKa, and blood flow to the various organ systems. For example, a lowering of the pH of a patient (increased acidosis) can prolong the action of a neuromuscular blocking drug. This potentiation of effect can be seen in the PACU.

Regional Anesthesia

Spinal

	Dose (mg)	Duration (minutes) Plain	Epinephrine (0.2 mg)
Lidocaine	50–100	45–60	60–90
Tetracaine	6–12	60–90	120–180

Drugs administered through either a 22- or 25-gauge spinal needle. Baricity and dose are major determinants of level of block.

Epidural

	Percentage	Duration (minutes)
Chloroprocaine	2.0, 3.0	60
Lidocaine	1.5, 2.0	50
Bupivacaine	0.25, 0.5	120

Drugs administered through 17- or 18-gauge needle or catheter. Volume is major determinant of level.

Peripheral nerve blocks

1. Brachial plexus block:
   Using the interscalene, supraclavicular, or axillary techniques requires 20 ml (interscalene) to 40 ml (axillary) of local anesthetic. Either lidocaine (1.5%), carbocaine (1.5%), or marcaine (0.25 to 0.5%) may be used.

2. Blocks of either upper or lower extremities may be accomplished using 3 ml (for radial, ulnar, or median nerve blocks) to 25 ml of local anesthetic (for sciatic nerve block). Blocks of the femoral, obturator, or lateral femoral cutaneous nerves may be accomplished using 10 ml of local anesthetic.

3. Sympathetic blocks:
   Stellate ganglion using 15 ml of 0.25 to 0.5% marcaine or 1.5% of lidocaine.
   Lumbar sympathetic block using 20 to 40 ml of local anesthetic.

4. Intravenous regional anesthetic (Bier block):
   Requires use of tourniquet, proper technique, and the use of 25 to 50 ml of local anesthetic (0.5% prilocaine or 0.5% lidocaine) for upper extremity or 100 to 200 ml of local anesthetic for lower extremity.

TABLE 6–4. COMMON ANESTHETIC DRUGS AND AGENTS

Drugs for Sedation	Remarks
Sedative-Hypnotics and Antianxiety Drugs	
Benzodiazepines	
Diazepam	Diazepam (Valium) duration of action 45 minutes.
Lorazepam	Average sedative dose 5 to 15 mg IV.
Midazolam	Plasma half-life of 30 hours but shorter duration of action due to degree of receptor site (protein) binding.
Flunitrazepam	
Chlordiazepoxide	Biotransformed to active metabolites.
	Dose of 1 to 1.5 mg/kg can produce general anesthesia.
	Diazepam can be titrated when used for conscious sedation (Verrill sign is ptosis of upper eyelid and is used as endpoint).
	Diazepam versus Lorazepam—Lorazepam is difficult to titrate. Effects develop 5 to 20 minutes after IV injection and produce a long duration of action (6 to 8 hours).
	In general, benzodiazepines are the best antianxiety agents, producing a low incidence of respiratory depression at low doses in younger patients.
Barbiturates	
Pentobarbital	Thiopental most commonly used for induction of anesthesia.
Secobarbital	Barbiturates produce a reversible depression of all excitable tissues including the CNS.
Methohexital	Half-life 3 to 8 hours, but short duration of clinical action due to redistribution of the agent.
Thiopental	Barbiturates do *not* obtund pain.
Thiamylal	Respiratory depression at higher doses.
Antihistamines	
Promethazine	
Hydroxyzine	
Narcotic Agonists	
Meperidine	Morphine is the prototypical narcotic agonist, effecting stereospecific receptors.
Morphine	

Alphaprodine
Fentanyl

Narcotics in general modify both components of the pain experience—perception of and reaction to pain. Narcotics can produce or cause analgesia, drowsiness, mood changes, mental clouding, miosis of pupil, nausea and vomiting, histamine release (morphine and demerol, not fentanyl), GI effects, and dose-dependant respiratory depression.

Narcotic Agonist/Antagonists
Pentazocine
Nalbuphine
Butorphanol

Narcotic Antagonist
Naloxone

Anticholinergics
Atropine
Scopolamine
Glycopyrrolate

Antidotal Drugs
Naloxone
Nalbuphine
Physostigmine
Procaine

Others
Innovar (droperidol with fentanyl)
Ketamine

Inhalation Agents
N_2O (nitrous oxide)
Halothane
Enflurane

Isoflurane

N_2O has a MAC of 105 volume percent.
MAC is the minimum alveolar concentration, or gas concentration in the alveoli, at which 50% of individuals will not move—and therefore 50% will move—in response to a painful cutaneous stimulation.
N_2O is an excellent analgesic but a poor anesthetic agent since a hypoxic mixture must be given to achieve one MAC.

(Continued)

TABLE 6–4. (Continued)

The pharmacologic properties of common intravenous anesthetic agents are summarized in Chart 6–1 for comparison.

Chart 6–1. Pharmacologic Properties of Intravenous Anesthetic Agents

	Thiopental	Methohexital	Diazepam	Ketamine	Propanidid	Althesin
Induction Dose	3–5 mg/kg	1–1.5 mg/kg	0.2–0.3 mg/kg	1–2 mg/kg, IV; 5–8 mg/kg, IM	3–5 mg/kg	50–60µl/kg
Excitatory Phenomena	0¹	++¹	0¹	++	+++	+ Feature of large doses
Respiratory System	Initial apnea	Initial apnea	Minimal depression	Hypoventilation at higher doses	Initial hyperventilation	Minimal depression
Cardiovascular System	Hypotension and tachycardia	Hypotension and tachycardia	Minimal effect	Elevated blood pressure and pulse	Depressed blood pressure at high doses	Hypotension and tachycardia
Duration	A few minutes	Shorter than with thiopental	Slow onset: 2–3 minutes	10–15 minutes	Short: 1–2 minutes	Similar to thiopental but more rapid recovery
Therapeutic Index (mice) LD_{50}/AD_{50}	6.9	7.4	About 100	8.5	8.1	30.6
Recovery Due To	Redistribution to fat and muscle	Redistribution to fat and muscle	Redistribution and metabolism	—	Metabolism	Metabolism and redistribution
Excretion	Hepatic metabolism	Hepatic metabolism	Slow metabolism and urinary excretion		Pseudocholinesterase destroys	All metabolized; mostly excreted via bile
Cumulation	Considerable	Some	Considerable after long-term administration	Some	Minimal	Some
Postoperative Status	Drowsy	Moderately drowsy	Patient may be drowsy	Patient drowsy, liable to	Mental clarity is marked	Slightly quicker and more lucid

recovery than
with thiopental

Minimal

More nausea and
vomiting than
with thiopental

unpleasant
dreams

Emergence
dreams, hal-
lucinations,
and delirium

for many
hours

Muscle relax-
ation by spinal
and limbic
system
interneuronal
inhibition

Antanalgesic

Antanalgesic

Side Effects

¹0 = Absent, + = rare, ++ = common, +++ = very common.

Chart 6–2 outlines the physical and pharmacologic properties of the three major inhalation agents used today.

Chart 6–2. Physical and Pharmacologic Properties of Three Inhalation Agents

Drug and Formula	Halothane $CF_3 \cdot CClBrH$	Enflurane $CClHF \cdot CF_2\text{-}O\text{-}CF_2H$	Isoflurane $CF_3\ CHCl\text{-}O\text{-}CF_2H$ (Note ether structure)
Properties			
Boiling point, °C	50.2	56.5	48.5
Saturated vapor pressure mm Hg	243	174.5	250
Solubilities: blood/gas	2.4	1.91	1.4
brain/blood	2.1	____	
oil/gas	224	98.5	99
MAC volume %	0.765	1.68	____
MAC × oil: gas × 1000/22.4	76.5	73.9	____
Other physical properties	Colorless, sweet nonirritating odor; nonflammable, nonexplosive	Clear, colorless, completely stable liquid; requires no stabilizers	Stable to soda lime; sweet odor; nonflammable, nonexplosive, stable, requires no stabilizers
Pharmacology			
Central nervous system	Depresses vasomotor and respiratory centers, cerebral vasodilator, poor analgesic, raises intracranial	Epileptic movements at deep anesthesia, enhanced by low PCO_2; poor analgesic	Smooth induction; no CNS activity as with enflurane; poor analgesic; postoperative vomiting

(Continued)

Chart 6–2. (Continued)

Drug and Formula	Halothane $CF_3 \cdot CClBrH$	Enflurane $CClHF \cdot CF_2\text{-}O\text{-}CF_2H$	Isoflurane $CF_3\ CHCl\text{-}O\text{-}CF_2H$ (Note ether structure)
	pressure (at normal PCO_2), spinal cord–generated muscular rigors during recovery		may occur.
Autonomic	Depresses sympathetic nervous system, mild ganglionic blockade	—	
Cardiovascular	Hypotension due to myocardial depression, ganglionic block, increased vagal tone, arteriolar dilatation, central vasomotor inhibition, raised baroreceptor discharge; nodal rhythm; ventricular extrasystoles more likely if epinephrine is injected	Transient hypotension during induction due to vasodilatation; with increase in PCO_2, cardiac output rises with occasional dysrhythmia	Progressive hypotension with anesthetic depth × skin + muscle vasodilatation; heart contractility depressed; stroke volume cardiac output maintained by tachycardia; no dysrhythmias with hypercarbia
Respiratory	Increased rate, lower tidal volume and hypoventilation; secretions not stimulated	Minimal secretions; respiratory reflexes depressed	Respiratory depressant
Muscular	No effect on myoneural junction; abdominal relaxation unsatisfactory	Effective relaxant; potentiates non-depolarizers	Better muscle relaxant than halothane; potentiates muscle relaxants
Kidney	No effect; increased antidiuretic hormone is suspected	No effect suggested	—
Liver	Possible allergic reactions to metabolic products of halothane cause hepatitis	Claimed to be harmless to liver	No hepatotoxicity yet metabolism minimal
Uterus	Uterine contractility diminished; increased bleeding in gravid uterus	—	
	Notes: Induction 3%, maintenance 0.5% to 2.0%, 20% metabolized		Blood glucose rises

TABLE 6–5. PROBLEMS ASSOCIATED WITH ANESTHETIC TECHNIQUES

Anesthetic Technique	Problems
Conscious Sedation and Deep Sedation	There are a few problems associated with this technique since patients remain conscious (see Table 6–1). Certain drugs may have a prolonged duration of action. Pain or anxiety in the PACU requires careful titration of additional drugs to relieve patient complaints. The duration of action and the interaction of drugs to be given in the PACU must be correlated with those agents already administered to the patient. Under sedation the patient is in stage I of anesthesia (under the influence of the drug but technically awake). *Respiration* should be normal. *Eye movements* are normal with *voluntary movements*. *Protective reflexes* are intact. *Amnesia* may or may not be present depending upon drugs or agents used to achieve the state of sedation, either conscious or deep.
General Anesthesia	Patients coming to the PACU will generally not be any deeper than plane I of stage III: surgical anesthesia. At stage III *respiration* should be regular, *muscular tonus* is lost, and *protective reflexes* are either absent or greatly diminished. This places the patient at risk of airway obstruction or aspiration. As patients emerge from stage III, plane I, they may pass through stage II: delirium. The patient may exhibit *excitement*, an *irregular pattern of respiration*, *exaggerated reflexes, muscular rigidity,* and an increased incidence of *laryngospasm*. Care must be taken to prevent blood, saliva, or foreign materials from reaching the level of the patient's larynx. Thanks to modern inhalation agents (with low blood-gas solubility coefficients) this stage is of short duration in most patients and requires only a watchful eye to make certain that the transition from unconsciousness to consciousness is without incident.
	Emergence from anesthesia may be marked by:
	1. Hypertension
	2. Tachypnea
	3. Hypoxemia
	4. Complaints of pain, nausea, and vomiting due to incision or site of surgery (increased incidence of nausea and vomiting in gynecological cases)
	5. Hypothermia
	6. Respiratory depression leading to hypoxemia and hypercarbia
	For these reasons, careful monitoring and documentation of the patient's vital signs (especially ECG, blood pressure, and temperature) and respiratory status (respiratory rate and tidal volume, vital capacity, and negative inspiratory force if intubated and extubation is planned) is mandatory.
Regional Anesthesia	Many patients who receive regional anesthesia will also receive conscious sedation, so the remarks listed under conscious sedation apply. In addition, the PACU nurse should:
	1. Be familiar with the type of regional anesthesia used and the specific areas of the body that were blocked. Take care to protect those areas.
	2. Observe the patient carefully for signs of regression of the block. To assess this adequately, the PACU nurse should

(Continued)

116

TABLE 6–5. (*Continued*)

Anesthetic Technique	Problems
	know the duration of action of the specific local anesthetic and if a vasoconstricting agent was added to the local anesthetic. Lack of regression of an epidural could be due to an epidural hematoma. This requires prompt treatment (laminectomy and decompression) before irreversible changes occur to portions of the spinal cord due to vascular compromise.
	3. Observe the patient for changes in hemodynamic stability such as orthostatic hypotension secondary to residual sympathetic blockade in a patient who received either a spinal or an epidural anesthetic. Watch for nausea and vomiting as an initial manifestation of hypotension.
	4. Beware of urinary retention following spinal or epidural anesthesia.
	5. Watch for casts or bandages that might be too tight and therefore be compromising the patient's circulation. The patient may not experience or verbalize pain due to residual sensory block.

TABLE 6–6. PROBLEMS ASSOCIATED WITH ANESTHETIC DRUGS/AGENTS

Drug or Anesthetic Agent	Problems
Diazepam	Contraindications include allergy, psychoses, and acute narrow angle glaucoma. Caution when used with other CNS depressants. May see transient drowsiness (respiratory depression may occur with low doses in the elderly), fatigue, or ataxia. Occasional paradoxical reaction (excitement rather than sedation).
Lorazepam	As of yet, there is no specific reversal agent (one is being developed). For now, try physostigmin. Duration of clinical action 6 to 8 hours. May see excessive sleepiness, restlessness, or hallucinations. In general, patients given this drug are sleepy in the PACU.
Thiopental	If repeated doses are used in the OR, may see "a very sleepy patient" in the PACU due to a prolonged duration of action. No effective reversal agent available and *no* analgesic properties. Supportive treatment if respiratory or cardiovascular collapse should occur.
Meperidine	Minimal but definite histamine release. Can increase heart rate. Blocks or attenuates the shivering response. Interaction with monamine oxidase (MAO) inhibitors. Equianalgesic dose: 100 mg of meperidine = 10 mg of morphine.
Morphine	The prototypical narcotic agonist, producing analgesia, drowsiness, and mood changes. Good for relief of dull, aching, continuous pain. Will see miosis, dose-related respiratory depression, histamine release, nausea and vomiting, and orthostatic hypotension in ambulatory patients. Clinical duration of 4 to 6 hours.
Fentanyl	Rapid onset, short duration of action, and potent (0.1 mg fentanyl = 10 mg morphine). Respiratory depression of longer duration than analgesic action. Produces less nausea and vomiting than other narcotics. May see miosis, bradycardia, and muscle rigidity.

TABLE 6–6. (*Continued*)

Drug or Anesthetic Agent	Problems
Narcotic Agonist/Antagonists	Agents like butorphanol have a small incidence of nausea, sweating, and headache in the PACU. May see an increase in heart rate and blood pressure. May see withdrawal symptoms.
Anticholinergics	Agents used to dry secretions and to block the muscarinic effects of prostigmin-like drugs (drugs used to reverse muscle relaxants). Vagolytic actions, tachycardia, and mydriasis may be seen in the PACU. Glycopyrrolate is a quarternary ammonium compound with no CNS effects (like those seen with scopolamine and atropine).
Naloxone	Stereospecific reversal agent affording direct, specific reversal of narcotic agonists in the PACU. Duration of action shorter than narcotic agents, so renarcotization may occur. Also, administration of naloxone in the PACU may result in a hypertensive response.
Innovar	A combination of two drugs, droperidol and fentanyl. When administered intravenously, this combination of drugs can produce a state of neurolept analgesia (patient is conscious) or neuroleptanesthesia (patient is unconscious). The latter state is usually attained by adding N_2O and O_2 to the Innovar. Duration of clinical action is 45 minutes for the fentanyl and 6 to 8 hours for the droperidol. Benefit for use in the PACU: droperidol in small doses is a powerful antiemetic; however, it can cause orthostatic hypotension in ambulatory patients.
Ketamine	Stimulation of cardiovascular system via stimulation of sympathetic nervous system. Therefore, may see hypertension and it may cause an increased intracranial pressure (ICP). Depending upon dose and route of administration, hallucinations may be seen in the PACU. No specific reversal agent (consider physostigmin). A drug not primarily used in the PACU.
Muscle Relaxants	
Depolarizing	Anectine (succinylcholine) provides rapid skeletal muscle relaxation and a short duration of clinical action. Is known to trigger malignant hyperthermia—a good reason to monitor temperature in the PACU. If used as a "drip," prolonged muscle paralysis may occur (a phase II block).
Nondepolarizing	Of primary importance to the PACU nurse is the assessment of the function of the neuromuscular junction to make certain that effects of the neuromuscular blocking agent have worn off or been properly reversed. Sustained head lift for 5 seconds or a normal response to Train of 4 monitoring are good tests of the function of the neuromuscular junction. Every PACU should have a nerve stimulator for this purpose. See Table 6–7.
Inhalation Agents	
Nitrous oxide	An inhalation agent used in the OR to reduce dosage (and MAC) of the more potent agents. With a blood-gas partition coefficient of 0.47, this drug has a rapid onset of action and is rapidly eliminated. High solubility makes it easy for N_2O to diffuse into body

TABLE 6–6. (*Continued*)

Drug or Anesthetic Agent	Problems
	cavities supplied by blood. For example, N_2O could double the size of a pneumothorax in 12 to 15 minutes.
Halothane	Has a high fat solubility coefficient (halothane in fat is 60.0 while N_2O is 1.0). This results in a prolonged uptake, which is important in the PACU when emergence and recovery from anesthesia is occurring. A long exposure time results in a slow wakeup time. Twelve percent of the inspired halothane is metabolized. Oxidation and dehalogenation occur in the liver microsomes, forming trifluoracetic acid, bromide, and chloride radicals. Frequent administration of halothane may result in a "sleepy" patient due to increased bromide levels. Reductive pathway metabolites may play a role in the "posthalothane hepatitis" picture. Postoperative hepatitis in a patient given halothane may be explained by either an allergic or a metabolic activation theory. Other causes for postoperative hepatitis are usually present, confusing the picture. Depression of the myocardium is directly related to the depth of halothane anesthesia, a dose-effect relationship. Vasodilation is produced. Both effects may be due in part to a block of the action of norepinephrine and an inhibition of uptake of calcium ions by the sarcoplasmic reticulum of cardiac muscle.
Enflurane	Has a 25–35 percent lower solubility in fatty tissue when compared to halothane, but this is *not* the reason for a faster rate of recovery from enflurane anesthesia. Rather, enflurane has a lower solubility in blood (1.8 versus 2.3 for halothane). 2.4 percent of inspired enflurane may be recovered from the urine. Serum inorganic fluoride levels in excess of 50 μM (a nephrotoxic threshold) would require greater than 9 MAC hours of enflurane anesthesia to achieve. High output renal failure due to excess inorganic fluoride levels has been reported. A few cases of postoperative hepatitis in patients receiving enflurane have been reported but the mechanism is unknown. As with halothane, a dose-related depression of myocardial contractility is seen.
Isoflurane	Has a relatively low blood-gas solubility coefficient of 1.4 at 37°, which suggests swift induction of anesthesia (a slightly pungent ethereal smell limits the rate at which the inspired concentration may be increased and thus slows the induction of anesthesia) and rapid emergence from anesthesia. The lower the blood-gas solubility coefficient, the faster levels of anesthesia can be altered. However, isoflurane is a weaker anesthetic than halothane (oil-gas partition coefficient is 98 while halothane is 244). The higher the oil-gas partition coefficient, the more potent the agent. Isoflurane is viewed by many in the field of anesthesia as a "close to ideal" anesthetic inhalation agent. It sustains myocardial contractility, does not sensitize the heart to epinephrine, maintains central venous pressure, and provides a relatively high margin of safety. Isoflurane enhances the action of both depolarizing and nondepolarizing muscle relaxants. Less than 0.2% of the inhaled isoflurane is found in the urine—a characteristic of major importance. Minimal metabolism is desirable since it means a markedly decreased production of toxic metabolites that may affect the kidney or liver. Greater stability and a lower blood-gas partition coefficient (lower than enflurane or halothane) make this agent a major consideration in formulating an anesthetic plan.

anesthesia. Remember, that the anesthesiologist or anesthetist often leaves the PACU before the patient has recovered and therefore misses seeing developing problems.

Another problem faced in the PACU is the patient who has undergone a major operation and will not be extubated immediately postoperatively. This patient will be intubated, probably ventilated, and may not have muscle relaxant drugs—if utilized intraoperatively—reversed. Such a patient may be semiawake in the PACU setting, and consideration of the mental status of the patient is necessary. Realizing that muscle relaxant drugs have no cortical activity, one should assess the need for appropriate and adequate sedation lest the patient remain paralyzed but unsedated and aware. Monitoring the autonomic nervous system activity (blood pressure and heart rate) and noting any attempts at respiration or diaphragmatic breathing ("bucking on the tube") may alert the nurse to this situation, which can and should be corrected. Appropriate drugs should be given to produce a desired level of sedation while the patient remains intubated and mechanically ventilated.

A final problem that occurs in the PACU is noted in patients having received a regional block, either spinal or epidural. Many times the anesthesiologist chooses a local anesthetic drug on the basis of its longer duration of action, or mixes local anesthetic drugs with vasoconstricting drugs to prolong their expected duration of action. This may be desirable if the need for pain control in the postoperative setting is anticipated. Although the goal of the anesthesiologist may be prolonged pain control, a prolonged stay in the PACU is an unnecessary cost if all vital signs are stable and the PACU nurse is waiting only for the complete return of the motor, sensory, and sympathetic nervous systems. The anesthesiologist or anesthetist should communicate his or her intentions to the PACU nurse, and the patient should remain in the unit only until signs of regression of the block are noted and documented in the PACU record. The anesthesiologist frequently makes a postoperative visit to the patient's room 2 to 3 hours after the operation to document the complete (or further) regression of the block. This is certainly less costly for patients than an extra 2 to 3 hour stay in the PACU, and allows patients to spend time in their own rooms with family and friends.

There is no doubt that multiple, potent drugs are used to induce and maintain the state of anesthesia. Review of each agent or drug by the PACU nurse with careful consideration of its pharmacology, duration of clinical activity, and effects good and bad on the physiology of the patient, will benefit the nurse tremendously. It will aid the nurse in knowing what to watch for, what to consider in the differential diagnosis, and how to treat the patient before irreversible events occur.

In summary, the following points, if adhered to, will aid PACU nurses in managing patients during a critical time—the emergence from anesthesia.

1. If the patient complains of pain, a carefully titrated narcotic is indicated. Watch the respiratory rate and depth and note the mental status of the patient. Allow time for the drug to work (know the time of onset and the time of peak effect, and titrate with these times—which are different—in mind). Also, consider newer methods of individualized pain control, such as epidural narcotics via epidural catheter, and patient-controlled analgesia (Cousins & Mather, 1984; Stenseth & Sellevold, 1985; White, 1984).

2. Know the anesthetic drugs and agents used and know their duration of action. Always be ready for a prolonged duration of action. For example, a muscle relaxant of intermediate duration may not reverse well and may have prolonged clinical activity in a patient who is hypokalemic and acidotic. Know the interaction of drugs with other drugs, disease states, and altered physiology (such as abnormal electrolytes or hypoalbuminemia).

3. Differential diagnosis is most important. For example, a patient with shallow respirations at a slow rate is brought to the PACU. Assessment of this patient requires a comprehensive drug review: residual inhalation agent, residual narcotics, and residual muscle relaxant drugs (Cullen, 1985; Goldberg & associates, 1985). Communication with the anesthesiologist or anesthetist who performed the case is mandatory before problems get out of control.

4. Use a nerve stimulator if there is a question of residual neuromuscular blockage; See Table 6-7 (Ali & Miller, 1986; Wellcome Trends in Anesthesiology, 1985).

TABLE 6–7. CRITERIA OF RECOVERY FROM NONDEPOLARIZING NEUROMUSCULAR BLOCKADE

I Clinical:
A Nonrespiratory Parameters:
1. The ability to open the eyes wide
2. Sustained protrusion of the tongue
3. Sustained hand grip
4. Sustained head lift for at least five seconds
5. The ability to cough effectively
B Respiratory Variables:
1. Adequate tidal volume
2. Vital capacity of at least 15–20 ml/kg^{-1}
3. Inspiratory force of 20–25 cm water negative pressure
II Evoked Responses:
1. Return of the single twitch to control height
2. Sustained tetanic response to high frequency stimulation
3. Recovery of the train-of-four to a ratio above 75%

5. Assessment of rate and depth of ventilation may be difficult and, in the final analysis, may require an arterial blood gas determination to assess adequacy of oxygenation (PaO_2), adequacy of ventilation ($PaCO_2$), and overall metabolic status (pH, bicarbonate, and base excess or deficit).

6. Review a dermatome chart. If a patient is brought to the PACU with a spinal sensory level of T_{10} and, after 30 minutes, has a spinal sensory level to L_1, the block is regressing. This regression check should be made for all spinals and epidurals and documented in the PACU record (Carron & associates, 1984).

7. Complaints of nausea and vomiting must include the following assessment.
   A. Check vital signs—blood pressure and heart rate.
   B. Determine site of surgery—there is an increased incidence in gynecological cases or when CO_2 is used.
   C. Check if drugs were administered that have an incidence of nausea and vomiting as a known side affect (not an allergic reaction).
   D. Assess fluid status: decreased fluids can cause an increased incidence of nausea and vomiting.
   E. Check for electrolyte imbalance (check Na^+ and K^+).
   F. Determine blood sugar.
   G. Find out if a mask was used (patient not intubated): gastric distension secondary to air entry into the stomach during ventilation may cause nausea and vomiting.
   H. Check ECG for rate or rhythm disturbances—PVCs and tachycardias may cause nausea and vomiting.
   I. Check for any medications that may have recently been given or are currently infusing—for example, was the patient digitalized intraoperatively or is/was an aminophylline drip running?

8. Monitor and control patient's temperature. Beware of malignant hyperthermia and prevent postanesthetic shivering (Gronert, 1986; Murphy & associates, 1985).

9. Be ready for the unexpected. Have suction, oxygen, means to provide positive pressure ventilation, and equipment to reintubate (laryngoscope and endotracheal tube) ready.

10. Don't distrust your monitors but do trust your senses (Gravenstein and Paulus, 1982). A dampened wave form noted on a monitor displaying a blood pressure of 50/30 should immediately prompt evaluation and correction of the monitoring device (not the patient!) if the patient is responding appropriately, has good color and a palpable, bounding bracheal pulse (Gallagher, 1984). Know your monitoring systems well and troubleshoot as needed, but never lose "touch" with the patient. Utilize your monitor to read drug effects—how successful is your NTG or nipride drip in controlling the patient's blood pressure?

REFERENCES

Ali HH & Miller RD: Monitoring of neuromuscular function. In RD Miller (Ed.), Anesthesia (2nd ed.). New York: Churchill Livingstone, 1986. chap. 26.

Attia RR & Grogono AW: Practical Anesthetic Pharmacology. New York: Appleton-Century-Crofts, 1978.

Carron H, Korbon GA, & Rowlingson JC: Regional Anesthesia. Orlando: Grune & Stratton, 1984.

Cousins MJ & Mather LE: Intrathecal and epidural administration of opioids. Anesthesiology 61:276–310, 1984.

Cullen DJ: Problems in the recovery room. Resident and Staff Physician, Feb., 1985.

Gallagher TJ: Monitoring for anesthesia: What and when? American Society of Anesthesiologists annual refresher course lectures 1–7, 1984, p. 209.

Goldberg M, Ishak S, et al.: Postoperative rigidity following sufentanil administration. Anesthesiology 63(2), August, 1985.

Gravenstein JS & Paulus DA: Monitoring Practice in Clinical Anesthesia. Philadelphia: Lippincott, 1982.

Gronert GA: Malignant hyperthemia. In RD Miller (Ed.), Anesthesia (2nd ed.), (vol. 3). New York: Churchill Livingstone, 1986. chap. 56.

Malamed SF: Sedation—A Guide to Patient Management. St. Louis: C.V. Mosby, 1985, p. 23.

Murphy MT, Lipton JM, et al.: Postanesthetic shivering in primates: Inhibition by peripheral heating and by Taurine. Anesthesiology 63:161–165, 1985.

Office of Medical Applications of Research, National Institute of Health: Consensus conference—Anesthesia and sedation in the dental office. Journal of the American Medical Association 254 (8), 1985.

Smith NT, Miller RD, & Corbascio AN: Drug Interactions in Anesthesia. Philadelphia: Lea & Febiger, 1981.

Stenseth R, Sellevold O, & Breivik H: Epidural morphine for postoperative pain: Experience with 1085 patients. Acta Anaesthesiologica Scandinavica 29:148–156, 1985.

Wellcome Trends in Anesthesiology/Symposium Perspectives 3(6), 1985.

White PF: Selection of narcotic and administration technique in class I and II patients. American Society of Anesthesiologists annual refresher course lectures 1–6, 1984, p. 505.

Chapter 7

Triage

Kay E. Fraulini

Current economic constraints have forced hospitals to keep nurse staffing at a bare minimum. In areas such as the PACU and SICU, nurse-to-patient staffing ratios are usually 1 to 2 or 1 to 1. Additionally, there appears to be a trend among major hospital centers toward becoming more surgically oriented and managing more complex and critically ill patients. The need for perioperative intensive care can only increase.

This combination of circumstances has led to frequent crowding in the PACU and the consequent need for triage. Triage refers to the sorting and allocation of treatment to patients according to a system of priorities designed to maximize successful outcome. A basic problem is finding bedspace in the PACU or, beyond that, in the ICU. The uncertain availabiity of ICU beds makes it necessary to assign priorities to patients requiring postanesthesia and surgical intensive care. It is clear that not every patient requires the same treatment in the PACU, nor does every patient require an ICU bed. Decisions must be made about who will be placed where in the PACU, who can be moved at a given time, and who is most ready to be moved to the ICU.

THE BASIS FOR INTEREST IN TRIAGE

Triage was developed by the military to maximize care for battlefield and disaster victims. It is used in hospital emergency departments, upon patient arrival, to determine the urgency of the problem and to designate the appropriate health care resources. The patient is then classified according to priority.

This would be a logical system to use in the PACU as well as in the emergency room. There are striking similarities between the two areas, in physical design, in the short term of patient stay, in the lack of control of the number and frequency of patient admissions, and in the unpredictability of the patient's course while in the unit.

The burden of triage often falls on the PACU nurse. Although not identified as a triage nurse, the responsibility for these functions is usually assumed by the head or charge nurse. As beds in ICU are eliminated because of lack of staff, postoperative patients may have to be diverted to floor care or await the forced triage of another patient in PACU. For these reasons, it is becoming necessary for PACU nurses to develop a thorough understanding of triage.

Nurses should take the lead in developing their role as triage personnel. They should attempt to use a problem-solving approach to making triage decisions. Benefits would include efficient and effective use of time, appropriate use of personnel and equipment, and most important, reduction of morbidity and mortality.

The central element of triage is a set of clinical algorithms used to train and guide the triage workers. (An algorithm is broadly defined as a step-by-step procedure for solving a problem or accomplishing some end. Clinical algorithms are simply rules for solving clinical problems.) Data exist to indicate which patients may be at greater risk for postanesthetic morbidity. This information can be used to develop the initial screen algorithm. Most PACUs have arbitrarily designated certain areas for certain patients—for example, patients having cystoscopies go against the wall with a lower nurse-to-patient ratio, patients who have had open-heart surgery have a specific area designated for their recovery, and a critical care module for equipment such as Swan-Ganz catheters and ventilators may be located where it is convenient to have a high nurse-to-patient ratio. It is a logical progression to formalize the sorting and allocation of all patients in the PACU based on the patient's preoperative condition and course in the operating room.

Figure 7-1 gives an untested initial screen algorithm for patients entering the PACU. Basic to this system is the need to designate certain areas of the room for specific patients. This, of course, is more difficult for the smaller PACU where space is always a problem. The authors have found it helpful to centralize sicker patients in critical care modules. Also, classifying these patients with a priority rating for ICU beds should allow more expedient transfer as space becomes available in the ICU. The designation of a resuscitation area will add yet another dimension to the wide spectrum of specialized care offered in the PACU. Hypothetically the area could also be used for patients triaged to the PACU from the radiology department, the pain clinic, after cardiac catheterization, or following physiologic crises or critical incidents.

In this era of ever-increasing specialization, it is no longer satisfactory

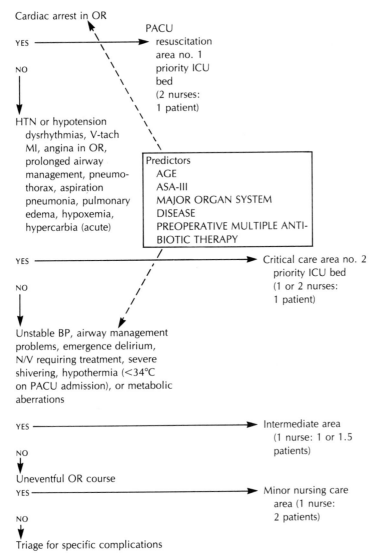

Cardiac arrest in OR

YES ———————————————▶ PACU
resuscitation
area no. 1
NO   priority ICU
bed
(2 nurses:
1 patient)

HTN or hypotension
dysrhythmias, V-tach
MI, angina in OR,
prolonged airway
management, pneumo-
thorax, aspiration
pneumonia, pulmonary
edema, hypoxemia,
hypercarbia (acute)

Predictors
  AGE
  ASA-III
  MAJOR ORGAN SYSTEM
  DISEASE
  PREOPERATIVE MULTIPLE ANTI-
  BIOTIC THERAPY

YES ———————————————▶ Critical care area no. 2
priority ICU bed
NO   (1 or 2 nurses:
1 patient)

Unstable BP, airway management
problems, emergence delirium,
N/V requiring treatment, severe
shivering, hypothermia (<34°C
on PACU admission), or metabolic
aberrations

YES ———————————————▶ Intermediate area
(1 nurse: 1 or 1.5
NO   patients)

Uneventful OR course
YES ———————————————▶ Minor nursing care
area (1 nurse:
NO   2 patients)

Triage for specific complications

Figure 7–1. Initial screen algorithm.

to allow the haphazard placement of patients in the PACU. Nurses working in the PACU may want to add other clinical dispositions in the algorithm presented in Figure 7-1.

Referral to a specific location in the PACU by the algorithm-directed screener is based on a brief history from the anesthetist or operating room nurse, preanesthetic nursing assessment history as it relates to predictors of the care urgency category and the level of care needed by the patient. It is reasonable to expect that patients referred to the critical care or resuscitation area may need the continued attention of the physician and that cardiologists, neurologists, or other specialists may need to be urgently summoned.

This has the potential of enhancing the quality of patient care concentrating patients requiring the same level of care in separate areas of the PACU, thereby increasing efficiency and concentration of valuable resources, supplies, and technology. For all these reasons, triage would be a cost-effective system.

In the past, triage has been forced upon nurses and physicians by the urgency of need and lack of staff, requiring them to make quick and often unplanned decisions about where to place patients in the PACU, who will go to the ICU, and which patients will be moved out of the ICU to the floor. This chapter proposes that PACU personnel make the triage system work for them. Patients can only benefit from a more sophisticated streamlined triage plan.

Cork and Gluck (1982) have proposed a recovery nursing care algorithm. They further examined this classification system for usefulness, and with discriminant analysis succeeded in classifying patients based on a minimum number of objective parameters availalbe on admission to the recovery room. Six variables were selected as discriminators:

1. Origin of patient   OR (OR = 1, non-OR = 0)
2. Presence of ET tube   TUBE (yes = 1, no = 0)
3. Presence of central line   CENT (yes = 1, no = 0)
4. Presence of A-line   ALN (yes = 1, no = 0)
5. Presence of ventilator   VENT (yes = 1, no = 0)
6. ASA physical status   ASA (1–5)

The following two discriminant functions were derived, with each variable entering the functions at $p < 0.05$ and total significance of the functions at $p < 0.001$:

$$\text{Function 1} = -2.1 \times OR - 0.8 \times TUBE - 1.0 \times CENT - 3.6 \times ALN - 1.5 \times VENT - 0.3 \times ASA + 3.1$$

$$\text{Function 2} = -7.8 \times OR + 0.1 \times TUBE + 0.3 \times CENT + 1.1 \times ALN - 0.6 \times VENT + 7.4$$

These two functions can be used to classify patients (see Figure 7-2) by the discriminant analysis package of SPSS (Statistical Package for the Social Sciences). With this system, 93.1 percent of cases are correctly classified.

This easily may be done by hand since all variables except ASA take 0 or 1 as a value. Figure 7-2 can serve as a guide or a programmable calculator can be used to input the values of the six discriminator variables for each patient and receive as output the proper group classification for nursing allocation.

Because this is a new idea for postanesthesia care units, there is little in the literature to guide the development of such a system. The authors

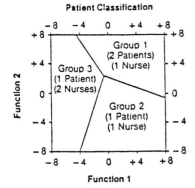

Patient Classification

Function 1

Figure 7–2. Recovery nursing care algorithm.

have attempted to implement a rudimentary form of triage in the PACU at Rush-Presbyterian–St. Luke's Medical Center. The results indicate the system has great possible benefit for the postanesthetic population.

The nurse assigned as the initial screener should be rotated as often as is necessary to prevent stress overload. This may not be more often than a weekly rotation. What is required next is a clarification of the role of screener or triage nurse. With that accomplished, further testing of triage systems will be possible. This is but one example of the challenges that face PACU nurses and the opportunities for creatively contributing to postanesthetic care.

BIBLIOGRAPHY

Cork RC & Gluck C: A recovery nursing care allocation algorithm. Anesthesiology 57 (A170), Sept., 1982.

Cullen DJ: Surgical intensive care: Current perceptions and problems. Critical Care Medicine 9 (4), April, 1981.

Estrada E: Triage systems. Nursing Clinics of North America 16:13–23, March, 1981.

Nursing Skill Books: Giving Emergency Care Competently. Philadelphia: Intermed Communications, 1978.

Pozen M, et al.: The usefulness of a predictive instrument to reduce inappropriate admissions to the coronary care unit. Annals of Internal Medicine 92 (part 1):238–242, 1980.

Stephenson HE (Ed.): Immediate Care of the Acutely Ill and Injured (2nd ed.). St. Louis: C.V. Mosby, 1978.

Vaughan RW, Vaughan MS, et al.: Predicting adverse outcomes during anesthesia and surgery by prospective risk assessment. Abstract of scientific papers, 1983 annual meeting. Anesthesiology 59, Sept., 1983.

Vickery DM: Triage: Problem Oriented Sorting of Patients. Bowie, Md.: Brady, 1975.

Warner CG: Emergency Care—Assessment and Intervention (3rd ed.), St. Louis: C.V. Mosby, 1983.

Chapter 8

Interface Between Anesthesiology and Nursing

Kay E. Fraulini

THE ANESTHESIOLOGIST–NURSE INTERFACE

It is essential that the PACU nurse and anesthesiologist work together. This chapter proposes some guidelines that could enhance that interaction.

The anesthesiologist-nurse interaction could also be termed *interface,* a systems theory term. It has been defined as the area of contact between one system or subsystem and another, or between a system and the environment. The boundaries are limitations or parameters that may be defined arbitrarily but must be observable. Although boundaries constitute a form of limit, they also permit passage of input and output from one side to the other.

An intriguing contemporary application of systems thinking is in the area of health care. Health care organizations, like most business entities, are complex organizations characterized by intensive technologies, openness to the environment, and interrelated and interdependent psychosocial relationships between health care personnel, patients, and others. Figure 8-1 gives a suggested model of the PACU nurse–anesthesiologist interface.

Various guidelines have been published concerning this interface.

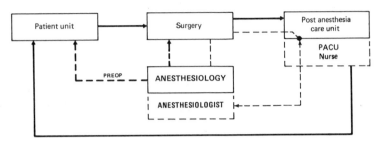

Figure 8–1. Anesthesiologist–PACU nurse interface. *(From Fraulini KE. Current Reviews for Recovery Room Nurses. 5(8), 1983. Reprinted with permission.)*

The Joint Commission on Accreditation of Hospitals states (in Standard IV) that there should be written policies relating to the delivery of anesthesia care. Concerning the PACU nurse–anesthesiologist interface, the policies at a minimum should provide that:

following the procedures for which anesthesia was administered, the anesthetist or his qualified designee(s) shall remain with the patient as long as required by the patient's condition relative to his anesthesia status, and until responsibility for proper patient care has been assumed by other qualified individuals. Personnel responsible for postanesthetic care should be advised of specific problems presented by the patient's condition.

The American Society of Anesthesiologists covers the interface in this way in *Guidelines for Patient Care in Anesthesiology* (1974):

A. Basic Guidelines for Anesthesia Care
. . .
c. Post-Anesthesia Care means:
    (3) Informing personnel caring for patient in immediate post-anesthetic period of any specific problems presented by each patient.
    (4) That the individual responsible for administering anesthesia remain with the patient as long as his presence appears necessary.

In an anesthesia practice advisory for the PACU, (ASA Newsletter, 1978), the ASA further recommends that:

. . . all patients transported to the recovery room should be accompanied by at least two individuals, one of whom must be a member of the anesthesia care team, or the person responsible for the administration of the anesthetic. A verbal report to recovery room [PACU] personnel should include what transpired during the procedure as well as pertinent preoperative data.

DATA COLLECTION FOR INTELLIGENT NURSING ASSESSMENT

PACU records should contain at least the following admission information:

- Documentation of the patient's general condition evaluating respiration, circulation, state of consciousness, color, and type of anesthesia.
- Special problems or precautions.
- Summary of all fluids received during surgery.

It is recommended that each patient be *formally* handed over to the PACU staff. The information transmitted should include:

1. Patient identification.
2. The nature of the operation, details of any drainage tubes or catheters, and whether suction is needed.
3. Type of anesthesia used, the anesthetic technique and its duration.
4. Estimated blood loss, and quantity and type of intravenous fluids given during the operation, with instructions for maintenance.
5. The condition of the patient at the end of the operation, including systolic blood pressure, pulse, and respiration rates.
6. Any complications encountered.
7. Any complications predicted for the immediate postoperative period.
8. Instructions about ventilation, recording of VS, administration of sedation, and extubation.

In return, the anesthesiologist should receive an acceptance of the patient from the PACU staff, should note vital signs on arrival in the PACU, and should not release the patient until both he or she and the PACU staff are satisfied with the patient's condition.

The American Society of Post Anesthesia Nurses gives detailed guidelines for health status data collection and assessment. These are quoted in the first appendix to Chapter 9.

What methodology can be used for collecting patient data? An effective tool is the PACU record. This should be an accurate record of the patient's course in the PACU. The record eventually becomes part of the permanent hospital record, and is of value to personnel who subsequently assume responsibility for the patient, since it provides a summary of the early postoperative period. It is desirable to code the record in a way that permits retrieval of data for retrospective research studies. In addition, since the PACU record is a legal document, it is imperative that times (arrival in the PACU, for example) and information are accurate and coincide with the anesthesia record.

Figure 8-2 shows one type of PACU record. When the anesthesiolo-

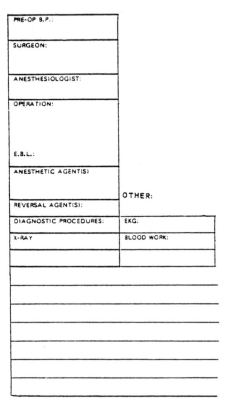

PRE-OP B.P.:	
SURGEON:	
ANESTHESIOLOGIST:	
OPERATION:	
E.B.L.:	
ANESTHETIC AGENT(S)	OTHER:
REVERSAL AGENT(S):	
DIAGNOSTIC PROCEDURES:	EKG:
X-RAY	BLOOD WORK:

Figure 8–2. Sample PACU record form. *(From Fraulini KE. Current Reviews for Recovery Room Nurses 5(8), 1983. Reprinted with permission.)*

gist arrives with the patient, it is convenient to go over, step by step, the boxes in the record. This assures collection of certain basic information and serves as an introduction to any special problems the patient may have developed intraoperatively or that were preexisting. The anesthesiologist tells the nurse who the surgeon is (this may or may not be apparent), and identifies the anesthesiologist ultimately responsible for this patient's anesthetic management (a qualified designee may accompany the patient to the PACU). Other items on the form are completed as follows:

- Operation—the surgical procedure performed and any unusual occurrences or complications.
- EBL—how much blood was lost during the procedure? In addition, what were the preoperative hematology values—specifically hemoglobin and hematocrit—and any blood dyscrasias that might affect the postoperative course.
- Anesthetic agents—type, and amount. In addition, was the patient intubated? Was there any difficulty with intubation or extubation? Was a hypotensive or hypothermic technique used? How was this achieved? If the patient is still intubated, why and what kind of

oxygen therapy, mechanical ventilation, T-piece? What is the plan for the endotracheal tube?

- Reversal agents—Did the patient receive naloxone, for example, and how much? Was physostigmine used? Which anticholinesterase drug and how much was used to reverse a nondepolarizing muscle relaxant? Which anticholinergic agent was used, and what was the dose? (Remember that the anticholinesterase may be more prolonged than the atropine and that the peripheral muscarinic effects that may occur, such as bradycardia, increased secretions, and bronchospasm, may require further treatment.) Also, administration of aminoglycosides in combination with nondepolarizing muscle relaxants should be communicated because acetylcholine release is affected, calcium is bound, and the effect of the neuromuscular blockade is increased. Table 8-1 lists some of the antibiotics to be aware of, especially if used intraperitoneally.
- Other—this area is used for any pertinent history. For example, indicate any previous myocardial infarctions, dysrhythmias, or cardiac medications, What was the cardiac rhythm intraoperatively? If there is a history of hypertension, what were the blood pressure parameters intraoperatively? Were vasopressors or antihypertensives required? Was the patient maintained on drugs preoperatively? Any previous surgeries? Any medical problems should be noted, such as diabetes, COPD, myasthenia gravis, congestive heart failure, sickle cell, and SLE. Is the patient drug-dependent as a result of this? IV fluids: how much and what type of fluid was administered intraoperatively?

It becomes apparent that pharmacology plays a large role in patient care in the perianesthetic period. The practice of anesthesia entails a daring

TABLE 8–1. ANTIBIOTIC–NONDEPOLARIZING MUSCLE RELAXANT INTERACTIONS

Antibiotic	Increase in Neuromuscular Block of D. Tubocurare
Neomycin	Yes
Streptomycin	Yes
Gentamicin	Yes
Kanamycin	Yes
Paromomycin-Humatin	Yes
Viamycin	Yes
Polymixin A	Yes
Polymixin B	Yes
Colistin	Yes
Tetracycline	Yes
Lincomycin	Yes
Clindamycin	Yes

From Fraulini KE. Current Reviews for Recovery Room Nurses 5(8), 1983. Reprinted with permission.

incursion into human pharmacology and pharmacodynamics. The anesthesiologist daily performs a complex experiment with drugs that profoundly affect patients essential functions, such as respiratory, cardiovascular, and neuromuscular activity. To achieve anesthesia speedily and effectively often requires many agents (six to ten on the average) in patients who may have been exposed to 20 or even more drugs in the preoperative period. There are few other branches of medicine in which polypharmacy is such a necessity and drug interactions such an inevitable consequence. The science of interactions is still in its infancy, but it constitutes an area of explosive development that is bound to affect many traditional therapeutic concepts (Smith, Miller, & Corbascio, 1981).

Knowledge of interactions is extremely important for the PACU nurse, who cannot be expected to remain current on all drugs but must be aware of the resources available—for example, the pharmacist. PACU nurses should become accustomed to consulting the pharmacy department as frequently as necessary to safeguard patients against possible negative interactions.

A final example of information that must be shared during this interface is allergies. If you are told, for example, that a patient is allergic to penicillin, try to find out what kind of reaction the patient has had. If it was an anaphylactic reaction and the patient has a cephalosporin ordered IV, you would want to watch this patient very carefully, because the incidence of crossreactivity is about 10 percent.

There are many other examples of the kinds of information that need to be reported during the nurse–anesthesiologist interface. The point in this chapter is that it is essential for the PACU nurse to have the patient history or data base, and the person to communicate these data is the anesthesiologist, especially if the nurse has not visited the patient preoperatively and personally taken a history. The patient, at this point, cannot give the nurse a history and also cannot tell the nurse what occurred intraoperatively.

Standard 1 of the American Nurses Association Standards for Medical-Surgical Nursing Practice (1974) calls for:

- Systematic and continuous collection of data about the health status of the patient. These data are to be communicated to appropriate persons, and recorded and stored in a retrievable and accessible system.
- Interview, physical examination, review of records and reports, and consultation are all to be employed to obtain data.
- Priority of data collection to be determined by the immediate physical condition of the patient.

Intelligent nursing assessment can be made only if the nurse has knowledge of the patient's history. Many of the problems encountered in the postanesthetic period can be attributed to events that occurred during

TABLE 8–2. PROBLEMS IN THE PACU

	Impaired Cardiovascular Performance		
Symptom	*Possible Cause*	*Symptom*	*Possible Cause*
Hypertension	Carbon dioxide retention Shivering Pain Use of ketamine Vasopressors Circulatory overload Following fentanyl Analeptics or narcotic antagonist Distension of bladder Respiratory obstruction leading to carbon dioxide retention	Hypotension	Bleeding Underreplacement of fluids Pain Sedation and persistent anesthesia Removal of stimuli Hypothermia Underventilation Hypoxia Alkalosis Myocardial depression or infarction Electrolyte disturbances Diuresis Hypoglycemia Reaction to blood transfusion Adrenal failure Gastric distension Pneumothorax Tamponade Aspiration of gastric contents

	Variations in Heart Rate		
Symptom	*Possible Cause*	*Symptom*	*Possible Cause*
Bradycardia (Pulse rate <60)	Consequent on the use of prostigmine Pain Vagal stimulation Nausea Heart block Hypoxia—especially in small children Cyclopropane and halothane	Tachycardia	Bleeding Dehydration Pyrexia Pain Carbon dioxide retention Atropine Tachyarrhythmia Myocardial infarction Thromboembolic accident Reaction to blood transfusion Heart failure Ether Aspiration of vomit
Cyanosis— peripheral	Vasoconstriction Congestion Hypothermia Polycythemia		
Cyanosis— central	Underventilation Respiratory obstruction Heart failure Over transfusion	Pallor	Bleeding Pain Nausea and vomiting Myocardial infarction Anemia Hypoglycemia Methoxyflurane

(Continued)

TABLE 8–2. (Continued)

Alterations in Respiratory Performance

Symptom	Possible Cause	Symptom	Possible Cause
Ineffective breathing pattern	Respiratory obstruction— lips, tongue Pulmonary edema Asthma Heart failure Central depression Residual paralysis Pneumothorax Laryngeal palsy Inhalation of vomit Anaphylaxis Air embolism Tamponade	Restlessness	Hypoxia, hypercarbia, or acidosis until proved otherwise Unrelieved pain, especially if barbiturate premedication has been used and no analgesic administered during surgery; particularly common in children Use of ketamine Following phenothiazine drugs Alcohol withdrawal Drug withdrawal Overdosage with narcotic antagonist, such as naloxone Full bladder

Sensory and Perceptual Alterations—Impaired Physical Mobility

Symptom	Possible Cause	Symptom	Possible Cause
Convulsions	Pyrexia Use of analeptics In the known epileptic After neurosurgery Cerebral tumor Hypoglycemia Eclampsia Decreased sodium	Pyramidal tract signs	Following phenothiazine drugs After droperidol
		Extensor plantor response is initially present in nearly all cases emerging from anesthesia.	
Dilated pupils	May mean neurological damage due either to circulatory arrest or air embolism. *Note,* however, that pupils will be dilated for several hours after ganglion blockage used for deliberate hypotension (e.g., arfonad).	Hemiplegia	Cerebral thrombosis occurring incidentally during anesthesia or following hypotension or cerebral embolism.
Constricted pupils	Use of narcotics during surgery. Pontine hemorrhage and following the use of meiotic eye drops in glaucomatous patients.	Sweating	Bleeding Pyrexia Hypoglycemia CO_2 retention Pain Nausea Vasovagal response Reaction to sedative, especially meperidine
Unequal pupils	Horner's syndrome: Unequal pupils after neck or upper chest surgery or following spinal or epidural anesthesia.		

(From Stark & Roberts, 1980)

surgery and anesthesia. Therefore, assessments and interventions are made possible and facilitated by the report given to the PACU nurse by the anesthesiologist. This can be illustrated by reviewing some of the problems encountered in the PACU, *focusing particular attention on the etiologies*. The nurse, in making her or his patient assessments, goes through a process that considers many possibilities. With a comprehensive report from the anesthesiologist, the nurse is able to retain certain possible causes of patient problems and discard others; the result is a nursing diagnosis. From this, further nursing and medical interventions are possible.

Table 8-2 lists examples of problems encountered in the PACU. The most common of these are discussed in more detail in Chapter 10.

The problems cited in Table 8-2 and other challenging situations require the best in diagnostic acumen and therapy. It is quite apparent that many of the problems encountered in the PACU are directly related to events both surgical and involving anesthesia that occur intraoperatively, as well as to conditions or situations that are preexisting.

BIBLIOGRAPHY

American Nurses Association: Standards for medical surgical nursing practice. Kansas City, Mo.: ANA, 1974.

American Society of Anesthesiologists: Guidelines for patient care in anesthesiology. Park Ridge, Ill.: ASA, 1974.

ASA Newsletter: Practice advisory for the recovery room. ASA Newsletter 2:1–7, May 1978.

Fraulini KE: The anesthesiologist–recovery room nurse interface. Current Reviews for Recovery Room Nurses 5(8):1983.

Miller RD: Antagonism of neuromuscular blockade. Anesthesiology 44:318–329, 1976.

Smith NT, Miller RD, & Corbascio AN: Drug Interactions in Anesthesia. Philadelphia: Lea & Febiger, 1981.

Stark DC & Roberts RB: Practical Points in Anesthesiology. (2nd ed.). Garden City, N.Y.: Medical Examination Publishing Co., 1980.

Chapter 9

Nursing Care of the Postanesthetic Patient

Kay E. Fraulini

TRANSFER FROM THE OPERATING ROOM TO THE PACU

It is customary for patients to be brought to the postanesthesia care unit by members of the anesthesia care and surgical teams. There is some controversy whether patients should be transferred on oxygen. Dripps and associates (1982, p. 41), propose that because recognition of cyanosis is unreliable and because PaO_2 is usually decreased, particularly in the elderly or after a major operation, patients should be transported to the PACU with oxygen given via mask and assisted ventilation. Portable oxygen cylinders are easily suspended from litter or bed.

Israel and DeKornfeld (1982, p. 87) point out that the PACU should be in close proximity to the operating rooms, meaning on the same floor as the operating room or where an available elevator is guaranteed for the exclusive use of postanesthesia patients. Transfer of a patient from the operating room to the PACU should require no more than 5 minutes. Oxygen, suction, resuscitation equipment, and appropriate monitoring equipment should be available during the transfer.

Chapter 8 discusses in some detail what should happen when patients are transferred to the PACU nurse. This chapter explores the nursing process as it applies to the postanesthetized patient.

DURATION OF POSTANESTHESIA MONITORING

One of the questions we can ask is when should anesthesia monitoring stop. The data that are generated by physiologic monitoring are essential to the PACU nurse's assessment. One cannot possibly develop a plan of care if one does not have information on the patient's condition. Vaughan (1982) points out that during operating room and postanesthesia care, critical incidences may occur related to anesthesia and surgery. Constant vigilance to identify and treat such physiologic alterations becomes the charge of operating room and PACU personnel. Prior to Vaughan's studies, data did not exist to characterize operating room and PACU critical incidences.

Vaughan's first study (1982) was designed to identify, compare, and quantify the type and frequency of commonly occurring critical incidences in these vital perioperative areas. Following Institutional Human Subjects Committee approval, data were accumulated prospectively on 425 adults by a double-blinded technique on randomly selected weekdays. All subjects for elective or emergency operations under general or regional anesthesia were included, except those under 18 years of age or those undergoing open heart operations. PACU critical incidents were defined, as modified from Cooper and associates (1978), as occurrences requiring intervention and included dysrhythmias, hypotension, (preoperative systolic blood pressure over 30 percent below normal), hypertension (preoperative systolic blood pressure over 30 percent above normal, hypoxemia, hypercarbia, electrolyte abnormalities, PACU airway maintenance, hypothermia (less than 34.0°C, core), or other cardiac and pulmonary abnormalities. Descriptive statistics were used.

The study sample (male/female = 183/242) included characteristics as follows (both the mean and the range are given): age 48.7 ±1.0 years (18–96); weight 71.4 ±0.9 kg (38–159); height 167.0 ±0.6 cm (109–193); surgery time 91 ±4 minutes (3–540); and anesthesia time 125 ±4 minutes (10–630). Anesthesia type included general (n = 334) or regional (n = 57). The remaining 34 subjects received combinations of general and regional anesthesia. Types of operations included intraabdominal (97), pelvic (107), peripheral (190), intrathoracic (5), and other (26). Twenty-four percent (101/425) of the sample experienced at least one critical incident in the operating room. Of these occurrences, abnormalities in blood pressure and dysrhythmias were most frequent (52 and 27 respectively). Thirty-one percent (139/425) of the sample experienced at least one critical incident in the PACU. Of these, prolonged airway management accounted for 39 percent and dysrhythmias for 16 percent. Sedation was the most frequently occurring reason for prolonged airway management (65 percent). Although premature ventricular contractions (greater than 5 per minute) were the most frequently occurring dysrhythmia in the operating room (50 percent), 63 percent of dysrhythmia occurring in the PACU were categorized as tachycardia (greater than 100/minute). No patients experienced pneumothorax, aspiration pneumonia, pulmonary embolus, pulmonary edema, ventricular tachycardia, myocardial infarction, angina, or mortality.

The researchers conclude that critical incidents (CIs) occur commonly both intraoperatively and during the immediate postoperative period. Specific CIs may differ between areas of the hospital, but their frequent occurrence mandates careful cardiopulmonary monitoring from anesthetic induction to PACU discharge. In addition to its use in monitoring the patient, a hard-copy 6-second rhythm strip—more as the patient's condition dictates—should be kept for the record. Although a common practice in critical care units, there has been some resistance to adopting this practice in PACUs.

THE POSTANESTHETIC RECOVERY SCORE

Another means of assessing the postanesthetic patient is with an objective scoring system. Aldrete and Kroulik (1970) proposed a method analogous to the APGAR score for collecting objective information on the physical condition of patients arriving in the PACU after anesthesia. They recognized that to be practical, a method of evaluation of postanesthetic patients had to be simple, easy to memorize, and applicable to all situations, whether a patient had received general, regional, or intravenous anesthesia. Only physical signs that are commonly observed were considered. A rating of 0, 1, or 2 was given to each sign, depending on its absence or presence. At the end of each evaluation, the numbers given to each sign were added up. A score of 10 indicated a patient in the best possible condition.

The initial report evaluated the following signs: activity, respiration, circulation, consciousness, and color. The scoring system gained popularity and has been widely used in PACUs. In its newsletter, the American Society of Anesthesiologists (1978) in referring to the Aldrete score stated that "it is highly desirable to have an objective scoring system to evaluate recovery from anesthesia."

However, certain parameters have been difficult to assess on the Aldrete score and it sacrifices some of its objectivity because of the need for individual interpretation. Further, recent scientific knowledge indicates that other parameters may be better predictors of recovery from anesthesia.

This prompted Fraulini and Murphy (1984) to develop a new postanesthetic score, the REACT scoring system (Table 9-1). The parameters evaluated are respiration, energy, alertness, circulation, and temperature. The previous use of color as a guide to recovery status was considered unsatisfactory. Although it has the merit of custom, color is a subjective evaluation and can be misleading. Some races have large quantities of melanin in their lips and nail beds, for example, which makes an assessment of adequate oxygenation difficult. Some lighting, particularly fluorescent lights, accentuate desaturated hemoglobin pigment excessively. Reproducing color evaluations consistently may be difficult.

Also, the measurement of respiratory adequacy according to the patient's ability to cough or breathe deeply proved confusing and perhaps inadequate. In an age where we rely heavily on accurate spirometric and blood-gas measurements to indicate the need for respiratory support, the score we accord to a patient should be one that reflects these measurements. When the patient has been given the proper degree of respiratory support, he or she can be scored appropriately.

Measuring temperature and scoring this feature was added to the system. Not a great deal of experience has been accumulated to indicate how vigorously we should treat the hypothermia that results from nearly every anesthetic. But temperature is a parameter that is depressed by anesthetics, is easily measured, and returns to normal as anesthetics effect wears off. These features alone make temperature an excellent yardstick of recovery. It is also well known that lower than normal temperatures slow recovery from anesthesia in the infant and the elderly, depress central nervous system function and renal function, and eventually promote a tendency toward cardiac dysrhythmias.

The REACT Table of Values

The parameters of the REACT scoring system are described in detail below and outlined in Table 9-1.

Respiration. This parameter is scored after the patient's respiratory deficiencies have been overcome with suitable pharyngeal airways or by the use of a ventilator. The withdrawal of the support very often is justified by spirometry or blood–gas measurement, and the patient's score is then upgraded.

Respiratory rate is assessed in the spontaneously breathing patient. With the advent and growing popularity of narcotic anesthesia, it is necessary to insure a respiratory rate of 10 per minute or greater.

Energy. A score of 2 is achieved with sustained head lift and movement of legs. The PACU nurse is concerned not only with evaluation of patients with subarachnoid or epidural blocks but with all patients who have received muscle relaxants. Data point to sustained head lift as being the most sensitive (Miller, 1976) and therefore the most conclusive clinical sign of reversal from muscle relaxant (in other words, the fewest number of ACh receptors, if any, are still occupied). If the patient can move his or her legs but cannot sustain a head lift, a score of 1 is given. A score of 0 is given to patients who cannot move their legs.

TABLE 9–1. THE REACT SCORING SYSTEM

(R)espiration		Score	0.	Ventilator essential.
			1.	Spontaneous respiration, not less than 10/minute, airway essential.
			2.	Spontaneous respiration, no support. RR 10/minute or greater.
(E)nergy		Score	0.	Does not move legs.
			1.	Moves legs, cannot sustain head lift.
			2.	Sustains head lift, moves legs.
(A)lertness		Score	0.	Awakens only with vigorous stimulation.
			1.	Awake only when stimulated, gently.
			2.	Awake, seldom dozes.
(C)irculation	*Adults*	Score	0.	BP less than 80 mm Hg or any weak pulse at the wrist.
			1.	BP 80 mm Hg systolic to preoperative resting level, full wrist pulse.
			2.	BP resting preoperative level or above. Full pulse.
	Infants	Score	0.	Carotid only reliable pulse palpable.
			1.	Axillary pulse felt but not wrist.
			2.	Pulse can be felt easily at wrist.
(T)emperature		Score	0.	Axillary temperature less than 95°F (35°C).
			1.	Temperature between 95–96°F (35–35.5°C).
			2.	Temperature more than 96°F (35.5°C).
Explanation		Score	10.	Patient fully recovered from narcosis, paralysis, and exposure. Safe to discharge.
			9.	Patient still shows residual anesthetic effect, such as mild drowsiness or moderate hypotension. Care must be exercised when transferring this patient to another unit.
			8.	It is doubtful if patients with this score or less should be moved out of the PACU unless they are transferred to an intensive care situation.

(From Fraulini KE & Murphy P. REACT—A new postanesthetic recovery score. Nursing April, 1984.)

Alertness. A patient who has had a spinal anesthetic is one of the few who will be fully alert. Most others will still be dazed by the anesthetic experience. A gentle touch on the face area is sufficient stimulus to persuade most patients to open their eyes as they awaken.

Circulation. Evaluation is offered in two parts. In the adult section, attention is drawn to the low score criterion. Any situation where the pulse at the wrist feels less than full in volume automatically scores a 0. The simpler system of assessing infant circulation works well in practice.

Temperature. The proposed temperature scores were considered appropriate following experience gathered in the PACU at Rush-Presbyterian– St. Luke's Medical Center. Axillary temperature is measured on all patients returning from the operating room. There are times, too, when vigorous steps have to be taken to bring the patient's temperature up to 96°F. Generous application of warmed blankets may be required, or heated humidification may be used.

Scoring systems are useful devices that are extensively used for various endeavors. In the case of the PACU, the REACT system can be used to:

1. Define objectively the trend toward recovery from anesthesia.
2. Offer a simple but consistent method of evaluating recovery status.
3. Facilitate the dissemination of information about the recovery status.
4. Provide an index of recovery that can be used to compare and evaluate different anesthetic techniques, drugs, their antidotes, and PACU nursing procedures.

Scoring systems enable us to summarize a group of ratings of closely related functions. We then elect to act according to the total as we do when adding up a bridge-bidding score or a scholastic grade-point average. If the REACT score reaches 9, we discharge the patient; and if it is less than 9, we continue to watch the patient's progress, transfusing or warming the patient until the score improves.

In addition to physiologic monitoring (described in detail in Chapter 11) and an objective scoring system to assess the postanesthetic patient, the PACU nurse can be expected to use physical assessment skills, the patient data base, lab values, consultation with other members of the health team, and subjective statements from the patient (see the ASPAN Guidelines for Standards of Care given in the first appendix to this chapter).

THE CARE PLAN

The next phase of the nursing process is developing the care plan. Table 9-2 shows a sample standardized care plan used in the PACU at Rush-Presbyterian–St. Luke's Medical Center. See also Appendix 9-2 for a sample nursing care plan for general anesthesia patients.

Implementing the Plan

The plan of care is implemented as outlined in nursing orders (Table 9-2). Additionally, physicians' standing orders may be used to implement the plan. Standing orders are not widely used but may be encountered with specific groups of surgical patients. For example, Table 9-3 gives a list of orders that may be used for postoperative open heart surgery patients.

EVALUATION

Two methods of evaluation will be discussed here: (1) evaluation of the plan for nursing care in relation to the patient's status for discharge, and (2) an ongoing quality assurance program that reviews the quality of care given.

Evaluation for Discharge

It is a good idea to duplicate on the PACU record the initial assessment as the discharge assessment (Fig. 9-1). This assures that the same parameters are being assessed and that changes will be noted. ASPAN has enumerated evaluation criteria in Section V of its "Guidelines" (given in Appendix 9-1).

It is generally accepted that patients may be discharged only after vital signs are stable and after an evaluation of the patient's condition by a responsible physician (anesthesiologist) or designee. Certainly, the condition of the patient on discharge should be indicated. This usually involves a checklist such as that in Figure 9-1, a narrative note by the primary nurse or designee, and an objective scoring system, such as REACT.

Israel and DeKornfeld (1982) state that only a physician can determine when the postoperative surveillance period ends. Length of stay is determined by the patient's condition and available space in the PACU (see Chapter 7). Most PACUs adhere to a minimum stay of 1 hour. Less time than this does not allow for sufficient data collection to show trends in the patient's condition. The anesthesiologist should discharge the patient by either a direct or indirect method. In the direct method, the anesthesiologist or another designated physician writes a note on the chart indicating that the patient's vital signs are stable and that the level of consciousness and muscular activity are acceptable; indicates whether there are complications and if so, how they should be managed; and makes any other pertinent remarks. The note should also state that the patient may be discharged from the PACU and give the destination, such as the hospital room, ICU, patient's home, and so on.

The indirect method of discharging a patient uses a scoring system to evaluate the patient. This has already been discussed. A minimum score for releasing the patient must be established by the physician and forms a part of the discharge criteria stated in the policy manual.

When the patient's evaluation score meets the discharge criteria, the nurse may release the patient. This does not excuse the physician from the responsibility of discharging the patient; rather, it allows the release of the patient without the physician's signature at that time. It also allows

TABLE 9–2. STANDARDIZED CARE PLAN: POSTANESTHESIA RECOVERY (PACU)

Date	Potential/Actual Patient Problems	Desired Patient Outcomes	Target Dates	Nursing Orders	Time
	1. Changes in cardiovascular status resulting from: Surgical procedure Anesthesia Blood loss	1. Maintain baseline vital signs as evidenced by: Reestablishment of pre-operative parameters	Upon discharge from PACU	1a. Check vital signs	Q 15 minutes and prn
				b. Monitor ECG	Continuously
				c. Assess color, temperature and circulation to skin	Upon admission, Q 30 minutes and prn
				d. Assess motion and sensation of all extremities	Upon admission, Q 30 minutes, and prn
				e. Assess LOC	Upon admission, Q 15 minutes, and prn
				f. Monitor drainage from surgical site with drainage tubes	Upon admission and prn
				g. Keep patient warm and comfortable	Continuously
				h. Check IV site for infiltration	Upon admission, Q 1 hour and prn

Problem	Objective	Nursing Orders	Time
II. Pulmonary complications resulting from: Anesthesia Incision Pain	1. Maintain ventilation and perfusion of lungs as evidenced by: Temperature <100° Respiratory rate >12 and <28 minutes Bilateral breath sounds		Upon discharge
		i. Monitor I & O	Upon admission and prn
		j. Observe for: S/s of shock Excessive drainage Swelling at surgical site	Continuously
		1a. Assess respiratory exchange, rate and quality	Upon admission, Q 15 minutes and prn
		b. Auscultate breath sounds	Upon admission and Q 30 minutes
		c. Suction airway and/or endotracheal tube	Prn
		d. Provide HHO_2 per face tent and/or T piece at 40% O_2	Prn
		e. Provide mechanical ventilator for patients requiring assisted and/or controlled ventilation	Prn
		f. Place patient on side until aware and has cough reflex (unless contraindicated by surgery)	Continuously
		g. Instruct patient to cough and deep-breathe (unless contraindicated by surgery)	Q 15 minutes
		h. Assess respiratory status, ability to speak and swallow prior to discharge	Upon discharge

TABLE 9–3. PHYSICIAN'S POSTOPERATIVE ORDERS FOR HEART SURGERY

1. NPO
2. Vital signs: Q 15 min until stable; then Q
              HR, BP, CVP, RR. I/O c sp gr, chest drainage and peripheral pulses
3. ECG monitor
4. Endo trach tube care (i) suction PRN; instill NS 5–10 ml prn for thick secretions
   MA-Bennett respiratory; T vol ml
                    O_2% rate
5. Chest tubes to suction, −25 cm H_2O
6. Arterial line maintenance: 5–10 ml prn with solution (500 ml NS c 1000 units heparin via
   Sorenson intraflow)
7. Semifowler's position; head up 30 degress
8. Oral hygiene
9. ECG stat and Q A.M. for 5 days
10. Chest x-ray; upright—45 degrees; stat _____, _____, _____, and Q A.M. for 5 days
11. Blood gases: stat at _____, _____, _____, _____, _____, _____, and Q A.M. for 48 hr
12. Na, Cl, K, CA, stat at _____, _____, _____, _____, _____, _____, and Q A.M. for 5
    days
13. Hb, hct, stat at _____, _____, _____, _____, _____, _____
14. CBC with diff. Q A.M. for 5 days
15. SGOT, SGPT, LDH, CPK, stat and Q A.M. for 5 days
16. BUN, creatinine, stat and Q A.M. for 5 days
17. Pacemaker battery at bedside
18. Pacemaker wires on chest; labeled and covered
19. Morphine sulphate; 2–4 mg IV Q 1 hour until 2 A.M. (then prn)
20. Phenergan; 25 mg IM, Q 6 hrs prn for 3 days
21. Tylenol supp; Gr _____ Q 4–6 hours for temperature over 101°F; if not controlled—alcohol
    sponge and cooling mattress
22. Keflin 2 Gms. IV Q 6 hours for _____ days.
23. IV fluids: (a) all with metriset in microdrip
             (b) change ALL IV tubings Q 24 hours
24. CVP line: 1000 ml 5% D/¼ NS with 40 mEq KCL at 60 ml/hr
25. Keep open line: 150 ml 5% D/W
26. Fresh frozen plasma: 2 units (each to run in 15 min)
27. Packed cells _____ units. Each in _____ hours
28. *KCL Replacement Schedule:*
    (i)   With urine output of at least 30–40 ml/hour
    (ii) ALWAYS to run per CVP line
    (iii) 1 unit; 20 meq KCL in 60 ml fluid to run in 1 hour per metriset
    If serum K is . . . . . .
    3–3.5 mEq/L. . . . . .infuse 3 units of KCL
    3.5–4 mEq/L. . . . . .infuse 1 unit of KCL
    4–4.5 mEq/L. . . . . .infuse 1 unit of KCL
    Repeat Serum K (a) after the last unit is infused
                   (b) if serum K is more than 6 mEq/L
                   (c) if serum K is less than 3 mEq/L
                   Digoxin: _____ mg IV
29. Nitroglycerin: 0.4 mg (1 ml IV Q 1 hour) to maintain BP less than 150 systolic
30. Isordil, 5 mg QID sublingually (10 days)
31. Start weaning patient off respirator at _____ A.M.
32. BEFORE weaning patient off ventilator:
    (a) Phenergan 25 mg IM
    (b) Suction the pharynx thoroughly
    (c) Deflate the cuff
    (d) Connect to T piece with 40% O_2
33. Blood gases drawn after 30 min and 2 hours off the ventilator with patient on T piece with
    humidified O_2 at 40% oxygen

INITIAL ASSESSMENT: _____

Signature

CONSCIOUS LEVEL	SKIN	BREATH SOUNDS	RESPIRATIONS	PULSE	IV
ADM.:	Warm____ Turgor ____	R Lung_____	Spont.____ Ventilator __	Reg. _____	R_____
KEY:	Cool____ Flushed ____	L Lung _____	Labored____ Rapid____	Irreg. _____	L_____
C = CONSCIOUS	Pale____ Moist ____	CL = Clear	Shallow _____	Full _____	Sub-Cl____
SC = SEMICONSCIOUS	Cyanotic____ Dry ____	CO = Congested		Thready __	CVP ____
UN = UNCONSCIOUS		Wheezing_____			Other____

SURGICAL SITE: ADM.:	AIRWAY	OXYGEN	TEMPERATURE	HEART
	Oral_____	HHO_____	Oral_____	Monitor_____
	Nasal_____	Mask_____	Rectal_____	Arrhythmias____
TUBES	ET _____	Nasal_____	Ax_____	
		Liter Flow_____		

N/G____ Jejunostomy____   Sumo____ Hemovac __
F____ Gastrostomy_____   Doolas____ Penrose____   **OTHER:**
Supra-Pubic____ Chest ___   Packing _____
Ureteral____ Trach._____   3-Way Foley Irrigation_
T____ Laryngectomy_____

_____ DISCHARGE ASSESSMENT

Signature

CONSCIOUS LEVEL:	SKIN	BREATH SOUNDS	RESPIRATIONS	PULSE	IV
DISCHARGE:	Warm____ Turgor ____	R Lung_____	Spont.____ Ventilator __	Reg. _____	R_____
KEY	Cool____ Flushed ____	L Lung _____	Labored____ Rapid____	Irreg. _____	L_____
C = CONSCIOUS	Pale____ Moist ____	CL = Clear	Shallow _____	Full _____	Sub-Cl____
SC = SEMICONSCIOUS	Cyanotic____ Dry ____	CO = Congested		Thready __	CVP ____
UN = UNCONSCIOUS		Wheezing_____			Other____

SURGICAL SITE: DISCHARGE:	AIRWAY	OXYGEN	TEMPERATURE	HEART
	Oral_____	HHO_____	Oral_____	Monitor_____
	Nasal_____	Mask_____	Rectal_____	Arrhythmias____
TUBES	ET _____	Nasal_____	Ax_____	
		Liter Flow_____		

N/G____ Jejunostomy____   Sumo____ Hemovac __
F____ Gastrostomy_____   Doolas____ Penrose____   **OTHER:**
Supra-Pubic____ Chest ___   Packing _____
Ureteral____ Trach._____   3-Way Foley Irrigation_
T____ Laryngectomy_____

Figure 9–1. Postanesthesia recovery record. *(Courtesy Rush-Presbyterian–St. Lukes Hospital, Chicago.)*

for telephone orders to discharge the patient from the unit. If this method is used, the physician must sign the discharge order at some later time.

There is one more notation on the chart to be made by the anesthesiologist—a postanesthesia note. It is to be written after the patient leaves the PACU and preferably within 24 hours after surgery. Obviously, this may not be possible in "short stay" cases, but it is expected for all others. A note written into the patient's medical record should indicate the presence or absence of anesthesia-related complications. A note written in the PACU does not constitute a visit.

In summary, the criteria for discharge should include:

1. Stable vital signs.
2. Orientation as to person, place, and time, or return to the pre-anesthetic level of consciousness.
3. Satisfactory airway.
4. Absence of significant bleeding.
5. Stabilization or resolution of any acute problem.
6. Movement of the extremities following regional anesthesia.

Once a collaborative decision has been made to discharge the patient, the primary nurse should phone the floor nurse to give a report on the patient. An exception to this protocol is the PACU that involves the nurse in transporting the patient back to his or her room. In this situation, the report can be given face-to-face. In all cases, it is the responsibility of the receiving nurse to review the intraoperative and PACU record. The question remains as to whether surgical nurses consistently study the intraoperative and postanesthetic record.

The patient who is being transferred to another critical care unit should be accompanied by a PACU nurse and such additional personnel as are necessary. Portable equipment—monitors, O_2 cylinders, ambu bags, and so on—should be readily available for such transfers.

Quality Assurance Program

The Joint Commission on Accreditation of Hospitals implemented quality assurance standards as of January 1, 1981, and will assess the quality assurance programs in the hospitals it surveys. These standards may be found in the Quality Assurance section of the Accreditation Manual for Hospitals published annually by the JCAH and should be reviewed as an initial step toward developing a quality assurance plan for the PACU.

Chapter 3 discusses external and internal quality review specific to the PACU. Concurrent and retrospective audits can serve as evaluative tools to measure nursing care quality. This requires a properly designed instrument and well-trained personnel to ensure that the data are correctly interpreted.

STANDARDS OF CARE

A professional association is an organization of practitioners who judge one another as professionally competent and who have bonded together to perform social functions which they cannot perform in their separate capacity as individuals (*ANA: Standards of Nursing Practice, 1973*).

A professional association must provide measures to judge the competency of its membership and to evaluate the quality of its services. Studies show that the tendency for self-organization and the establishment and implementation of standards unique to the organization is characteristic of professions.

Follet (Metcalf & Urwich, 1942) points out that professional associations have one function above all others:

The members do not come together merely for the pleasure of meeting others of the same occupation; nor do they meet primarily to increase their pecuniary gain; although this may be one of the objects. They join in order to better perform their functions. They meet to:

- Establish standards
- Maintain and improve standards
- Keep members up to standard
- Educate the public to appreciate standards
- Protect the public from those who have not attained standards or who willfully do not follow them
- Protect individual members of the profession from each other

A profession's concern for the quality of service constitutes the heart of its responsibility to the public. The more expertise required to perform the service, the greater is society's dependence upon those who carry it out. A profession must seek control of its practice in order to guarantee the quality of its service to the public. Behind that guarantee are the standards of the profession that provide the assurance that the guarantee will be met. This is essential both for the protection of the public and the profession itself. A profession that does not maintain the confidence of the public will soon cease to be a social force.

DATA COLLECTION

Most of the data that should be collected on the postanesthetic patient have already been described. The logical tool for data collection, as previously mentioned, is the PACU record. The design of this form should meet the needs of the individual unit, hospital, and patient population. For example, one might expect to see different records in a small community hospital as compared to a large university medical center. The goal for each, however, is to collect all pertinent data and make certain it is recorded, retrievable, continuous, and communicated.

DOCUMENTATION OF CARE

Groah and Reed (1983) suggest that we use the nursing process as a basis for planning and documenting. The nursing process is appropriate because it is a systematic approach to problem-solving techniques and provides a structure to enable us to identify and follow through on problems.

In review, the assessment step prepares the nurse to focus in on the patient's problem, which results in a nursing diagnosis. Assessment is purposeful. Groah and Reed propose that we collect data or information about the patient, sort the data for what is relevant to the surgery, interpret the data, and then identify a nursing diagnosis.

A nursing diagnosis focuses on a patient's physical or behavioral response to a problem. In contrast, a medical diagnosis centers on the disease process. Over the last decade, the nursing profession has worked toward standardizing nursing diagnoses. There is a growing list of accepted nursing diagnoses (Table 9-4). Developed in a series of national conferences, these are intended to be conditions that nurses diagnose and treat. The goal is to develop a standard nomenclature for nursing diagnoses so that all nurses will be using the same terminology in describing patient problems. The list is amended and revised every few years.

Nursing diagnoses are used in planning care by identifying goals or expected outcomes for the patient. The goal is written so that it is measurable. Goals are ranked according to priority and nursing actions are prescribed. The evaluation determines how well nursing care assisted the patient in meeting the goal.

The three basic types of documentation are written records, observation, and reports. Each type validates in some way that nursing intervention took place.

Written Records
Probably the type of documentation that is most familiar, written records simply mean data recorded on the patient's chart. The reader is reminded of the previous discussion of record-keeping in Chapter 4.

In addition to the nursing care plan, several other methods can be used to record patient care: the narrative note; the problem-oriented medical record (POMR); the subjective, objective, analysis, and plan (SOAP) or, with the addition of implementation and evaluation, SOAPIE, note; or the assessment, plan, implementation, and evaluation (APIE) note. All of these formats can be used to record the same patient information (Groah & Reed, 1983).

TABLE 9–4. ACCEPTED NURSING DIAGNOSES

This is a list of all nursing diagnoses approved as of 1980 after four national conferences. The list continues to evolve as nurses refine categories and definitions. An example is "anxiety," which formerly was a separate diagnosis. In this list, it is considered a defining characteristic of a new category, "fear."

Airway clearance, ineffective
Bowel elimination
  alteration in: constipation
    diarrhea
    incontinence
Breathing pattern, ineffective
Cardiac output, alteration in: decreased
Comfort, alteration in: pain
Communication, impaired verbal
Coping, ineffective individual
  ineffective family: compromised
    disabling
  family: potential for growth
Diversional activity, deficit
Fear
Fluid volume deficit, actual
  potential
Gas exchange, impaired
Grieving, anticipatory
  dysfunctional
Home maintenance management, impaired
Injury, potential for; poisoning, potential
  for; suffocation, potential for;
  trauma, potential for
Knowledge deficit (specify)
Mobility, impaired physical
Noncompliance (specify)
Nutrition
  alteration in: less than body requirements
    more than body requirements
    potential for more than body require-
      ments
Parenting
  alteration in: actual
    potential
Rape-trauma syndrome: rape trauma, com-
  pound reaction, silent reaction
Self-care deficit (specify level): feeding,
  bathing/hygiene, dressing/grooming,
  toileting

Self-concepts, disturbance in: body image,
  self-esteem, role performance, per-
  sonal identity
Sensory perceptual alteration: visual, audi-
  tory, kinesthetic, gustatory, tactile,
  and olfactory perceptions
Sexual dysfunction
Skin integrity
  impairment of: actual
    potential
Sleep pattern disturbance
Spiritual distress (Distress of the human
  spirit)
Thought processes, alteration in
Tissue perfusion, alteration in: cerebral, car-
  diopulmonary, renal, gastrointestinal,
  peripheral
Urinary elimination, alteration in patterns
Violence, potential for

*Diagnoses "accepted" without defining char-
    acteristics*
Cognitive dissonance
Decision making, impaired/ineffective (decisions made by client produce results
  other than or less than desired)
Family dynamics, alteration in
  developmental transition
  dysfunctional coping
  family role changes/shifts
  situational transition
  stress management patterns
Fluid volume, alteration in, excess: potential
  for
  memory deficit
  rest-activity pattern, ineffective
  role disturbance
  social isolation

Informal surveys indicate that few recovery room nurses use SOAP charting, nor does any one system predominate. Bonner (1982) proposes that POMR is particularly suited to the detailed, time-consuming analysis and resolution of chronic disease and complex disorders. Its practical application in the environment of the PACU or SICU has, however, been delayed because of special requirements of the critically ill surgical patient, who often demands life-saving intervention before a detailed data base can be constructed. Compulsive attention to the construction of a data base may detract from immediate needs of the patient. Alternate approaches to data management and medical records have included the mission-oriented medical system and organ systems approach. As a consequence, no universal flowsheet or method of record keeping, whether generated by hand or computer, has satisfied all requirements of the unit specializing in care of the critically ill surgical patient.

Observation

We can validate a nursing intervention by having someone witness it. Observation is considered a type of documentation because it is proof an act was performed. A good example of this is observation during process audit.

This type of documentation has disadvantages, however. First, the information is not retrievable. Second, the data may be skewed by the judgments, values, biases, or limited perspective of the observer.

Reporting

Reports may be either oral or written. Oral reports are useful because they provide an opportunity to expand on the written record and to pass on information or observations that would not ordinarily be included in written documentation. Examples are change-of-shift reports, especially reports held at the beginning of the day shift; relief reports at break or lunch times; and transfer reports to the floor nurse. The disadvantages of oral reporting are that, as with observation, the data are not retrievable, and the report receiver may misinterpret the content.

Written reports—such as the PACU log book, morbidity and mortality records, and incident reports—are different than written *records*. Reports are not part of the patient's permanent medical record. They are designed to communicate patient care information, either within the department or to other areas of the hospital.

Groah & Reed (1983) summarize patient documentation with the following points:

- Base written records of nursing care on the nursing process.
- Include all essential patient care information, regardless of the format.
- Try to record any information obtained by observation or oral report so it is retrievable.
- Keep in mind that written reports communicate patient information to other nurses and departments.

REFERENCES

Aldrete AJ & Kroulik D: A post anesthetic recovery score. Anesthesia and Analgesia 49:924–934, 1970.

American Nurses Association: Standards of Nursing Practice. Kansas City, Mo.: ANA, 1973.

American Society of Anesthesiologists: Anesthesia practice advisory for the recovery room. ASA Newsletter 2:7–8, 1978.

Bonner JT: Medical records and flow sheets in the surgical I.C.U. Anesthesia Review 9(4):39–42, 1982.

Borchardt A & Fraulini K: Hypothermia in the postanesthesia patient. AORN Journal 36(4):648–669, 1982.

Buchan RF: The problem of the problem-oriented record. New England Journal of Medicine 288:1133, 1973.

Cooper JB, Newbower RS, Long CD, et al.: Preventable anesthesia mishaps: A study of human factors. Anesthesiology 49:399–406, 1978.

Cullen DJ: Surgical intensive care: Current perceptions and problems. Critical Care Medicine 9(4):295–297, April, 1981.

Dripps RD, Eckenhoff JE, & Vandam LD: Introduction to Anesthesia. The Principles of Safe Practice (6th ed.). Philadelphia: Saunders, 1982.

Fraulini KE & Murphy P: REACT—A new postanesthetic recovery score. Nursing April, 1984.

Groah L & Reed E: Your responsibility in documenting care. AORN Journal 37(6):1174–1188, May 1983.

Israel J & DeKornfeld T: Recovery Room Care. Springfield, Ill.: Chas C Thomas, 1982.

Merton RK: The functions of the professional association. American Journal of Nursing 58(50): 1958.

Metcalf HC & Urwich L (Eds.): Dynamic Administration: The Collected Papers of Mary Follet. New York: Harper, 1942, p. 136.

Miller RD: Antagonism of neuromuscular blockade. Anesthesiology 44:318–329, 1976.

Vaughan MS: When should anesthesia monitoring stop: Selected abstracts for the 8th Postanesthesia Care Symposium for RR nurses presented by the Illinois Society of Anesthesiologists, May 6–8, 1982, Chicago.

Waisbren BA: Care of the critically ill: The system method. Hospital Medical Staff 1, 1972.

Waisbren BA: Toward a mission-oriented medical system. Critical Care Medicine 1:261–266.

Worthley LG: A system-structured medical record for intensive care patient documentation. Critical Care Medicine 3:188–191, 1975.

Guidelines for Standards of Care in the Postanesthesia Care Unit*

I. ASSESSMENT

Health status data are collected. These data are recorded, retrievable, continuous, and communicated. Data are obtained by physical exam, review of records, and consultation.

1. Assessment factors include but are not limited to:
    a. Relevant preoperative status, including electrocardiogram, vital signs, radiology findings, laboratory values, allergies, disabilities, drug use, physical or mental impairments, mobility limitations, and prostheses (including hearing aids).
    b. Anesthesia technique (general, regional, local), effect of preop medications.
    c. Anesthetic agents, muscle relaxants, narcotics, and reversal agents used.
    d. Length of time anesthesia administered.
    e. Type of surgical procedure.
    f. Estimated fluid/blood loss and replacement.
    g. Complications occurring during anesthetic course, treatment initiated, response.
2. Initial physical assessment to include the documentation of:
    a. Vital signs.
        1. respiratory rate and competency, airway patency, type of artificial airway, mechanical ventilator and settings.
        2. blood pressure—cuff or arterial line.
        3. pulse—apical, peripheral—cardiac monitor pattern.
        4. temperature—oral, rectal, axillary, digital through dermal sensors.
    b. Pressure readings—central venous, arterial blood pulmonary artery wedge.
    c. Position of patient.
    d. Condition and color of skin.

*(*Courtesy of the American Society of Post-Anesthesia Nurses (ASPAN), 1983.)*

    e. Circulation—peripheral pulses and sensation of extremity(ies) as applicable.
    f. Condition of dressings.
    g. Condition of suture line, if dressings are absent.
    h. Type and patency of drainage tubes, catheters, and receptacle.
    i. Amount and type of drainage.
    j. Muscular response and strength.
    k. Fluid therapy, location of lines, type and amount of solution infusing (including blood).
    l. Level of consciousness.
    m. Level of comfort.
3. Numerical score if used.

II. NURSING DIAGNOSIS

Nursing diagnosis is a concise statement and represents analysis of the data collected during the assessment phase.

1. Nursing diagnosis is consistent with current scientific knowledge.
2. Nursing diagnoses are based on identifiable data as compared to established norms or previous conditions.
3. Nursing diagnoses include but are not limited to:
    a. Altered level of consciousness.
    b. Alterations in comfort.
    c. Anxiety.
    d. Alterations in cardiac output.
    e. Alterations in fluid volume (both excess and deficity).
    f. Impairment of mobility (including decrease in muscle strength).
    g. Potential for physical injury.
    h. Respiratory dysfunction.
    i. Impairment in skin integrity.
    j. Abnormal tissue perfusion.
    k. Alterations in urinary elimination.

III. CARE PLAN

The plan for nursing care describes a systematic method for achieving the goal of postanesthesia nursing care—to assist the patient in returning to a safe physiological level after an anesthetic.

1. The plan includes setting priorities for appropriate nursing actions.
2. The plan is based on current scientific knowledge.

3. The plan is developed with and communicated to the patient, family, and/or significant others and appropriate health care team personnel.
4. The plan is formulated in conjunction with preoperative, intraoperative, and current postanesthetic health status assessment.
5. The plan includes but is not limited to the following nursing actions:
   a. Identification of the patient.
   b. Monitor, maintain, and/or improve respiratory function.
   c. Monitor, maintain, and/or improve circulatory function.
   d. Promote and maintain physical and emotional comfort.
   e. Receive report from operating room nurse, anesthesiologist and/or anesthetist.
   f. Monitor surgical site.
   g. Interpretation and documentation of data obtained during assessment.
   h. Documentation of nursing plan, action, and/or interventions with outcome.
   i. Notify family and/or significant others of patient's arrival and discharge from the PACU.
   j. Notify patient care unit of any needed equipment.
   k. Notify patient care unit when patient is ready for discharge from the PACU.
   l. Outpatient surgicals—discharge planning with patient and family.

IV. IMPLEMENTATION

The plan for nursing care is implemented to achieve the goals as stated under the Care Plan (above).

1. Nursing actions remain consistent with the written plan to provide continuity of care in accordance with established policy and procedure.
2. Comfort, safety, efficiency, skill, and effectiveness are reflected in nursing actions.
3. Nursing decisions and actions regarding patient care reflect upholding the dignity of the patient and family.
4. The plan may be altered to meet the changing needs of the patient.

V. EVALUATION

The plan for nursing care is evaluated.

1. Current assessment data are collected and recorded to evaluate the patient's status for discharge:
   a. Airway patency and respiratory function.
   b. Stability of vital signs, including temperature.

    c. Level of consciousness and muscular strength.

    d. Mobility.

    e. Patency of tubes, catheters, drains, intravenous lines.

    f. Skin color and condition.

    g. Intake and output.

    h. Comfort.

2. The nurse informs the family and/or significant others and health care team personnel of the patient's status.

VI. DISCHARGE

The postanesthesia nurse shall discharge the patient in accordance with written policies set forth by the Department of Anesthesia and also in accordance with the criteria and data collected through the use of nursing process. A final nursing assessment and evaluation of the patient's condition will be performed and documented. If a numerical scoring system is used, the discharge score will be recorded to reflect the patient's status. The postanesthesia nurse arranges for the safe transport of the patient from the PACU to his or her room.

APPENDIX 9–2

Grant Hospital of Chicago Nursing Care Plan: Postanesthesia Care Plan—General Anesthesia

PRIMARY MEDICAL DIAGNOSIS _____

SECONDARY MEDICAL DIAGNOSIS _____

Date Initiated	Actual/Potential Patient Problems	Expected Patient Outcomes	Deadlines Checkpoints	Nursing Interventions	Outcomes Achieved & Initial

	Problem List:
	I. Potential for Shock
	II. Pain
	III. Postoperative anxiety
	IV. Sensory disturbances
	V. Pulmonary complications/ Disturbance of pulmonary function
	VI. Potential residual muscle relaxants
	VII. Resuscitation of the general anesthesia patient
	VIII. Potential for abnormal temperature regulation
	  A. Hypothermia
	  B. Malignant hyperthermia
	IX. Potential for untoward effects of anesthesia drugs
	X. Potential complication or injury while medicated and anesthetized
	XI. Potential for fluid and electrolyte imbalance
	XII. Infection (wound)				

I. Potential for shock due to:	Regain normal cardiac function, circulation, and blood volume, evidenced by stable vital signs	By discharge from PACU	Note preoperative pulse and blood pressure
Postanesthetic depression			Assess patient for previous complications following anesthesia
Hypovolemia	Free of preventable complications or have them quickly recognized and controlled		Assess patient for history of anemia, abnormal bleeding times and/or clotting factors, cardiac disease, elevated blood loss
			Assess changes in vital signs and report significant changes
			Note and record color of nail beds, lips, and oral mucosa
			Note condition of skin:
			Compare with preoperative description
			Report significant changes
			Cyanosis
			Cold
			Clammy skin
			Diaphoresis
			Observe cardiac monitor for dysrhythmias; report significant changes
			Observe incision, dressing and drains frequently every 15 minutes; notify MD if unusual amounts of bleeding noticed
			Avoid changing patient's position rapidly or moving patient suddenly
			Have emergency equipment available

(Continued)

Date Initiated	Actual/Potential Patient Problems	Expected Patient Outcomes	Deadlines Checkpoints	Nursing Interventions	Outcomes Achieved & Initial
	I. Potential for shock due to: Hypovolemia (Cont.).			If shock occurs: Have anesthesiologist called Initiate or continue O_2 Increase rate of IV fluid Elevate legs (modified Trendelenberg) Identify source of bleeding (if present) and apply pressure as indicated Monitor continous vital signs Have emergency equipment available Administer emergency drugs as ordered Facilitate prompt performance of diagnostic procedures (ABGs, ECG, blood cultures, etc.) Apply warm blankets prn or institute cooling measures as ordered Follow hospital policy Follow hospital policy and procedure for blood transfusion administration and transfusion reaction when indicated Observe and report signs of return to consciousness	

Problem	Expected Outcome	Time Frame	Nursing Interventions
II. Pain	Verbal or nonverbal expression of reasonable comfort	PACU discharge	Assess level of discomfort by subjective and objective evaluation Provide comfort measures: Position comfortably, ask patient for suggestions Provide environment conducive to comfort Offer pain medication if ordered by anesthesia Check type of anesthesia and preoperative medication prior to administration of pain medication Evaluate and record the effectiveness of pain medication after each dose
III. Postoperative anxiety due to: Fear of an unfamiliar environment	Verbal expression of anxiety (patient expressing feelings, thoughts, questions, and concerns)	PACU discharge	Listen to patient, allowing adequate amount of time for patient to express him/herself Clarify questions and concerns Establish eye contact Speak slowly and quietly Allow coping mechanism, such as crying
Fear of an uncertain outcome of surgical procedure and its effect on prognosis	Verbal indication patient can identify reasons for anxiety		Follow through on MD information to patient and family, communicate fears and concerns of patient to MD as necessary
Pressure of pain	Verbal expression of ability to understand reasons for pain and availability of pain medication		Administer pain medication as ordered by anesthesia See problem II

(Continued)

Date Initiated	Actual/Potential Patient Problems	Expected Patient Outcomes	Deadlines Checkpoints	Nursing Interventions	Outcomes Achieved & Initial
	III. Postoperative anxiety due to: (Cont.) Lack of understanding of postoperative course	Verbalized understanding of effects of procedures, correct knowlege of limitation for type of procedure and necessity of treatments to be performed		Explain specific procedures Give clear, concise explanations Repeat as often as necessary Explore concerns about limitations of treatments, etc.	
	Separation from family or significant others	Verbal expression when visitation permitted Communication with family or significant others regarding patient's progress		Communicate with family about patient's discharge time Be available to family or significant others for explanations and clarifications Praise supportive behavior	
		Absence of panic situation		If panic situation occurs: Stay with patient and provide privacy Use breathing exercises to reduce anxiety Consult anesthesiologist Use ancillary departments as necessary	
	IV. Sensory disturbances	Regain and maintain sensory equilibrium (the patient will be able to perceive and describe the components of his environment in an oriented, nondisturbed manner)	Before discharge	Assess level of consciousness and support reorientation process: Speak directly to patient Inform patient of his/her location on arrival to PACU and prn Speak to patient at regular intervals Assess ability to follow simple command: Cough and deep-breathe Lift head off of cart	

V. Pulmonary complications/
Disturbance of pulmonary
function due to:
Anesthesia
Immobility
Abdominal incision
Age
Narcotic
Thrombus formation

Maintains satisfactory pulmonary
ventilation and perfusion as evidenced by:
Respiratory rate above 12 and
below 24 per minute
Lungs clear on auscultation
Temperature below 100°F
Respiratory pattern equal to
preop status
ABGs within normal (preoperative) limits

Assess order of ascending de-
pression of CNS:
Medullary center
Spinal cord
Basal ganglia and cerebellum
Cortical and psychic centers
Offer explanations verbally when
performing nursing duties
Promote active participation in re-
covery (use interpretors when
necessary) by encouraging pa-
tient to:
Identify location, day, time
Ask questions
Engage in short conversations
Assume position of comfort,
where indicated
Prevent sensory overload: Control
levels of light, noise, odors and
levels of activity in area when
possible
Provide privacy for patient

Prior to PACU
discharge

Identify patients susceptible to respiratory complications by history of lung disease, smoking
habits, thoracic surgery, chest
tubes, prolonged anesthesia
Assess respiratory status every 15
minutes and prn:
Check rate and quality of respiration every 15 minutes and
prn
Check temperature on admission, discharge and prn

(Continued)

Date Initiated	Actual/Potential Patient Problems	Expected Patient Outcomes	Deadlines Checkpoints	Nursing Interventions	Outcomes Achieved & Initial
	V. Pulmonary complications/ Disturbance of pulmonary function (Cont.).			Auscultate lungs on admission and prn Notify MD of significant change Provide respiratory care: Cough and deep-breathe on admission and prn Employ use of yawning and inspiratory hold prn Splint surgical area prn Suction prn Check lab values as ordered by anesthesiologist Report significant lab values to anesthesiologist	
		No signs or symptoms of pulmonary emboli evidenced by absence of: Increased restlesness Sudden onset of chest pain Cough productive of bloody sputum Tachycardia Rapid shallow respiration		Assess for signs and symptoms of PE on admission and prn Notify MD immediately of presence Administer or continue oxygen as ordered Administer and record narcotic analgesics as ordered	
	VI. Potential residual muscle relaxants	Provide mechanical venilatory support until patient is able to adequately ventilate by self	Prior to PACU discharge	Provide mechanical ventilatory support and care: Utilize mechanical ventilator as ordered by anesthesia Assess breath sounds on admission, after moving patient, and prn	

| VII. Resuscitation of the general anesthesia patient | Restoration of stable cardiovascular status following cardiac arrest | During resuscitation | Assess tidal volume of patient as indicated
ABGs if indicated by anesthesia
Suction prn to maintain patency of airway and just prior to and after extubation
Continual assessment of returning muscle strength of patient
Chest x-ray if indicated to check tube placement
Assess need for resuscitation:
Level of consciousness, spontaneous respiration
Assess presence of pulses:
Carotid, femoral
Cardiac rhythm
Vital signs
Begin cardiac pulmonary resuscitation in absence of stable cardiac rhythm, with absence of carotid pulse, lack of spontaneous respiraton, significant change in vital signs and decreased level of consciousness:
One-man rescue:
Two breaths followed by 15 sternal compressions
Two-man rescue:
Initial two breaths followed by 5 sternal compressions continued as advised by AHA cardiac pulmonary resuscitation protocol |

(Continued)

Date Initiated	Actual/Potential Patient Problems	Expected Patient Outcomes	Deadlines Checkpoints	Nursing Interventions	Outcomes Achieved & Initial
	VII. Resuscitation of the general anesthesia patient (Cont.).			Call for anesthesiologist and surgeon stat to PACU (7 A.M.–3 P.M. code blue/after 3 P.M. stat 2222), notify attending if other than surgeon, call for appropriate stat team members: Cardiologist if consulted ECG Respiratory therapy Pastoral care Supervisory nursing personnel Communicate with family or significant other Administer emergency medication as ordered and document Continuous cardiac monitoring with rhythm strips for documentation	
				Defibrillate patient if ordered, and document Intubation of patient by anesthesia if necessary with mechanical ventilatory support Lab work as ordered: ABGs Electrolyte Blood glucose Lactic acid levels Other	

			Have emergency equipment at bedside (i.e., ambu bag, crash cart defibrillation, etc.)
			Have temporary pacemaker available
			Have Swan-Ganz catheter available
			Continue CPR until patient revived or effort stopped by MD
			Provide safe transfer of patient to indicated intensive care unit
			If expired, follow policy and procedures of death in operating room and postmortem care
VIII. Potential for abnormal temperature regulation Hypothermia Fluid and electrolyte imbalance from: Increased urinary output	Maintains fluid and electrolyte balance as evidenced by: Serum K+ of 4.0–5.4 mEq/L Serum calcium of 9–11 mg% Serum sodium of 136–142 mEq/L	Continuously with VS	Assess fluid and electrolyte imbalance: Obtain serum electrolyte levels and check results
Decreased sodium reabsorption	CVP 5–15 or as ordered Output correlates with intake appropriately	Prn	
		Continuously	Monitor and measure input and output; check CVP
Vasoconstriction	Absence of apathy, seizures, confusion arrhythmias	Every hour as ordered	Observe level of consciousness monitor cardiac status
Hyperglycemia resulting from history:	Exhibits no sign of hyperglycemia as evidenced by:	Continuously	Assess for signs and symptoms of hyperglycemia:

(Continued)

Date Initiated	Actual/Potential Patient Problems	Expected Patient Outcomes	Deadlines Checkpoints	Nursing Interventions	Outcomes Achieved & Initial
	VIII. Potential for abnormal temperature regulation (Cont.). Diabetic, insulin withheld Decreased insulin production	Urine negative for sugar, stable level of consciousness Blood glucose within normal limits	As ordered	Check urine for sugar and notify physician as ordered Assess level of consciousness, obtain blood glucose levels and report results.	
	Dehydration resulting from: Increased urinary output Hypovolemia and insensible fluid loss Increased basal metabolic rate (BMR) (shivering)	Exhibits adequate hydration as evidenced by: Decreased secretions Moist mucous membranes Elastic skin turgor CVP 5–15 or as ordered Vital signs within limits	Prn	Assess for signs of dehydration Measure input and output Check skin turgor and mucous membranes Check CVP Monitor VS	
	Decreased level of consciousness resulting from: Electrolyte imbalance Decreased metabolism of drugs Decreased BMR	Maintains adequate level of consciousness as evidenced by: Appropriate responses to verbal commands Oriented to person able to maintain own airway	Continuously	Assess level of consciousness Assess patient orientation, reorient when necessary, check electrolytes, ABG's as ordered Check for signs and symptoms of hypoxia, airway obstruction, ventilation	
	Systemic hypertension resulting from: Vasoconstriction Shivering Hypoxic agitation	Maintains blood pressure within a normal range systolic 90–180 diastolic 50–90 or as ordered	Immediate and change prn Prn Prn Prn	Apply measures to maintain a normal blood pressure and to monitor blood pressure: Apply warm blankets around head, feet, and body to rewarm and dilate vessels Elevate head of bed Encourage deep breathing Insert oral/nasal airway	

Impaired peripheral perfusion resulting from: Vasoconstriction	Maintains adequate perfusion of peripheral tissue as evidenced by: Absence of mottling, cold extremities Good capillary refill of nailbeds Presence of dorsalis pedis, posterior tibial, and radial pulses	Provide O_2 therapy as ordered Intravenous rate to keep vein open Assess peripheral perfusion and apply nursing measures for improvement: Apply warm blankets to aid in vasodilation of peripheral vessels Assess extremities for color, temperature, capillary refill and presence or absence of appropriate pulses
Acidosis (metabolic) resulting from: Impaired peripheral perfusion (anaerobic metabolism)	Maintains arterial blood gases within normal limits for patient as evidenced by: ph 7.35–7.45 pCO_2 35–45 mm Hg HCO_3 21–29 mEq/L pO_2 80–100 mm Hg O_2 saturated, 95% or greater BE − 3 to + 3 or gases that are consistent with preoperative baseline	Assess for signs of acidosis: Check for rapid, deep breathing, stupor, weakness
Increased O_2 consumption		Obtain arterial blood gases and report results
Increased BMR (shivering)		
Coagulation defects resulting from: Increased blood viscosity Decreased platelets	Maintain normal electrolyte status Exhibits no signs or symptoms of coagulation defects as evidenced by: Absence of calf pain/burning sensation Absence of unequal leg temperature	Monitor electrolytes Assess for signs and symptoms of coagulation defects: Assess peripheral circulation until no longer hypothermic Observe for signs and symptoms of pulmonary emboli

Immediately as per MD

(Continued)

Date Initiated	Actual/Potential Patient Problems	Expected Patient Outcomes	Deadlines Checkpoints	Nursing Interventions	Outcomes Achieved & Initial
	VIII. Potential for abnormal temperature regulation (Cont.).	Negative Homan's sign Absence of spontaneous bleeding or bruising Normal coagulation test results		Obtain coagulation profile and chest x-ray results	
	Malignant hyperthermia manifested by: Tachycardia Tachypnea Fever over 40°C (104°F) Arrhythmias Cyanosis Dark venous blood Red urine Hot skin Prolonged generalized skeletal muscle rigidity Lab findings: Metabolic and respiratory acidosis Hypoxemia Hyperkalemia Hypomagnesemia Myoglobulinemia Elevated lactate Myoglobinuria Hypocalcemia Impaired blood coagulation Elevated serum enzymes SGOT, LDH, SGPT CPK Acute renal failure	Return patient to normal metabolic status, as evidenced by: Temperature ABGs Electrolytes	Throughout PACU course	Assess for history of previous anesthesia complications Assess what agents were used in administering anesthesia, such as: Halothane Succinylcholine Routine monitoring of electrical activity of the heart and body temperature ABGs and other lab work as ordered and report results I & O Hyperventilation with 100% Dantrolene (Dantrium) 1–2 mg/kg IV could be requested every 5–10 minutes for a total dose of 10mg/kg if ordered. IV administration of Na barcarbonate (2 to 4 mEq/kg) to correct acidosis Prompt measures to control temperature by rapid external and internal cooling: External cooling methods:	

Packing the patient with ice
Use of hypothermia blankets
If possible, immersion of patient in an icewater bath
Internal cooling methods:
  Rapid IV infusion of cold fluids
  Gastric, wound and rectal lavage
  Possible use of extracorporeal cooling with the heart-lung bypass machine
  IV injections of diuretics (furosemide and mannitol)
  IV drip of pronestyl for treatment of arrhythmias
Hyperpotassemia treated by infusion of buffers and dextrose with insulin
Secure monitoring lines:
  ECG continuously
  Temperature continuously
  Foley catheter
  Arterial line
  CVP lines
  Lytes

IX. Potential for untoward effects of anesthesia drugs
Thiopental sodium (sodium pentothal) as evidenced by:

On admission to PACU and prn

Assess for allergies
Assess for history of complications from anesthesia drugs

(Continued)

Date Initiated	Actual/Potential Patient Problems	Expected Patient Outcomes	Deadlines Checkpoints	Nursing Interventions	Outcomes Achieved & Initial
	IX. Potential for untoward effects of anesthesia drugs (Cont.).				
	Prolonged somnolence Retrograde amnesia Myocardial depression Arrhythmias Bronchospasm Laryngospasm			Ascertain what agents were utilized for anesthesia Contraindicated in absence of suitable veins for IV administration, hypersensitivity to barbiturates, status asthmaticus, respiratory depression, shock and intracranial pressure Check if atropine was given as a premedication to prevent spasms of vocal cords Have resuscitative equipment and O₂ ready	
	Succinylcholine chloride (anectine) as evidenced by: Bradycardia Tachycardia Hypertension Hypotension Prolonged respiratory depression			Maintain patent airway Have mechanical ventilatory equipment available Airway must be established when administered Monitor vital signs every 15 minutes and prn Assess amount used and length of operation (no effective antagonist) Assess presence of reflexes and muscle strength Encourage coughing and deep breathing	

Pancuronuin Bromide (pavulon) as evidenced by:
Tachycardia, hypertension
Transient skin rash
Excessive sweating and salivation
Prolonged dose-related apnea
Residual muscle weakness

Assess if used in patient with history of renal failure
Monitor vital signs every 15 minutes
Assess presence of reflexes and muscle strength
Assess K$^+$ level
Assess for history of myasthenia gravis
Have atropine available, if ordered by anesthesiologist

Fentanyl (sublimaze) as evidenced by:
Hypotension
Bradycardia
Nausea
Vomiting
Urinary retention

Assess if MAO inhibitors have been given within the last 14 days (contraindicated)
Use caution in head injury, COPD, Addison's disease, CNS depression
Monitor vital signs every 15 minutes and prn
Have narcotic antagonist and resuscitative equipment available

Innovar (fentanyl droperidol) as evidenced by:
Emergence delirium
Hallucinations
Nausea, vomiting
Blurred vision
Respiratory depression
apnea or arrest
Laryngospasm

Assess for previous reaction or allergies
Maintain patent airway
Vital signs every 15 minutes and prn
Have narcotic antagonist and resuscitative equipment available
Assess for history of liver disease (broken down in liver)

(Continued)

Date Initiated	Actual/Potential Patient Problems	Expected Patient Outcomes	Deadlines Checkpoints	Nursing Interventions	Outcomes Achieved & Initial
	IX. Potential for untoward effects of anesthesia drugs (Cont.).				
	Twitching				
	Shivering				
	Neostigmine bromide (prostigmin) as evidenced by:			Assess for history of bronchial asthma	
	Dizziness			Monitor vital signs every 15 minutes and prn	
	Muscle weakness			Observe closely for side effects, may indicate toxicity	
	Mental confusion			Position patient for easy breathing	
	Respiratory depression			Have atropine available	
	Sweating				
	Increased salivation				
	Bradycardia				
	Hypotension				
	Atropine sulfate as evidenced by:			Assess for narrow-angle glaucoma—DO NOT GIVE	
	Disorientation			Assess for coronary artery disease	
	Restlessness			Monitor I & O	
	Irritability			Monitor vital signs every 15 minutes and prn	
	Palpitations			Assess for allergies	
	Tachycardia				
	Blurred vision				
	Dilated pupils				
	Vomiting				
	Dryness of mouth				
	Constipation				
	Narcan (naloxone):			Assess for allergy	
	Nausea and vomiting			Use cautiously in cardiac irritability and narcotic addiction	
				Monitor respiratory depth and rate	

Doxapram hydrochloride (dopram) as evidenced by:
Headache
Dizziness
Apprehension
Disorientation
Pupillary dilatation
Bilateral Babinski sign
Chest pain and tightness
Variations in heart rate
Nausea, vomiting
Diarrhea
Coughing
Laryngospasm
Bronchospasm
Hiccups
Rebound hypoventilation

Monitor vital signs every 15 minutes and prn
Have oxygen, ventilation and other resuscitative equipment available
Assess for allergies
Assess for adequate airway before administering drug
Prevent aspiration of vomitus
Monitor blood pressure, heart rate, deep tendon reflexes
Arterial blood gases should be taken before giving drug and prn if ordered
Assess for signs of overdose:
Hypertension
Tachycardia
Arrhythmia
Skeletal muscle hyperactivity
Dyspnea
Discontinue if patient shows signs of increased carbon dioxide or oxygen tension or if mechanical ventilation is started
Have anticonvulsant available
Report all significant findings or changes to anesthesiologist

Inhalation Agents
Halothane
Myocardial depression
Arrhythmia- producing drug
Sensitizes the myocardial conduction system to

Assess for history of necrosis of the liver
Assess admission temperature, use warming techniques as necessary

(Continued)

Date Initiated	Actual/Potential Patient Problems	Expected Patient Outcomes	Deadlines Checkpoints	Nursing Interventions	Outcomes Achieved & Initial
	IX. Potential for untoward effects of anesthesia drugs (Cont.).				
	action of catecholamines			Continue cardiac monitoring	
	Toxic to liver			Administer supplemental O_2 as ordered; maintain patent airway	
	Causes lowering body temperature			Assess level of consciousness	
	Forane (isoflurane)			Assess cardiovascular system	
	Depresses cardiovascular system			Assess for impaired renal function	
	Shivering			Assess length and amount used	
	Possibility of acute or delayed injury to liver			Assess temperature and provide warm blankets or heated aerosol	
				Continue cardiac monitoring	
				Administer supplemental O_2 as ordered; maintain patent airway	
				Assess level of consciousness	
				Assess cardiovascular system	
	Nitrous oxide		On admission to PACU and prn	Assess length and amount used	
	Requires low oxygen concentration for the surgical level of anesthesia			Assess temperature and provide warm blankets or heated aerosol	
	Weak anesthetic			Provide continous cardiac monitoring	
	No muscular relaxation			Administer supplemental O_2 as ordered; maintain patent airway	
	Possible bone marrow aplasia and fatal agranulocytosis			Assess cardiovascular system	
	Changes in middle ear mechanics				
	X. Potential complication or injury while medicated and anesthetized	A safe and protected post-anesthetic environment during emergence from general anesthesia	Throughout PACU stay	Assess level of consciousness upon arrival to PACU	
				Keep side rails of cart up at all times	

(Continued)

Keep ECG monitoring cables and O$_2$ tube free from around patients neck

Utilize only safety-checked electrical equipment with appropriate grounding prongs, if indicated

Keep patient and equipment free from water or wet area

Inspect ECG monitoring electrodes; change if soiled or wet

Keep patient's chest clean and free of excess monitoring conduction jelly

Restrain if necessary

Orient frequently and reinforce as necessary

Assist patient when voiding

Patient discharged from PACU in an injury-free condition

Throughout PACU stay

Assess history of the present illness including weight, body functions and I & O during the illness

Assess perioperative medications that would alter renal functions:
Diuretics
Chronic user of antacids or laxatives
Antibiotics—such as neomycin

To maintain the interior environment within physiologic limits

XI. Potential for fluid and electrolyte imbalance
Volume depletion (water and Na)
Gastrointestinal losses
Diarrhea
Vomiting
Bowel fistulas (colostomy, ileostomy)
Gastric or small bowel drainage (T tubes)
Renal losses
Diuretics
Osmotic diuresis
Chronic renal failure (renal disease)
Adrenal dysfunction

Date Initiated	Actual/Potential Patient Problems	Expected Patient Outcomes	Deadlines Checkpoints	Nursing Interventions	Outcomes Achieved & Initial
	XI. Potential for fluid and electrolyte imbalance (Cont.). (Cushing's disease, aldosteronism) Post obstructive nephropathy Diuretic phase of acute tubular necrosis			Assess vital signs: Narrowing of pulse pressure, possibly indicating slowly occurring fluid deficit A drop in blood pressure which could indicate rapid volume loss Heart rate: Tachycardia, possibly indicating hypovolemia Heart sounds: Change to more muffled sound Temperature: Assess for elevation in temperature secondary to peripheral vasoconstriction Respiration: Assess rate and depth Skin: Assess color and temperature (feel to touch) Assess skin turgor	
	Skin losses Burn Sweating	Adequate fluid replacement			
	Third space losses related to: Ascites Free fluid in the bowel Intestinal edema			Observe for secondary water loss without electrolyte deficits producing thirst, furrows in the tongue, folds in the skin, for moderate dehydration; observe for sunken eyes and signs of shock	

Adequate fluid replacement as evidenced by:
Vital signs
Output
CVP

Assessment:
  Assess preoperative Na$^+$ and K$^+$ and serum osmolality
  Lab work as ordered and report
  Check hematocrit for changes in blood volume and extracelluar volume
  Observe urine specific gravity
  Check for sugar in urine acting as osmotic diuretic contributing to water loss
Replacement therapy:
  Check time fluid replacement was begun or needed amount was calculated (i.e., when NPO started)
  Assess for surgical procedure (if large amount of raw surface was exposed during procedure)
  Assess for losses due to evaporation and inhalation of dry anesthetic gases
  Administer plasma to increase volume if ordered
  Catheterize patient if ordered
  Hourly I & O as needed
  Administer blood or albumin per policy and procedure, if ordered

Potassium and calcium deficiencies

ECG:
  Observe ECG for reflection of potassium and calcium

(Continued)

Date Initiated	Actual/Potential Patient Problems	Expected Patient Outcomes	Deadlines Checkpoints	Nursing Interventions	Outcomes Achieved & Initial
	XI. Potential for fluid and electrolyte imbalance (Cont.).			Change in K^+ concentrations Hyperkalemia: Flattened P wave Widened QRS complex Peaked T wave Hypokalemia: Flat or inverted T wave Presence of U wave Calcium alternations Hypercalcemia: Shortened QT interval Hypocalcemia: Prolonged QT interval Give supplement if ordered	
	XII. Infection (wound) due to: Interruption of skin integrity secondary to surgical incision.	Good healing and absence of signs and symptoms of infection as evidenced by: Temperature below 100°F orally. Incision free of erythema, edema, tenderness, warmth, induration, foul odor, or purulent drainage. Absence of dehiscence. Approximation of wound edges.	Throughout PACU stay	Assess for signs and symptoms of wound infection and notify MD if present Initial dressing change by MD unless otherwise ordered Change dressing as ordered Good hand washing techniques Use aseptic technique when changing dressing: Inspect operative area at time of dressing change and document	

Reapply sterile dressing only
when edges become un-
sealed or dressing soiled
Secure sterile dressing with all
edges sealed

(Courtesy of Duggan S & Wentzloff J, Grant Hospital of Chicago.)

Chapter 10

Postanesthetic Problems

Anne C. Borchardt
Kay E. Fraulini

Anesthetic agents alter levels of consciousness, which is the purpose of their administration. But anesthesia can also alter other normal physiological processes. It is not always a harmless and reversible insensibility. The hazards of receiving anesthesia can be just as great as the risks of undergoing surgery. As one authority observed, the anesthesized state "must be considered as a comatose state produced by severe drug poisoning" (Luckmann & Sorenson, 1974).

Recognizing the deleterious effects anesthetics can produce, Vaughan and Vaughan performed a prospective risk assessment on 451 operative and postanesthetic adult patients. They developed an anesthesia related consequence (ARC) classification system to predict unfavorable outcomes. Less serious ARCs included unstable blood pressure, airway management problems, emergence delirium, electrolyte disturbances, nausea and vomiting requiring treatment, severe shivering, and hypothermia. Serious pulmonary ARCs were cited as prolonged airway management, pneumothorax, aspiration pneumonia, pulmonary edema, hypoxia, and hypercarbea. Hypertension, hypotension, arrhythmias, angina, and myocardial infarction were considered serious cardiac ARCs. Cardiac arrest and mortality were classified as worst ARCs.

Results indicated that at least one ARC of any type was found in 46.6 percent of operating room and 38.6 percent of PACU patients. Serious cardiac ARCs occurred in 45.2 percent of operating room patients and

20.8 percent of PACU patients. Worst cardiac ARCs were experienced by two operating room and one PACU patient (Vaughan and associates, 1981b).

The data illustrate the fact that anesthesia can produce unfavorable and even fatal consequences. Anesthetics can disturb or suppress almost all physiologic functions. They can produce complications that can make the immediate postoperative period discomforting or actually dangerous to the patient.

The remainder of this chapter is devoted to describing postanesthetic problems that can occur in the PACU. Appropriate nursing interventions are given; in addition, a number of case studies provide specific examples.

ALTERATIONS IN MENTAL STATUS

Sensory Perceptual Alterations

The purpose of general anesthesia is to produce a state of oblivion so that surgery can be performed without sensation. Consciousness is obliterated. Often such an absence of perception, however, extends into the immediate postoperative period. General anesthesia can produce significant alterations in sensory function and perception.

The unconscious patient cannot see, hear, feel, touch, or taste. But as consciousness returns, hearing becomes one of the first senses to reappear. For all practical purposes, the patient may appear to be sleeping—may not open the eyes, move about in bed, or speak—but may be able to hear.

The PACU nurse should keep this in mind when performing care. Initially, patients should be told that the surgery is over and that they are in the PACU. They should also be informed before any nursing measures are undertaken. Conversation at the bedside should be subdued. And a patient's condition should not be discussed, no matter how sleepy the patient seems.

The patient who has received spinal anesthesia faces a different sort of sensory deficit. Although awake and oriented, the patient feels no sensation from the level of the spinal down to the lower extremities. The absence of surgical pain may be pleasantly surprising to the patient, but the immobility and lack of sensation experienced can be frightening.

Nursing care is aimed at reassurance and repeated explanations about the temporary nature of spinal anesthesia. Providing the patient with diversionary activities, such as reading materials, may also decrease his or her level of anxiety. Since sensation is absent or greatly reduced, the patient may not experience cold or discomfort. Warm blankets and proper positioning can prevent further postoperative complications.

Case Study

Thirty-one-year-old Joan Valez underwent an exploratory laparotomy, total abdominal hysterectomy, bilateral salpingo-oopherectomy, and omentectomy. The preoperative diagnosis of adenocarcinoma had been accurate.

The patient appeared very sleepy in the PACU. She was difficult if not impossible to arouse. Shortly after admission, several physicians and nurses stood at her bedside, discussing the tragedy of her situation.

Thirty minutes later, the patient awoke, crying hysterically. She was very upset about her prognosis and the fact that she could never have a child.

Analysis

The patient's surgical procedure and prognosis should not have been discussed at her bedside. Even though the patient appeared sleepy and oblivious to external stimuli, she could hear. Although such news would have been devastating at any time, a more appropriate moment certainly could have been found.

Alterations in Levels of Consciousness

As stated previously, the primary purpose of general anesthesia is the elimination of perception and pain during surgery. Toward this end, anesthetics and adjuncts to them are valuable and beneficial agents, producing unconsciousness and obtunding reflexes. Unfortunately, however, the effects of anesthesia last long past the intraoperative period itself. The postanesthetic patient frequently displays prolonged somnolence, emergence delirium, or the central anticholinergic syndrome. Such alterations in levels of consciousness depend on the type and concentration of the anesthetic agent, intraoperative time, drug metabolism, and the individual's specific response to anesthesia.

Prolonged Somnolence. Somnolence can be prolonged when a high concentration of an agent is used over a long time period, or when a combination of anesthetics is used. Also, some agents such as Ativan and diazepam increase sleep times significantly. The patient may be semiconscious or may be unarousable to verbal or external stimuli. Pain may be the only means to elicit a response.

Sleep times can also be increased when drug metabolism is prolonged. Normally, metabolism and excretion of anesthetics occur via the kidney, liver, or lungs, depending on the agent used (see Table 10-1). Polar drugs and drug metabolites are rapidly cleared by the kidney, while lipid-soluble drugs are made polar and water-soluble by the liver and excreted in the urine (Orlandi 1972). For the most part, inhalants are excreted by the respiratory system, while intravenous agents are metabolized by the liver or kidney. Anesthetics themselves can decrease renal function, hepatic blood flow, and respiratory performance, altering nor-

TABLE 10–1. METABOLISM AND EXCRETION OF ANESTHETIC AGENTS

Agent	Primary Route of Metabolism and Excretion
Diazepam (Valium)	Liver
Droperidol (Inapsine)	Liver
D-Tubocurarine (DTC)	Kidneys
Enflurane (Ethrane)	Lungs
Fentanyl (Sublimaze)	Liver
Isoflurane (Forane)	Lungs
Halothane	Lungs*
Ketamine	Liver
Thiopentone (Pentothal)	Liver

*A halothane metabolite may be responsible for the development of hepatotoxicity.

mal metabolism and excretion. But the presence of renal, liver, or pulmonary disease can prolong these processes even further. Conditions such as renal failure, hepatitis, cirrhosis, and COPD can lengthen sleep times significantly (Table 10-2).

Emergence Delirium. Emergence delirium is another alteration in level of consciousness frequently observed in the PACU. Patients may be somnolent, only to suddenly awake and become restless and agitated. They may thrash about in bed, trying to pull out tubes or airways, and talk incoherently. Emergence delirium is a state of postanesthetic excitement characterized by such increased motor activity, disorientation, and vocalization. This condition can be produced by one or a combination of agents, but fortunately its duration is usually brief. The patient may relax and drift off to sleep, only to awake alert and oriented.

The Central Anticholinergic Syndrome. After the administration of anticholinergic agents, the patient may display excitement, thought impairment, drowsiness, or even coma. He or she may thrash about in bed, hallucinate, and express paranoid ideations. Or the patient may be very difficult to arouse, displaying prolonged somnolence. Atropine and hyoscine (Scopolamine), as well as diazepam, are particularly likely to create this syndrome, which tends to occur in the elderly more often than in the young (Atkinson, 1982).

TABLE 10–2. CONDITIONS THAT CAN PROLONG DRUG METABOLISM AND EXCRETION

Age	Cirrhosis
Diabetes	Chronic Pyelonephritis
Renal failure	Hydronephrosis
Obstructive jaundice	Nephrotic syndrome
Hepatitis	COPD

Nursing Intervention

Nursing care is first aimed at accurate assessment of the postanesthetic patient's level of consciousness. Is the patient awake, alert, and oriented? Or awake but incoherent and restless? Is the patient sleepy but easily arousable and cooperative while awake? Or is he or she very difficult to arouse? Such observations should be made and recorded on admission and during the patient's stay in the PACU.

Nursing measures then correspond to the patient's level of consciousness. The awake and oriented patient requires emotional support and explanation of all procedures. The restless patient may be experiencing emergence delirium or the central anticholinergic syndrome. Efforts should first be directed toward orienting and calming patients and then toward preventing them from harming themselves. The type of anesthesia and premedicant agent should then be examined. Emergence delirium is usually of short duration. But administration of physostigmine (Antilirium), an anticholinesterase that can cross the blood–brain barrier, may become necessary when the patient displays the central anticholinergic syndrome. A dose of 1–2 mg intravenously can reverse this condition rapidly. Note: Physostigmine is contraindicated in the bradycardic or asthmatic patient due to the peripheral muscarinic effects of the drug.

The sleepy and the unconscious patient may also be experiencing the central anticholinergic syndrome. Again, physostigmine is the treatment of choice. Prolonged somnolence, however, can also be attributed to the length of action of anesthetics or to prolonged metabolism and drug excretion. Continued assessment of vital signs is necessary. Patient positioning is also important to promote airway clearance, prevent aspiration, and facilitate circulation. Frequent stimulation and encouragement of ventilatory efforts are other vital nursing actions. If narcotics are responsible for such prolonged somnolence, naloxone administration may prove necessary.

Case Study

Thirty-five-year-old Ron Sanders underwent a lumbar laminectomy. Premedication was Demerol and atropine, and anesthesia consisted of enflurane, fentanyl, and diazepam. The patient was extubated on admission to the PACU, as he awoke coughing and gagging on the endotracheal tube. Shortly after extubation, the patient became very sleepy and began obstructing, and a nasal airway was inserted. Continuous stimulation became necessary to maintain adequate respiration. Narcotic reversal proved ineffective. Ninety minutes later, physostigmine was administered. The patient awoke 10 minutes afterwards, alert, oriented, and demanding pain medication. Pain medications were withheld until it was determined that the patient would remain awake.

Analysis

Mr. Sanders' prolonged somnolence was the result of the central anticholinergic syndrome. The premedicant atropine and intraoperative diazepam he received created this condition. Physostigmine administration became necessary to reverse this syndrome.

Increased Incidence of Pain

The patient who has undergone a surgical procedure of almost any kind will experience some degree of pain. The sensory organs of pain—naked nerve endings—are present in almost every tissue of the body. These nerve endings signal the cerebral cortex when an unpleasant stimulus is present.

Surgically induced pain is, of course, a very unpleasant stimulus. The patient will offer frequent complaints of pain in the immediate postoperative period. Sympathetic nervous system activity and catecholamine release will also be heightened by such acute discomfort, resulting in restlessness, anxiety, tachycardia, and hypertension. Pain can adversely affect the patient physiologically, especially if he or she has a significant preoperative history. Emotionally, the experience can be devastating.

A variety of factors can influence the patient's degree of postoperative pain. The type of surgical procedure is obviously a factor. The incisional pain produced by a thoracotomy is much more severe than the pain of a node biopsy. The anxiety level of the patient can also affect the severity of pain. Patients who are more anxious about the operation and its outcome may be more uncomfortable. Inadequate preoperative teaching can also influence pain and anxiety; if the patient has received insufficient instruction, he or she will be more fearful and anxious about surgery and hospitalization.

Pain tolerance is another factor that influences the patient's degree of pain. Certain ethnic groups as well as personality types have a higher pain tolerance than do others. A history of preoperative drug abuse can also affect sensations of pain.

Finally, the type of anesthesia administered during the surgical procedure can influence pain. Patients will remain relatively pain-free long after spinal and epidural anesthesia have been given. Narcotics such as morphine and fentanyl have both anesthetic and analgesic properties, depressing the central nervous system and alleviating sensations of pain and anxiety. Unfortunately, patients who have received inhalant anesthesia will experience the greatest degree of immediate postoperative pain. Halothane, enflurane, and isoflurane are potent anesthetics but have relatively poor analgesic properties. They are also more rapidly eliminated from the body. Finally, patients who have received narcan will be acutely aware of sensations of pain.

Nursing Intervention

Whatever its cause, the presence of pain can prevent the performance of effective postoperative care. Patients may not cooperate in turning in bed, coughing, and deep breathing if they are likely to experience pain during such maneuvers. The response of the sympathetic nervous system to pain also makes its presence undesirable.

Judicious use of pain medications is thus especially important in the immediate postoperative period. The type of anesthesia patients have received and their level of consciousness should first be ascertained. Many postanesthetic patients will awake and complain of pain, only to drift off to sleep and even require active stimulation soon after. Anesthetics themselves cause hypoventilation. Since analgesics can also produce respiratory depression, the quality and quantity of respirations should be accurately assessed prior to administration of analgesics. Heart rate and blood pressure should be determined as well; if the patient is bradycardic or hypotensive, pain medications should not be administered.

Because of their duration of action and the acuity of postoperative pain, intravenous analgesics are safer and more rapid acting than are intramuscular. Narcotics such as Demerol and morphine should be given in small increments. Epidural analgesia is another method of pain relief that has become increasingly popular (see "Epidural Morphine Infusion" in Chapter 12), although it can produce hypotension and respiratory depression. An epidural drip is usually administered with an infusion pump to control the rate.

Besides the judicious use of pain medications, other measures can be taken to alleviate sensations of pain and discomfort. Explanations of all procedures and emotional support may decrease the patient's anxiety level and reduce pain. Alterations in position may also make the patient more comfortable. Even a cool cloth to the head or a wet sponge to the mouth may help.

Unfortunately, if narcan is given, none of these measures will prove effective. The effects of intravenous narcan last approximately one hour; intramuscular duration is longer. Pain medications are usually not administered during this time. Emotional support is the most important nursing measure after narcan administration.

Case Study

Emily Jones underwent a right mastectomy with axillary node dissection. Anesthesia included fentanyl 5 cc and forane; 1 cc of fentanyl was administered 30 minutes before the completion of the procedure.

The patient was very upset upon admission to the PACU. Blood pressure, heart rate, and respiratory rate were increased; 4 mg of morphine was given immediately. Twenty minutes later, the patient was very sleepy and difficult to arouse. Respiratory rate and blood pressure were decreased as well. Narcan 0.1 mg IV was administered, and the patient became immediately responsive, complaining of severe pain.

Analysis

This example illustrates the injudicious use of analgesics. Many patients awake in the PACU and complain of pain, only to fall asleep minutes later. If the patient had been observed for a short time after admission, pain medication might not have been necessary, nor would the use of narcan.

ALTERATIONS IN RESPIRATORY PERFORMANCE

Respiratory complications are some of the most frequent and potentially serious conditions anesthetic agents can produce (see also Chapter 12). The ability of anesthesia to obtund normal reflexes can result in airway obstruction and inadequate ventilatory exchange. Besides interfering with airway clearance, anesthetics by their nature are potent respiratory depressants, creating hypoventilation, hypoxia, and hypercarbia. The use of muscle relaxants can also alter normal respiratory function significantly. Harrison found that anesthesia-related deaths accounted for about 2 percent of overall surgical mortality. The most frequent causes included respiratory depression following neuromuscular blockade, complications of intubation, and inadequate postoperative care and supervision (Atkinson, 1982).

The importance of protecting the patient from the adverse respiratory effects of anesthesia seems obvious. Inadequate airway performance and hypoventilation can place the postanesthetic patient in jeopardy. Even respiratory arrest can result. The process of surgery and anesthesia can also produce life-threatening states such as pulmonary embolism and pneumothorax.

Ineffective Airway Clearance
Obstruction by the Tongue. After anesthesia is administered, the tongue frequently falls backward and obstructs air passages, resulting in inadequate ventilation. This condition is particularly common in the PACU after the patient has been extubated but is not awake.

Obstruction Above or at the Glottis. Such a condition is usually due to foreign material that must be removed by suctioning or gravity. Emesis, saliva, secretions, a tooth, or bloody drainage can cause this obstruction.

Laryngospasm. Severe spasm of the larynx may be produced by the irritating effects of inhalant anesthesia or from an allergic reaction to the anesthetic. Suctioning, airway manipulation, and the presence of oral or nasopharyngeal airways may also cause laryngospasm (Cullen & Cullen, 1975).

Bronchospasm. Severe spasm of the bronchus can be observed during the immediate postoperative period. Such a condition may be due to airway obstruction or irritation, as well as a preoperative history of smoking, bronchitis, or asthma. As the patient attempts to overcome airway resistance, ventilation becomes increasingly difficult and bronchospasm results.

Signs and symptoms of ineffective airway clearance include noisy, shallow respirations, skin color and temperature changes, chest retraction, increased abdominal movements, and use of accessory respiratory muscles. Blood pressure and heart rate will be elevated. Level of consciousness will vary from lethargy to extreme anxiety, depending on the type of obstruction.

Nursing Intervention

Effective nursing intervention consists of immediate recognition of such signs and symptoms. The patient whose tongue is obstructing the airway may require only changes in positioning or stimulation to facilitate respiration. Chin lift may also be effective in promoting airway clearance. If such measures fail, an oral or nasopharyngeal airway should be inserted, and auscultation should then be performed to ascertain proper exchange. Respiratory rate, rhythm, and depth should be assessed frequently.

Besides actively maintaining airway clearance, proper patient positioning can promote drainage of secretions and removal of foreign material, preventing obstruction and aspiration. The patient should be positioned on his or her side with the neck extended or hyperextended. Suctioning may become necessary, but should be used sparingly as it can precipitate laryngospasm or bronchospasm.

Treatment of the patient in laryngospasm consists of sitting the patient upright and applying a bag with 100 percent oxygen. Ventilation with racemic epinephrine or intravenous Decadron administration are also effective. If such measures prove fruitless, however, succinylcholine administration may be necessary to break the spasm and relax the larynx (Benumof, 1983).

Bronchospasm may be arrested by mere removal of an endotracheal tube. Aminophylline administration may also ease the spasm. Bronchosol treatments are also effective if the patient can maintain spontaneous respiration. If the patient cannot, intravenous infusions of epinephrine or Isuprel will be necessary to reduce bronchospasm successfully (Cullen & Cullen, 1975).

Case Study

Thirty-eight-year-old Vanessa Redmond received a combination of diazepam, fentanyl, and Halothane anesthesia during the mastectomy she underwent. Even though she remained unresponsive, she was extubated shortly after admission to the PACU. She immediately began obstructing; an oral airway was inserted with little effect. Chin lift was then performed repeatedly, and she finally began ventilating and swallowing effectively.

Analysis
The patient should probably not have been extubated until her level of consciousness increased (see Appendix 10-1, Criteria For Extubation). Airway obstruction by the tongue resulted. Nursing measures were appropriate, however, in promoting effective ventilation.

Case Study

At 78 years of age, Ted Williams had a TURP performed. Anesthesia consisted of enflurane and valium. The patient was extubated, awake, and comfortable on admission to the PACU; vital signs were stable. Approximately 30 minutes later, Williams suddenly displayed very noisy, shallow respirations. The monitor showed a sinus tachycardia of 130; blood pressure was elevated as well. The patient was awake and extremely anxious. Color was flushed and skin very diaphoretic. Williams was in laryngospasm. He was bagged by mask with 100 percent oxygen. The spasm broke soon after this maneuver.

Analysis
The irritating nature of the inhalant enflurane, as well as intraoperative intubation, most probably precipitated the development of laryngospasm. In Williams' case, simply bagging with high oxygen concentrations broke the spasm.

Ineffective Breathing Patterns
Hypoventilation, involving decreased air movement in and out of the alveoli, can be the result of insufficient airway clearance. However, anesthetics themselves have the ability to alter normal respiration. Loss of consciousness will produce some degree of respiratory depression. But anesthetics can depress the central respiratory center and desensitize the patient to the stimulating effects of CO_2. Respiratory rate and tidal volume will be decreased, resulting in hypoxia and hypercarbia.

Inhalants such as Halothane, enflurane, and isoflurane decrease tidal volume significantly. The slight increase in respiratory rate produced by these agents does not compensate for the decreased depth of respiration. Hypoxia and hypercarbia result, leading to the development of respiratory and metabolic acidosis.

Narcotics such as fentanyl and morphine affect respiratory rate rather than depth. Tidal volume remains normal, while respiratory rate decreases. High-dose fentanyl may actually terminate involuntary breathing; only with stimulation will the patient initiate respiration.

Neuromuscular blockade can alter both respiratory rate and tidal volume if it has not been adequately reversed. Muscle weakness will make respiratory efforts difficult if not impossible. Respirations will be shallow and irregular, and further reversal or ventilatory assistance may be necessary.

Assessing the Patient for Residual Block

Obviously the most sensitive test stresses the neuromuscular junction the most. Sensitivity depends on both the intensity and duration of the stress applied. Miller organized data from several studies to correlate tests of ventilation and neuromuscular function with estimated receptor occupancy (Table 10-3). Even when the result is normal, none of these tests assures that all of the receptors are free of relaxant. The data suggest that the sensitivities of the tests in detecting the residual block are, starting with the most sensitive:

1. Head lift.
2. Hand grip.
3. Inspiratory force.
4. Inspiratory and expiratory flow rates.
5. Sustained contraction in response to a tetanic stimulus (30 Hz) and normal vital capacity.
6. Normal tidal volume and normal twitch height.

This sensitivity scale assumes that applications of these tests in all studies are identical, which is probably not true (Miller, 1976).

Clearly the use of tidal volume (TV) alone as a test for residual block is not reliable and by itself should not be used as a criterion for extubation.

Anesthetics as potent respiratory depressants can decrease ventilation, producing hypoxia and hypercarbia. But the ability of anesthetics to reduce cardiac output, create hypothermia, alter levels of consciousness, and promote hypotension can also create hypoxic and hypercarbic states.

Normal signs and symptoms of hypoventilation include restlessness, hypertension, tachycardia, cardiac arrhythmias, tachypnea, and dyspnea. These may be altered, however, by the presence of anesthetic agents, making recognition much more difficult.

TABLE 10–3. SUGGESTED CORRELATIONS BETWEEN TESTS OF NEUROMUSCULAR TRANSMISSIONS

Peripheral Nerve Stimulation	Ventilation	Estimated Receptors Occupied (%)
Reduced twitch height and sustained tetanus at 30 Hz	Normal tidal volume	75–80
Normal train-of-four	Normal expiratory flow rate and vital capacity	70–75
Sustained tetanus at 100 Hz	Normal inspiratory force	50
Sustained tetanus at 200 Hz	Normal head-lift and grip test	33

(From Miller RD, Antagonism of neuromuscular blockade. Anesthesiology 44:318–329, 1976.)

Accurate assessment of respiratory status is thus essential in the postanesthetic patient. After administering oxygen to the patient, rate, rhythm, and character of respirations should be assessed by visual observation and by auscultation. A look at the anesthesia record will reveal the type of anesthesia and any reversal agents that the patient has received. Most anesthetics will produce some degree of respiratory depression. Whether such depression can be reversed depends on the agent in question. Narcotics are easily reversed by naloxone, but inhalants cannot be reversed. Muscle relaxant reversal is not always effective or adequate.

Actually, blood-gas analysis is often the only accurate determinant of hypoventilation in the postanesthetic patient (see Appendix 10-2). If the patient is hypoventilating, stimulation may be the only necessary measure. Asking the patient to take a deep breath periodically is an important nursing intervention. If the patient is unarousable, or muscle relaxant remains in effect, reversals should be administered. Reintubation and ventilatory assistance will be required if such measures fail.

Case Study

Mary Becker, 22 years old, underwent a spinal fusion with iliac bone graft. During the procedure, 22 cc of fentanyl was administered and muscle relaxant reversal was achieved. The patient was awake and responsive on admission to the PACU. Respiratory rate was 12; respirations were regular and deep. Not long after admission, however, she drifted off to sleep, displaying a decreased rate of 6 to 8 breaths per minute. With frequent stimulation, the patient would deep-breathe, but she would not sustain an adequate rate. Blood gas analysis revealed respiratory acidosis, and naloxone 0.1 mg IV was administered. Although the patient became uncomfortable, respirations improved significantly.

Analysis

Fentanyl is a potent respiratory depressant, depressing the central respiratory center and desensitizing the brain to the stimulating effects of CO_2. While Becker was awake, respirations were adequate. But as somnolence ensued, conscious efforts at ventilation were decreased. Frequent stimulation was not totally effective, and narcotic reversal became necessary.

Respiratory Arrest

Respiratory arrest can be due to airway obstruction or to central respiratory depression. In either case, treatment is aimed first at reestablishing the airway and then ventilating the patient. Only after such maneuvers is the cause examined and appropriate treatment initiated.

Prolonged Apnea Following Succinylcholine. Succinylcholine (anectine) is broken down by pseudocholinesterase within 2 to 3 minutes, when its relaxant effect also disappears. But relaxation is greatly prolonged under certain conditions:

1. A so-called dual block. This means that the mode of action changes from depolarizing into nondepolarizing after large doses of succinylcholine. Neostigmine will not reliably act as antagonist because it counteracts the nondepolarizing effect but strengthens the depolarizing component. The mechanism of dual block is not fully understood, but an alteration in the structure of the receptor proteins is suspected. It becomes clinically manifest when doses exceed 10 mg/kg body weight. Apnea lasts for 20 to 30 minutes.

2. Delayed breakdown due to lack of pseudocholinesterase. This occurs in patients with latent or manifest liver damage and in those with severe burns. The same symptoms occur when eyedrops are used for glaucoma that contain a cholinesterase inhibitor (e.g., echothiophate iodide). Numerous reports of this complication exist. It is, therefore, imperative that during the preoperative interview of the patient who is about to undergo anesthesia for any surgical procedure, the anesthesiologist ask about the recent use of eyedrops.

   Note: More commonly encountered than echiothiophate in the patient with open-angle glaucoma is timulol, a recently introduced beta-adrenergic receptor blocking agent. Among the problems noted are bradycardia, hypotension, syncope, exacerbation of bronchial asthma, and worsening of congestive heart failure (Orkin & Cooperman, 1983).

   In pure pseudocholinesterase deficiency, succinylcholine apnea lasts about 30 minutes. Therefore, it is not seen when only one dose is given for intubation for prolonged operations.

3. Failure of breakdown due to presence of atypical pseudocholinesterase. This enzyme variant causes no manifestations but it is unable to break down succinylcholine. Even a small dose remains active for hours and can cause correspondingly long apnea. But in spite of this, the patient may show some slight muscle activity. Total muscle paralysis which, according to the literature, is said to go with apnea, is not always seen. Patients with homozygotic atypical pseudocholinesterase are relatively rare (0.04 percent); the heterozygotic form, which contains typical as well as atypical pseudocholinesterase, is somewhat more frequent (3.8 percent). Atypical pseudocholinesterase can be determined by dibucain inhibition (dibucain number): hydrolysis of benzoyl choline by normal pseudocholinesterase is inhibited in vitro by dibucaine (10^{-5} m solution) up to 60 to 100 percent (dibucaine number 60–100). In the atypical heterozygotic form, the inhibition is of the order of 20 to 60 percent (dibucain number 20–60), and in the atypical homozygotic form it is less than 20 percent (dibucain number below 20).

In the presence of atypical pseudocholinesterase, biochemical results show reduced general activity besides a low dibucaine number. But succinylcholine-induced apnea is far more marked than in analogous findings with a normal dibucaine number.

For succinylcholine-induced respiratory disturbances it is typical that the diaphragm is more affected than other muscles (in contradistinction to the nondepolarizing relaxants, which spare diaphragm and muscles of respiration). Therefore, the patient who is paralyzed by succinylcholine often breathes with his or her intercostal muscles. An inverted pendulum-like situation develops; in inspiration the chest rises and the abdomen sinks in; in expiration the abdomen becomes prominent and the chest sinks in.

Relaxation by succinylcholine shows no fading—that is, there is no weakening of paretic muscles. Once muscular activity is resumed, it continues, and undesirable movements continue unabated until another relaxant dose has been given.

Apnea from succinylcholine is always reversible, but one must be familiar with the syndrome and ventilate until efficient respiration has been attained. There can, of course, be no reversal by neostigmine (Tschirren, 1980).

Note: Myoglobinuria is occasionally seen after administration of succinylcholine. This phenomenon belongs to the same symptom complex as muscle pain and rise in potassium, and is presumably also caused by damage to muscle fibers from depolarization contractions. It was also observed in connection with muscular rigidity and hyperpyrexia (Tschirren, 1980).

Pulmonary Embolism

Pulmonary embolism is yet another significant respiratory complication that can occur in the operative, recovery, and postoperative periods. The usual onset is from 2 to 14 days after surgery (Atkinson, 1982). However, if bed rest has been maintained prior to surgery, the possibility of thrombus formation and subsequent pulmonary embolism during the operative and immediate postanesthetic period increases significantly.

Orthopedic procedures tend to place the individual at greater risk for the development of pulmonary embolism. Other predisposing factors include oral contraceptive use, previous history of thrombophlebitis, age, and obesity.

The patient will suddenly complain of severe chest pain or tightness and shortness of breath. He or she will display tachycardia, hypotension, pallor or cyanosis, restlessness, and anxiety. Depending on its size, pulmonary embolism may be minor to severe. Mortality rate has been estimated at 38 percent (Luckmann & Sorenson, 1974).

Preventive nursing measures include passive and active range-of-motion exercises, TED hose application, and low-dose heparin administration if predisposing factors are present. Assessment of the lower extremities for thrombus formation is also important.

Nursing intervention for the patient who has developed pulmonary embolism includes oxygen administration, frequent determination of vital signs, and proper positioning. The head of the bed should be elevated. Emotional support is also essential during this time. After a definitive diagnosis of pulmonary embolism has been made by chest x-ray and blood-gas analysis, anticoagulant therapy and analgesic administration will prove necessary.

Pneumothorax

Pneumothorax, a collection of air or gas in the pleural cavity, can occur after thoracic surgery and with the use of brachial plexus and intercostal blocks. Accidental puncture of the pleura causes air to escape into the pleural space, and the lung collapses.

The onset of pneumothorax is sudden and severe. Signs and symptoms include severe sharp chest pain, shortness of breath, decreased or absent breath sounds on the affected side, uneven chest expansion, rapid pulse, and hypotension.

When pneumothorax is suspected, clinical care includes calming the patient and sitting him or her upright in bed. Oxygen should be administered to relieve dyspnea. Respirations, heart rate, and blood pressure should be recorded at frequent intervals. Respiratory quality should also be assessed. The physician, of course, should be notified immediately. A chest x-ray—the best diagnostic indicator of the condition—should be ordered. Blood gas analysis may also be made to determine the patient's respiratory status.

A small pneumothorax may require only bed rest and oxygen therapy. If the pneumothorax is large, however, chest tube insertion will become necessary.

Case Study

Narcotics would not alleviate the postoperative pain Bobby Miller was experiencing after an exploratory laparotomy and cholecystectomy had been performed. An intercostal block was subsequently done. Shortly after the procedure, the patient became tachycardic, dyspneic, and diaphoretic. Blood presure decreased to 80 systolic. Auscultation revealed absent breath sounds on the right. A chest x-ray confirmed the presence of pneumothorax, and a chest tube was inserted.

Analysis

The intercostal block performed to alleviate pain produced a severe pneumothorax. A chest tube became necessary.

DISTURBANCES IN ORAL INTAKE AND GI FUNCTION

Increased Sensations of Thirst

Thirst is common after surgery and anesthesia. In the surgical patient, preoperative water deprivation and hypovolemia can activate the sensation of thirst. Anesthetics can also make the patient thirsty. Inhalants such as enflurane and Halothane dry the patient's oral mucous membranes. Premedicant anticholinergic agents like atropine and antiemetics such as Vistaril and Phenergan also cause dryness of the mouth and activate the sensation of thirst.

The postanesthetic patient will frequently complain of thirst and demand fluids, but water should not be given routinely. It is best to provide the patient with wet sponges, glycerin swabs, or mouthwashes. Sips of water and small amounts of ice chips may be administered only if the patient remains alert and oriented and denies complaints of nausea and vomiting.

Nausea and Vomiting

The incidence of postoperative nausea and vomiting in the PACU is fairly high. Preoperative fluid deprivation and premedicant anticholinergic agents have not prevented this condition. Why is the postoperative patient so susceptible to nausea and vomiting?

The use of general anesthesia and anesthetic adjuncts is generally responsible. Volatile anesthetics such as halothane, enflurane, and isoflurane may cause postoperative nausea and vomiting by irritating the mucous membranes of the stomach, thus stimulating the vomiting center in the medulla oblongata. Nitrous oxide is another agent that can cause emesis.

Narcotic analgesics can also precipitate nausea and vomiting. Given before and after surgery, incidence of vomiting can be as high as 30 percent (Atkinson, 1982). A study by Stephen revealed an even greater incidence; in selected surgical patients, 46 percent of those receiving morphine and 36 percent of those receiving Demerol experienced nausea and vomiting (Luckmann & Sorenson, 1974).

Nausea and vomiting after morphine administration is due to stimulation of the chemoreceptor zone in the medulla, not the vomiting center itself. But morphine has also been shown to sensitize the vomiting center to vestibular movements. Slight changes in patient positioning may trigger nausea and vomiting (Atkinson, 1982).

Certain reversal agents can also trigger nausea and vomiting. Physostigmine can produce nausea and vomiting by increasing peristalsis. Abrupt reversal of narcotic depression by naloxone may also result in nausea and vomiting. Still another agent, pyridostigmine (Regonol), can produce the condition.

The type of surgery the patient has undergone is another factor that may make him or her more susceptible to gastric distress. Major abdominal surgery, with extensive manipulation of the viscera, may result in nausea and vomiting. Atkinson (1982) finds that "vomiting is most frequent after laparotomy and especially after operation on the GI tract."

Other types of surgical procedures, such as tonsillectomy, adenoidectomy, and cleft palate repair, may also precipitate nausea and vomiting. The swallowing of bloody drainage is usually the cause.

The presence of airways and nasogastric tubes can also promote the development of nausea and vomiting by stimulating the gag reflex and increasing secretions.

Finally, the incidence of nausea and vomiting seems to be related to age, sex, and anxiety level. From the authors' clinical observations, anxious young women seem particularly susceptible.

Nursing Intervention

Nursing intervention is both preventive and palliative. Since postoperative thirst is extremely common, the patient will often request oral fluids. These should not be routinely administered. As mentioned previously, mouthwashes and swabs are a much better way to combat the dry mouth produced by anesthesia and surgery. Dehydration and fluid replacement, of course, should be resolved by intravenous fluid therapy as opposed to oral fluid administration. It is essential that the stomach remain empty to prevent nausea and vomiting.

Patient positioning is also vital. The patient who is initially recovering from anesthesia has a decreased level of consciousness. The patient may not be able to express or identify the fact that he or she feels nauseated. The patient's airway may also be unprotected. Patients who vomit may aspirate, inhaling stomach contents into the lungs. So serious a complication can be easily prevented by a bit of foresight. Positioning the sleepy patient on his or her side is an important nursing measure. The supine position greatly increases the likelihood of aspiration.

It is also important to remember, however, that rapid or frequent position changes can increase the incidence of nausea and vomiting in postoperative patients. Moving the patient slowly in bed may decrease the chances of inducing nausea. Since anxiety has been shown to trigger gastric distress, explanation of all procedures and emotional support should be given.

If the patient is severely nauseated and vomiting is frequent, an antiemetic drug should be administered. A number of medications are available by physician's order. Phenothiazine agents such as prochlorperazine (Compazine), chlorpromazine (Thorazine), and promethazine (Phenergan) reduce the incidence of vomiting significantly. Droperidol, a butyrophenone derivative, acts specifically on the chemoreceptor zone in the medulla to prevent vomiting. Miscellaneous agents such as trimethobenzamide (Tigan) and anticholinergic agents such as atropine and hyoscine (Scopolamine) are also effective.

Antiemetics will not relieve nausea, however, if obvious causes of the problem are ignored. If a patient is awake and gagging on an airway, it should be removed. Oral secretions or bloody drainage should be kept at a minimum by suctioning or positioning.

Case Study

> Pam Schultz, a 29-year-old woman who underwent a vaginal hysterectomy, came to the PACU in stable condition. Shortly after admission, however, she was awake and anxious, complaining of severe nausea. She had received morphine as a premedicant; general anesthesia consisted of enflurane and muscle relaxant. After several episodes of vomiting, Compazine 10 mg IM was administered.

Analysis

Nausea and vomiting was most probably due to the premedication and anesthesia the patient received. Volatile anesthetics such as Ethrane and narcotic analgesics precipitate postoperative nausea and vomiting. In addition, the patient's age and sex placed her in the group most susceptible to the development of this condition.

Aspiration

Inhalation of stomach contents, bloody drainage, or other foreign material into the lungs is another adverse process that can occur after the administration of anesthesia. Normal reflexes are obtunded, resulting in the passive passage of foreign material into the respiratory tract. Individuals particularly susceptible to aspiration include those with excessive or considerable stomach contents, the obese, and the pregnant patient, as well as patients who have limited mobility after operation. Such patients consist of those with decreased levels of consciousness, paralyzed individuals, patients who must lie supine, or individuals who have undergone head and neck surgery. The presence of oral airways may also produce aspiration.

Initially, aspiration can cause acute airway obstruction and result in difficulty breathing. Laryngospasm can even occur. Pneumonia and atelectasis are later consequences of aspiration.

Nursing Intervention

Nursing care of the postanesthetic patient demands foresight in the prevention of aspiration. Patient positioning is particularly important. Patients with decreased levels of consciousness should be placed in side-lying positions to promote drainage of emesis and foreign material. The patient who must lie flat or has limited head and neck mobility should be observed closely. Complaints of nausea in such individuals should not go unheard. Suctioning equipment should always be available at the bedside. Appropriate antiemetics may also be administered. Oral airways should be removed as the patient becomes awake and responsive.

Once aspiration has occurred, nursing measures are aimed at relieving airway obstruction and preventing hypoxia. Suction and gravity should be employed to decrease obstruction, and oxygen should be administered. Chest x-ray and blood-gas analysis are valuable diagnostic tools when aspiration is suspected. Occasionally, bronchoscopy may be necessary.

After respiration has been fully restored, treatment includes antibiotic and steroid administration, chest physiotherapy, and continued oxygen therapy. Close monitoring of respiratory status should be continued by both observation and auscultation. Temperature should be taken at intervals as fever may develop.

Case Study

Fifty-nine-year-old Ben Keats underwent a cervical fusion, receiving a combination of inhalant-narcotic anesthesia. A cervical collar remained in place on admission to the PACU. Level of consciousness and vital signs were determined; the patient was awake and stable.

Shortly after admission, the patient complained of nausea. He was told to relax and take a few deep breaths. As the nurse left the bedside, assuming the nausea had been controlled, Keats proceeded to vomit. Unable to turn his head, vomitus entered his airway and he aspirated.

Analysis

A little more attentiveness and foresight would have prevented the development of aspiration in this patient. Understanding that Keats had limited mobility, the nurse should have remained at the bedside, ready with suction equipment should vomiting occur.

IMPAIRED PHYSICAL MOBILITY

Postanesthetic patients will frequently display alterations in mobility. Their usual ability to perform independent movements is reduced or eliminated. Factors that impair physical mobility include anesthesia and the surgical procedure itself.

General anesthetics can decrease mobility by reducing levels of consciousness. The patient's sensorium is altered; often, arousal is difficult. Such patients do not actively move about or change position when they are uncomfortable. They are oblivious to sensations of pain and discomfort.

Spinal anesthesia also alters normal mobility. It involves a temporary interruption of nerve impulses produced by injection of a local anesthetic into the subarachnoid space (Greene, 1976). This causes a sympathetic blockade, its extent depending on the number of nerve fibers blocked and the segmental level of the blockade. The spinal obliterates both patient sensation and mobility.

Many factors affect the extent and the duration of spinal anesthesia. Immobility may be brief or prolonged depending on the volume, concentration, and temperature of the local anesthetic; the site of injection; the patient's position during and after injection; and the force and rate of injection.

Muscle relaxation is yet another type of anesthetically produced immobility. It involves the deliberate paralysis of a patient by the interruption of neuromuscular transmission at the synapse, the junction between one neuron and the next. The depolarizing muscle relaxant succinylcholine has a very brief duration of action; 2 to 4 minutes of paralysis will be achieved. Nondepolarizing agents such as pancuronium (Pavulon) and D-tubocurarine (DTC) are relatively longer acting; their duration of action is 40 to 60 minutes. Unlike succinylcholine, these agents can be reversed. Neostigmine (Prostigmine) is the agent of choice (Feldman, 1973).

A variety of factors, however, can prolong muscle relaxation even if reversal is administered. Metabolic acidosis, hyponatremia, disordered potassium metabolism, renal or hepatic disease, and hypothermia can potentiate muscle relaxation and make reversal ineffective. The aminoglycoside antibiotics, such as neomycin, gentamicin, and tobramycin, can also prolong muscle relaxation (Atkinson, 1982).

Obviously, anesthetic agents can greatly alter and impair normal mobility. The fact that the patient underwent surgery also influences the degree of postoperative immobility. The type of operation as well as the pain and anxiety the patient experiences determine voluntary patient movements. External devices such as traction, irrigations, multiple tubes, and IVs can also produce immobility.

Nursing Intervention
Nursing care of the patient with a decreased level of consciousness consists of frequent position changes and proper body alignment to promote oxygenation, facilitate circulation, and preserve skin integrity. Such patients should be turned and repositioned at intervals to maintain airway performance and to prevent postoperative pneumonia and atelectasis. Thrombus formation can also be prevented by such maneuvers, as well as by performance of passive range-of-motion exercises.

The patient who has received spinal anesthesia is often awake but immobilized. On admission to the PACU, vital signs should be taken and the sensory level of the spinal ascertained. Continuing assessment of vital signs, sensation, and mobility should subsequently be made.

The spinal's length of action frequently produces anxiety. Even though patients are given preoperative instruction, they may feel helpless and frightened, often verbalizing fears about their immobility and its duration. Emotional support is very important at this time. Reinforcement about the temporary nature of spinal anesthesia may also help to alleviate anxiety.

Primarily, nursing care of the patient who has received muscle relaxants involves both accurate assessment and prompt intervention. Muscle strength should be determined shortly after admission to the PACU. Head lift, hand grasps, and movement of extremities should be examined. Chest expansion and ventilation should also be assessed. If the patient is intubated, respiratory parameters such as tidal volume and minute ventilation should be measured. If the patient is not intubated, shallow or rapid respirations and complaints of shortness of breath may indicate reversal has been inadequate or ineffective. Further reversal or ventilatory support may then become necessary.

Nursing care of the patient whose mobility is impaired by muscle relaxants includes frequent position changes and proper body alignment. Emotional support is also essential. Being paralyzed is, no doubt, a terrifying experience. The patient cannot actively move about, communicate, or perhaps even breathe alone. Communication is important during this time. Explanation of all impending procedures and reassurance that this state is temporary may help alleviate some of the fear.

When considering mobility impaired by the operative procedure, the nurse should consider the type of surgery the patient has undergone. Orthopedic and neurological procedures can limit mobility significantly. The pain produced by major abdominal operations and thoracic surgeries can also reduce voluntary movement. Judicious use of pain medications is essential. The rationale for the presence of external devices such as tubes and IVs should also be explained to the patient.

Case Study

Robert Haley, 59 years old, underwent a TURP with spinal anesthesia. Vital signs were stable and sensory level was determined at T10 on admission to the PACU. The patient appeared comfortable and relaxed.

Forty-five minutes later, the patient suddenly became restless and extremely anxious, crying out "what have they done to me?" He could not be calmed even after repeated explanations and support by a nurse and anesthesiologist. Sedation with Valium 5 mg IV became necessary.

Analysis

Spinal anesthesia can be a terrifying experience. Preoperative and postoperative explanations of the procedure did not alleviate the patient's anxiety. Fears that immobility was permanent were overwhelming.

Case Study

Surgery for 63-year-old Helen Barrett consisted of an exploratory laparotomy, lysis of adhesions, and drainage of abdominal abscess under narcotic-inhalant anesthesia. Muscle relaxation was achieved by DTC and reversed with neostigmine and atropine.

The patient remained sleepy and intubated on admission to the PACU. Respiratory rate was 16 and regular, blood pressure 116/80, and pulse 88 and regular. Axillary temperature was recorded as 91.8. Twenty minutes later, the patient seemed more awake and responsive, opening her eyes and moving her extremities. Heart rate increased to 110 and BP to 154/90. The anesthesiologist was at the bedside and decided to extubate the patient.

After extubation, respiratory rate increased to 36, and Barrett complained that she was "not getting enough air." Assessment of muscle strength by the nurse revealed weak hand grasps and inability to perform a head lift. The anesthesiologist was notified and further reversal was administered. This proved ineffective, however. The patient was reintubated and placed on a ventilator. Only after several hours did her muscle strength return.

Analysis

Because her muscle relaxant had been reversed at the end of surgery, it was assumed that the patient had normal muscle strength and ventilatory capacity. Such assumptions should not be made. Hypothermia in this patient potentiated the action of DTC, prolonging muscle relaxation and making reversal ineffective. An accurate assessment of muscle strength and respiratory parameters should have been made by the nurse and anesthesiologist prior to extubation.

ALTERATIONS IN NORMAL BODY TEMPERATURE

Normal body temperature measured in the oropharynx ranges from 35.9 to 37° C, or 96.6 to 99° F (Borchardt & Fraulini, 1982). Usually, the body can maintain this normothermic range, balancing heat production by muscles, liver, and glands and heat loss through the skin and lungs. The process of surgery and the administration of anesthetics, however, can produce alterations in such homeostasis. Inadvertent hypothermia and malignant hyperthermia may result.

Hypothermia

Hypothermia, a clinical state of subnormal body temperature with a core temperature of less than 35° C (95° F), can be deliberately or inadvertently induced (Borchardt & Fraulini, 1982). The condition is deliberately induced during cardiac surgery with cariopulmonary bypass. It is a means to lower metabolism and reduce the dangers of hypoxia. Such hypothermia is controlled.

Inadvertent hypothermia, unfortunately, occurs during surgery and with the use of anesthesia. The cool temperatures of the operating room, body surface area exposure, cold irrigations, IV fluids, and intraoperative time can all produce drastic reductions in body temperature.

Anesthetics themselves can create hypothermia in several ways. Primarily, they reduce patient sensitivity to cold. With their level of consciousness altered, patients are oblivious to sensations of cold or helpless to warm themselves.

Another way anesthetics inadvertently induce hypothermia is their reduction of voluntary movement. Motion is a means of heat production. The movements of the patient who has received muscle relaxant are often restricted. Inhalants such as enflurane and isoflurane can also produce muscle relaxation or enhance the action of the nondepolarizing agents. Muscle relaxants can also prevent shivering, a normal homeostatic mechanism used to combat cold.

Shivering can increase an adult's metabolism and heat production by as much as 20 to 50 percent (Maclean & Emslie-Smith, 1977). It can actually prevent hypothermia despite large drops in environmental temperature. But the patient who has received muscle relaxants and is cold may not be able to shiver.

Finally, anesthetics can produce hypothermia by causing vasodilation. They increase the diameter of blood vessels, resulting in increased exposure of circulating blood and subsequent heat loss. Halothane, spinal, and epidural anesthesia are particularly effective in causing such vasodilation.

It is unfortunate that conditions in the operating room and anesthetic administration can create such hypothermic states. When muscle relaxants are used, hypothermia can actually potentiate their action and prevent shivering. If shivering does occur, however, oxygen demands can be increased by as much as 400 to 500 percent (Vaughan, 1981a). The patient with cardiac or respiratory disease may have difficulty adapting to a hypothermic state. Cardiac output and oxygen uptake must be drastically increased or ischemia and metabolic acidosis will result.

Vaughan recognized the significance of postoperative hypothermia. In a 1981 study, she examined frequency and duration of hypothermia in 198 adult PACU patients. Defining hypothermia as a temperature below 36° C, data indicated that 60 percent of the patients displayed subnormal temperatures on admission to the PACU. Type of surgery, age, and anesthesia were all indicative of hypothermia. And in spite of an average 82-minute stay, 13 percent of the patients were discharged still hypothermic (Vaughan, 1981a).

Awareness of the incidence of hypothermia in postoperative patients can prevent or at least decrease the severity of the condition. Gases and cold body solutions administered in the operating room should be warmed. Surgical drapes should be changed to avoid evaporative heat loss. In the PACU, heated oxygen and warm blankets should be applied;

hot water bottles may also be used. Special attention should be given to covering the patient's head and feet, as a great deal of heat loss can occur from these areas. As in the operating room, body fluids such as blood and irrigation solutions should be warmed. Patients may be anxious because they feel so cold. Reassuring them that this condition is only temporary may alleviate the fears.

Temperatures should be closely monitored throughout the surgical procedure and during the postoperative period. Axillary temperature is often the most direct and accurate route, unless a continuous temperature probe remains in place.

Case Study

Fifty-nine-year-old Melissa Adams underwent an exploratory laparotomy, lysis of adhesions, total abdominal hysterectomy, and partial omentectomy. The procedure lasted 5 hours. Anesthesia included isoflurane, fentanyl, and DTC; muscle relaxant was reversed. Estimated blood loss was 700 cc; the patient received two units of PRBCs in the operating room.

Temperature on admission to the PACU was 90.7° axillary. The patient was very sleepy and did not shiver. Her skin was cool and slightly dusky; vital signs were stable.

Heated oxygen and warming blankets were initially applied. After 2 hours, the patient was more awake, but temperature remained only 92.4° axillary. Five hours after admission, the patient was finally normothermic at 97.5° axillary, and discharged from the PACU in stable condition.

Analysis

Melissa Adams was the victim of hypothermia. The length of the surgical procedure, the injection of cold body fluids, the type of surgery the patient underwent, and the administration of anesthesia were all factors in the development of this condition.

Perhaps her temperature should have been more closely monitored in the operating room. The gases, blood, and irrigations she received were obviously not warmed prior to their administration. The admission temperature of 90.7° axillary was a complication that could have been avoided. Hypothermia placed her at greater risk and prolonged her stay in the PACU.

Chapter 12 offers a nursing care plan for hypothermic patients developed by Borchardt and Fraulini (1982). It is important to stress that effective treatment of inadvertent hypothermia and shivering in adults remains elusive. PACU heat-transfer treatments of radiation (heat lamps) and conduction (warmed thermal and cotton bath blankets) do not increase core (TM) body temperature or decrease the duration of hypothermia compared to nonheat-treated (no external heat) patients (Vaughan, 1980). Interestingly, several investigators (most recently Bourke & associates, 1984) have used a reflective blanket for intraoperative heat conservation. The material, TYVEK type 1443, is used as lining in survival apparel and apparently reduces radiant heat loss.

The hypothesis of changing the gradient between peripheral and core body temperature and thus decreasing shivering by application of radiation or conductive heat is not verified by controlled clinical studies.

Overall body temperature increases can be demonstrated in all PACU patients simply by maintaining ambient temperature (21° to 23°), humidity (55 ± 10 percent), and cessation of anesthesia and operation. The former affects the gradient for heat loss from the body, while the latter principally affects heat loss (i.e., vasodilation, heat loss by radiation, conduction, convection, and evaporation). In addition, normal homeostatic mechanisms (motor activity, shivering and nonshivering thermogenesis) operant in the homeotherm influences the return of the postoperative hypothermic patient to normothermia.

Heat-transfer treatments, such as warming blankets and radiant heat, which may be effective in increasing body temperature in infants, cannot be expected to maintain thermal balance in adults. Further, clinicians have hypothesized that external heat application (radiation) can cause peripheral vasodilitation and redistribution of blood flow from core body organs to the periphery, resulting in increased body heat loss (Vaughan, 1982).

The use of blankets may have merit in eliminating further body heat loss by reducing body surface area exposure. Also, from the standpoint of psychological benefit to the patient and staff, application of warmed blankets initiates a positive nursing approach to patient care and may contribute to the patient's overall feeling of well-being.

Postanesthetic Shivering (PAS)

Clinical interpretation of research regarding shivering is limited by the lack of uniform definitions, reliability and validity checks, and multiple raters, by nonrandomization of research groups, and subjective measurements. Nevertheless, PACU studies have allowed a general differentiation of type and incidence of shivering as well as identification of a time sequence seen in the patient recovering from anesthesia (Vaughan, 1982).

Spastic Shivering.   The term *shivering* has generally been applied to any muscular tremor observed in patients recovering from both general and regional anesthesia. Recently, however, two distinct types of shivering have been identified in patients recovering from general anesthesia. The first, spastic shivering, is defined as sustained muscular hypertonicity often observed in the masseters, platysma, pectorals, upper limb flexors and extensors, and abductors of the lower extremities. This type of shivering occurs in the first 15 minutes of anesthetic recovery and has an average duration of 6 to 7 minutes. Spasticity decreases with increasing levels of consciousness. Reported incidences of spastic shivering follow halothane (Fluothane); nitrous oxide, enflurane (Ethrane); nitrous oxide, and nitrous oxide; narcotic general anesthesia. However, no statistically significant differences can be identified among general anesthetic types (Vaughan).

Hypothermic Shivering

The second shivering differentiation can be described as rhythmic contractions of muscle groups ranging from mild to severe in intensity with irregular, intermittent periods of relaxation. This type, hypothermic shivering, relates to regaining thermal balance, and is one of three major heat-gain mechanisms (behavioral activity, shivering, and nonshivering thermogenesis). Such muscle activity is characterized as an "on or off" rather than a graded response. Hypothermic shivering initiates a metabolic response and is induced by a temperature gradient between peripheral and core body temperatures. Arterial blood oxygen tension measurements taken during hypothermic shivering have been reported in the range of 50 to 60 torr.

Recent data demonstrate that, regardless of age or sex, hypothermic patients shiver significantly more than do normothermic patients at 30 and 45 minutes after admission to the PACU. However, hypothermic patients do not differ significantly in incidence of shivering from normothermic patients on PACU admission or at 15 minutes after PACU admission. This evidence indicates that different types of shivering (spastic and hypothermic shivering) occur at different times during emergence from anesthesia. Further, shivering observed at 30 and 45 minutes after PACU admission signals a continuing hypothermic state.

The clinical implications of observed shivering must be evaluated in terms of type and duration of shivering coupled with the patient's level of consciousness and preoperative physical status. Nursing care can be planned using the knowledge that PAS is differentiated into types having a characteristic time sequence.

MALIGNANT HYPERTHERMIA

Malignant hyperthermia is another type of thermal imbalance that can be directly related to the administration of anesthesia. It is a rare anesthetic hazard characterized by the sudden onset of extremely high body temperature after the patient has received anesthesia. During this state of accelerated metabolism, body temperature may increase by as much as 1° C every 5 minutes (Gronert, 1980).

Besides the extreme elevations in body temperature, tachycardia, tachypnea, blood pressure fluctuations, restlessness, sweating, and muscle rigidity are characteristic signs and symptoms of malignant hyperthermia. Metabolic and respiratory acidosis develop rapidly. Unless the syndrome is recognized and treatment begun, malignant hyperthermia will prove fatal.

According to Gronert, malignant hyperthermia is due to "an inability to control calcium concentrations within the muscle fiber; it may involve generalized alterations in membrane permeability." Calcium release in the muscle fiber is increased and sustained, leading to greater heat production and oxygen consumption (Gronert, 1980).

Rodgers cites the incidence of malignant hyperthermia at one per 50,000 adult anesthesized patients (Rodgers, 1983). Research indicates the tendency to develop the syndrome is inherited. Susceptible patients often display minor muscle abnormalities such as cleft palate, hernia, muscle cramps, ptosis, and curvature of the spine (Zahorian, 1981). Preoperative CPK levels may be moderately elevated in such patients Unfortunately, muscle biopsy may be the only reliable determinant of a patient's susceptibility to the condition. (Gronert, 1980).

Studies have shown that men are more prone to developing this hypermetabolic state, and that the 16 to 30 age group is most susceptible (Thomas, 1981). Inhalants, succinylcholine, tricyclic antidepressants, MAO inhibitors, and phenothiazine agents have all been implicated in the production of malignant hyperthermia. Despite increasing knowledge and awareness of the condition, the mortality rate was estimated at 28 percent in 1976 (Gronert, 1980).

Successful treatment of the condition rests upon immediate intraoperative recognition. Surgery should be stopped and anesthesia discontinued when malignant hyperthermia is suspected. In the PACU or the intensive unit, every effort to monitor the patient closely and decrease his or her body temperature should be made. The patient should initially be placed on a cardiac monitor and receive high concentrations of oxygen. Continuous and accurate monitoring of temperature and vital signs should be performed. A cooling mattress, sponge baths, and ice packs should be utilized to reduce temperature, and immediate blood gas and serum electrolyte analysis should be performed. Often the physician will order several amps of sodium bicarbonate even before blood gas results return, as the development of respiratory and metabolic acidosis is rapid.

Currently, dantrolene sodium is the only drug used to actively combat malignant hyperthermia. Acting directly on muscle calcium movements, the drug is initially prescribed in intravenous doses of 1 mg/kg.

Case Study

Beth Jones, 28 years old, underwent what was supposed to be a routine D&C and tubal ligation. Significant preoperative history was essentially negative; the patient's only problem was occasional episodes of muscle cramping, for which she took Tylenol.

Halothane and succinylcholine were administered preoperatively. Since the procedure was short, temperature was not monitored during the intraoperative period. On admission to the PACU, Jones was noted to be diaphoretic, very warm to touch, tachycardic, and tachypneic. Muscle rigidity was also displayed. Temperature was recorded as 39° C.

Analysis

As a young woman with a history of muscle cramps, Jones was susceptible to the development of malignant hyperthermia. Inhalant and succinylcholine triggered the rare syndrome.

IMPAIRED CARDIOVASCULAR PERFORMANCE

The stress of surgery and the administration of anesthesia can produce a number of alterations in cardiovascular performance. Cardiac arrhythmias, hypertension, or hypotension may be witnessed in the postanesthetic patient. And if the patient has a significant preoperative cardiac history, angina, myocardial infarction, congestive heart failure, and pulmonary edema may result.

Cardiac Arrhythmias

Cardiac arrhythmias associated with anesthesia and operation were first reported by Levine in 1920 (Atkinson, 1982). Sixty-five years later, advanced medical research and knowledge has created a multitude of anesthetic agents and surgical procedures, many of which can alter normal cardiac rate and rhythm in the operating room and in the PACU (see Table 10-4).

Bertrand examined the incidence of supraventricular and ventricular dysrhythmias in 100 patients undergoing surgery with general anesthesia. Results revealed that 84 percent of the patients in his study displayed some sort of arrhythmia intraoperatively, while 47 percent had alterations in cardiac rhythm during the recovery period itself. Supraventricular arrhythmias consisted of premature atrial contractions, premature nodal contractions, nodal rhythms, nodal tachycardia, and supraventricular tachycardia.

The incidence of supraventricular arrhythmias was similar in patients with or without preexisting cardiac disease. Ventricular arrhythmias, however, occurred with much greater frequency in patients with a history of cardiac disease. These included unifocal and multifocal premature ventricular contractions and three instances of ventricular tachycardia. The incidence of sinus tachycardia and bradycardia was not considered in the study (Bertrand, 1971).

These findings illustrate the ability of anesthesia and operation to alter normal cardiac rate and rhythm. The patient may display sinus tachycardia, sinus bradycardia, supraventricular, and ventricular arrhythmias in the immediate postoperative period.

TABLE 10–4. ANESTHETIC AGENTS AND
DISTURBANCES IN CARDIAC RHYTHM

Agent	Arrhythmia
Atropine	Sinus tachycardia
Doxapram	Sinus tachycardia
Enflurane	Sinus bradycardia, sinus tachycardia, nodal rhythm, PVCs, PACs, AV dissociation
Fentanyl	Sinus bradycardia
Glycopyrrolate	Sinus tachycardia
Halothane	Sinus bradycardia, nodal rhythm, PVCs, AV dissociation, ventricular tachycardia, ventricular fibrillation
Inapsine	Sinus tachycardia
Isoflurane	Sinus tachycardia
Ketamine	Sinus tachycardia
Naloxone	Sinus tachycardia, PVCs, ventricular tachycardia, ventricular fibrillation
Pancuronium	Nodal rhythm
Physostigmine	Sinus bradycardia
Pyridostigmine	Sinus bradycardia
Thiopentone	Sinus tachycardia

Sinus Tachycardia. A rapid heart rate of greater than 100 beats per minute with impulses originating in the sinoatrial node is considered sinus tachycardia. Internal and external stimuli activate the sympathetic nervous system to release catecholamines, thereby stimulating the heart to increase its rate (Hudak, 1973).

Sinus tachycardia as a physiological response to stress is probably the most common arrhythmia witnessed in the PACU. Pain and discomfort can increase heart rate significantly. Anxiety can also trigger tachycardia. Heart rate, too, will increase during the presence of emergence delirium or the central anticholinergic syndrome.

The hypovolemia resulting from operation will also produce tachycardia. And anesthesia's ability to alter normal respiratory and metabolic processes will increase heart rate as well. Hypoxia, hypercarbia, and malignant hyperthermia can produce tachycardia.

Anesthesia and anesthetic adjuncts can also create tachycardic states. Thiopentone increases heart rate significantly but briefly. Ketamine, a sympathetic nervous system stimulant, has been shown to increase preoperative heart rate by as much as 33 percent (Bruce, 1980). Heart rate may also be increased when the inhalants enflurane and isoflurane are administered. These agents decrease stroke volume, and the heart attempts to compensate and maintain cardiac output by increasing rate.

Supplemental anesthetic agents such as nalbuphine (Nubain) and droperidol (Inapsine) can also induce tachycardia. Narcotic and muscle relaxant reversal agents can increase heart rate as well. Narcan increases heart rate by heightening sensations of pain and discomfort. The anticholinergic agents atropine and robinul can also cause increases in heart rate. Still another agent that can produce tachycardia is the respiratory stimulant doxapram (Dopram).

Nursing Intervention

The sinus tachycardia produced by anesthetic agents is usually self-limiting. Heart rate will gradually return to normal limits as the action of the anesthetic decreases and metabolism of the drug occurs. Treatment is seldom necessary.

In other instances, sinus tachycardia is a signal of an underlying clinical problem. Treatment is aimed at recognizing and correcting the disorder that precipitated the arrhythmia. Astute nursing assessment is essential.

Finally, the pain, anxiety, and confusion that can elevate heart rate should be alleviated. Emotional support and explanation of all procedures should be given. Pain medications should be administered judiciously. And repeated attempts at reorientation should be made if the patient is confused.

Sinus Bradycardia. A heart rate of less than 60 beats per minute, with impulses originating from the sinoatrial node, is considered sinus bradycardia. This arrhythmia is a product of excessive parasympathetic nervous system activity.

Vagal stimulation can produce sinus bradycardia. Common postoperative activities such as gagging, vomiting, straining, and breathholding stimulate the vagus nerve and the parasympathetic nerve to the heart, and the rate of impulse formation by the sinoatrial node is decreased.

The administration of anesthesia can also lower heart rates considerably. Spinal anesthesia involves a sympathetic blockade, interrupting nerve impulse transmission. If any of the nerve roots carrying sympathetic cardiac accelerator fibers are blocked, as in high spinals above T4–5, heart rate will be slowed. The Bainbridge effect is another cause of bradycardia. Blood pressure is lowered in the right atrium because of decreased venous return, and slower pulse rates result (Atkinson, 1982).

Intravenous anesthetic agents such as fentanyl and morphine can also produce bradycardia. Inhalants such as nitrous oxide and halothane reduce heart rate as well. Halothane has actually been shown to decrease the heart's rate of spontaneous beating by as much as 16 percent (Prys-Roberts, 1980). Reversal agents can also decrease pulse rate significantly. Physostigmine, pyridostigmine (Regonol), and neostigmine all have bradycardia-producing effects. Atropine or robinul is usually administered with the muscle relaxant reversals to counteract such bradycardia.

Nursing Intervention

Continuous monitoring and assessment are important in the bradycardic postoperative patient. Bradycardia can reduce blood pressure as well as precipitate more serious arrhythmias such as ventricular dysrhythmias. Slower heart rates may be benign in the healthy young adult, but the older patient or the patient with underlying cardiac disease may be in jeopardy.

Anesthesia-induced bradycardia is sometimes prolonged, as in the case of the spinal. Frequent vital signs and assessment of skin color and temperature will determine the patient's response to such bradycardia. Heart rates below 50 often require treatment. Atropine is often the agent of choice.

Bradycardia due to reversal agents and vagal stimulation is usually brief and self-resolving. The patient with limited cardiac reserves, however, may be at risk if vagal stimulation persists. Nursing care is then directed at relieving the frequent or prolonged vomiting, gagging, straining, and breathholding that have precipitated the problem.

Supraventricular Arrhythmias. Supraventricular arrhythmias involve impulse formation from either an ectopic atrial focus or from the atrioventricular node. Heart rate and rhythm will vary depending on the location of this new pacemaker. In the postanesthetic patient, supraventricular arrhythmias include premature atrial contractions, premature nodal contractions, nodal rhythm, and supraventricular tachycardia. Stress, surgical stimulation, underlying heart disease, and anesthetic agents can all precipitate the development of such rhythm disturbances.

Surgical stimulation can evoke a hypertensive response leading tc parasympathetic excitation (Price & Ohnishi, 1980). Vagal nerves are stimulated and acetylcholine is released. This hormone both decreases the rate and rhythm of the sinoatrial node and lowers the excitability of the atrioventricular junctional fibers (Guyton, 1971). Impulse transmission decreases, and an ectopic atrial focus or the AV node may become the new pacemaker. Supraventricular arrhythmias will result.

Anesthetic agents may also impair conduction. The volatile anesthetics Halothane and enflurane decrease sympathetic nervous system activity and catecholamine release. Conduction of the SA impulse becomes progressively delayed as concentrations of these agents are increased. A variety of supraventricular rhythms, particularly nodal rhythm, may result.

Supraventricular tachycardia has been reported to occur most frequently in patients over 70 years of age; individuals undergoing intraabdominal, intrathoracic, or major vascular procedures; and patients who display rales preoperatively. The presence of underlying cardiac or pulmonary disease does not necessarily predict the incidence of SVT (Goldman & associates, 1982).

Such arrhythmias include atrial fibrillation or flutter, paroxysmal atrial tachycardia, and nodal tachycardia. Besides age, surgical procedure, and preoperative rales, underlying conditions can precipitate the development of SVT. Potassium imbalance, hypoxia, hypotension, acidosis, anemia, or infection may be responsible for the development of SVT in the postanesthetic patient. Myocardial ischemia, congestive heart failure, pulmonary embolism, and pericarditis have also been cited as causative factors (Goldman & associates, 1982).

Nursing Intervention
Nursing care of the patient displaying supraventricular arrhythmias demands accurate determination of the arrhythmia and assessment of its effect on the patient. Premature atrial contractions, premature nodal contractions, and nodal rhythms are usually benign, resolving as the effects of surgery and anesthesia decrease. If such arrhythmias persist, however, the patient may become hypotensive, dyspneic, and diaphoretic. Atropine is usually the agent of choice in such cases.

Such prolonged supraventricular arrhythmias, as well as certain physiological states, may result in the development of SVT. Treatment of the underlying condition may correct the arrhythmia. Propranolol, Verapamil, and Digoxin administration may also prove necessary.

Ventricular Arrhythmias. The most serious and life-threatening disturbances in cardiac rate and rhythm are ventricular arrhythmias. Unfortunately, the process of surgery and the administration of anesthesia can produce premature ventricular contractions, ventricular tachycardia, and even ventricular fibrillation.

Premature ventricular contractions (PVCs) are contractions arising from one or more ectopic foci in the ventricle. They can be unifocal, multifocal, and patterned. PVCs are the most common of all arrhythmias, and can occur in any age group, regardless of the presence of heart disease (Hudak, 1973).

Ventricular tachycardia is the result of one ectopic focus emitting rapid and regular impulses. Atrial contractions are totally dissociated from the ventricular contraction.

PVCs or ventricular tachycardia sometimes lead to the development of ventricular fibrillation, which involves rapid, irregular ventricular contractions that are incapable of maintaining perfusion.

Walton examined the intraoperative incidence of ventricular arrhythmias during anesthetic induction, intubation, and extubation. She found that 33 percent of her control group displayed ventricular arrhythmias, older patients suffering from such disturbances in heart rate much more frequently than the young. From these observations, she was able to identify certain risk factors that could precipitate ventricular arrhythmias. These included a history of cardiac disease, hypertension, drug interaction, and electrolyte disturbances (Walton & associates, 1982).

These factors can precipitate the development of ventricular arrhythmias in the operating room and in the PACU. Potassium imbalance is of particular significance, even in patients with no previous history of cardiac disease. Nasogastric suctioning, vomiting, and prolonged antihypertensive and diuretic therapy can deplete potassium reserves and produce ventricular arrhythmias. Hypokalemia, according to Surawicz, "increases automaticity of Purkinje fibers, transforms nonpacemaker fibers into pacemaker fibers, prolongs terminal repolarization, and increases the differences between action potential durations of Purkinje and ventricular fibers" (Surawicz, 1984).

Hyperkalemia can be a product of overzealous treatment of hypokalemia or of acidosis, as well as preexisting renal dysfunction. Elevated potassium levels can produce ventricular arrhythmias by slowing conduction and depressing pacemaker activity.

Hypoxia and hypercarbia, fairly common states created by anesthesia, can also precipitate ventricular arrhythmias. The presence of an endotracheal tube, pain, and emotional irritability can alter normal cardiac rhythm as well. And anesthetics themselves can create ventricular arrhythmias by impairing normal conduction. The presence of hypoxia and hypercarbia, especially, can increase ventricular irritability if anesthetics are used.

Unfortunately, the inhalant Halothane is particularly effective in altering cardiac rate and rhythm. The arrythmias most commonly observed include nodal rhythms, premature ventricular contractions, and ventricular bigeminy. Such ventricular excitation can lead to the development of more serious arrhythmias, such as ventricular tachycardia and fibrillation. Halothane also sensitizes the myocardium to catecholamines, and drugs such as epinephrine should be avoided or used with caution.

Nursing Intervention

Nursing care of the patient who displays ventricular arrhythmias involves immediate recognition and prompt intervention. Rare unifocal PVCs are usually benign. If the monitor reveals frequent unifocal or multifocal PVCs, patterned PVCs, or the R-on-T phenomenon, however, treatment should be initiated. A lidocaine bolus may prove effective in abolishing such ventricular irritability until the underlying cause can be determined.

Vital signs, skin color, and temperature should be ascertained. Any subjective complaints by the patient should also be considered. Blood gas and serum potassium levels should be drawn. While awaiting such results, the patient should be stimulated and encouraged to deep-breathe, particularly if the level of consciousness is decreased. The monitor should also be closely observed for the frequency of ventricular ectopic beats, as well as for presence of a U wave or a narrow, peaked T wave, which may indicate the presence of hypokalemia or hyperkalemia.

Frequent PVCs can lead to the development of ventricular tachycardia and fibrillation. It is important to prevent the development of these arrhythmias because of their serious and life-threatening nature. Ventricular tachycardia will require more vigorous antiarrhythmic drug therapy, while CPR and countershock will be necessary when ventricular fibrillation occurs.

Case Study

Twenty-nine-year-old Barbara Adams underwent an exploratory laparotomy and splenectomy, receiving fentanyl 11 cc, isoflurane, and diazepam 10 mg during the procedure.

The patient was sleepy but easily arousable on admission to the PACU. The monitor showed a normal sinus rhythm in the 80s without ectopy. Thirty minutes later, however, the patient suddenly went into ventricular bigeminy. Lidocaine 100 mg IV was administered with temporary eradication of the PVCs. Unfortunately, they recurred about 20 minutes later. Blood-gas analysis revealed the patient was hypercarbic; frequent stimulation and efforts at increasing ventilation resulted in the disappearance of the arrhythmia. The patient remained PVC-free for one hour before her discharge from the PACU.

Analysis

The ventricular bigeminy displayed by this patient was the result of hypoventilation. The anesthetic agents the patient had received decreased her respiratory rate and depth, and desensitized her to CO_2 buildup. Such action resulted in the development of ventricular arrhythmias.

Case Study

For an exploratory laparotomy and hemicolectomy, 58-year-old Martha Edwards received a combination of narcotic-inhalant-relaxant anesthesia during the procedure. The patient was stable on admission to the PACU. The cardiac monitor showed a sinus rhythm in the 90s without ectopy.

One hour after admission, the nurse noted that the patient's nasogastric tube had been putting out large amounts of material. She also observed the patient's pulse to be very irregular. A look at the monitor revealed frequent multifocal PVCs. A lidocaine bolus was administered and a potassium level drawn. Results indicated the patient was hypokalemic. Potassium was 2.8.

Analysis

The hypokalemia produced by excessive loss of gastric secretions can result in the development of ventricular arrhythmias. Such was the case with this patient.

Case Study

Charles Lindsay underwent a right thoracotomy and lower lobectomy under Halothane anesthesia. He appeared awake and uncomfortable but stable on admission to the PACU; BP was 124/80, heart rate 96 and regular, and respiratory rate 24 and shallow. The patient was encouraged to deep-breathe after pain medication was administered.

Such stability proved only temporary, however. The patient became progressively hypotensive, tachycardic, and tachypneic. The monitor revealed a sinus tachycardia of 130 with intermittent episodes of supraventricular tachycardia. The pleurevac was putting out large amounts of sanguineous material; hemoglobin and hematocrit tests confirmed that the patient was hemorrhaging. Blood administration and a return to the operating room became necessary.

Analysis
Because this patient underwent intrathoracic surgery and also developed hypovolemia and hemorrhage, he was at greater risk for the development of SVT in the postanesthetic period.

Alterations in Blood Pressure
The level of blood pressure is the end result of many factors. It is dependent on total peripheral resistance, stroke volume, heart rate, and blood volume. The stress of surgery and the administration of anesthesia can affect blood pressure by altering any of these variables. Hypertensive and hypotensive states will result, and are probably among the most frequent complications the postanesthetic patient will experience.

Hypertension. Hypertension involves an increase in peripheral resistance due to sustained vasoconstriction throughout the body. High arterial pressure after operation and anesthesia is usually the result of increased sympathetic nervous system activity and catecholamine release in response to stress, although other factors, such as fluid overload, age, preexisting renal disease, and preoperative history of hypertension are also contributory.

The vasomotor center in the pons and medulla simultaneously stimulates sympathetic nerve fibers to vasoconstrict and the adrenal medulla to secrete the catecholamines norepinephrine and epinephrine. Norepinephrine and epinephrine are potent vasoconstrictors, increasing peripheral resistance and blood pressure. Hypertension will result.

A variety of factors can elicit this response. The reaction to surgical stimulation is one of stress. And pain and anxiety increase sympathetic nervous system activity significantly. Anesthetic-induced alterations in mental status, such as emergence delirium and the central anticholinergic syndrome, are other conditions that can elevate blood pressure. Difficulty in micturition, too, may be a factor.

Many anesthetics inhibit sympathetic nervous system activity. But use of the dissociative anesthetic ketamine can trigger hypertension. Ketamine is a sympathetic nervous system stimulant, elevating both heart rate and blood pressure. Reversal of narcotic anesthesia by the agent naloxone can also increase blood pressure significantly.

Hypoxemia and hypercarbia are other anesthetic-related occurrences that can precipitate blood pressure elevations. Carotid and aortic bodies contain chemoreceptors sensitive to O_2 and CO_2 fluctuations. As oxygen levels decrease and carbon dioxide levels increase, chemoreceptors excite the vasomotor center, and vasoconstriction and hypertension result (Guyton, 1971).

Nursing Intervention
Nursing care of the patient with hypertension involves accurate assessment to determine the underlying cause. Is the patient restless and confused? Is he or she anxious? Does the patient complain of severe pain? Physostigmine, sedation, or analgesic administration may be necessary to calm the patient and reduce blood pressure.

Bladder distention and difficulty voiding can also produce hypertension. The patient's bladder should be checked. If it seems distended, the patient should be encouraged to void. Catheterization will be necessary if the patient cannot.

The type of anesthesia the patient has received should also be considered. If ketamine has been administered, blood pressure will probably return to normal limits without treatment. Volatile anesthetics and narcotics, however, are potent respiratory depressants that can produce hypoxemia and hypercarbia and elevate blood pressure. Inadequate muscle relaxant reversal can also make ventilation poor. Treatment is aimed at frequent stimulation of the patient to deep-breathe, thereby increasing oxygen levels and expelling CO_2. Muscle strength should be determined as well. If hypoventilation persists, reversal or ventilatory assistance may be necessary.

Hypertension as a response to the stress of surgery may or may not require treatment. Patients with a history of hypertension or cardiac disease may display elevated blood pressure long after operation has been completed. Administration of antihypertensive agents may become necessary, depending on the severity of the hypertension. The other factors that can elevate blood pressure should be examined, however, before such treatment is initiated.

Case Study

Ninety-year-old Elma Jones had an exploratory laparotomy and cholecystectomy. Enflurane was the main anesthetic agent used during the procedure; muscle relaxation was achieved by DTC administration and reversed.

The patient remained intubated and difficult to arouse on admission to the PACU. Although she had a history of hypertension, blood pressure was dangerously high at 220/120. Daily antihypertensive medication had been withheld prior to surgery. Spirometry revealed low tidal volumes and irregular respiration. Ventilatory assistance became necessary. Blood pressure still remained quite high, however, and hydralazine 10 mg IV was administered. This placed blood pressures at more acceptable, though still elevated, ranges.

Forty-five minutes after admission, the patient was more awake and maintaining adequate respirations. She was extubated and immediately complained of pain. Blood pressure increased to 190/120. Pain medication was then administered, and blood pressure dropped to the patient's preoperative range of 170/90.

Analysis

Several factors made Elma Jones more susceptible to the development of hypertension in the immediate postoperative period. Her age and her history of hypertension predisposed her to the condition. The fact that antihypertensives were withheld prior to surgery also placed her at greater risk.

The stress of major abdominal surgery and the hypoventilation produced by anesthesia were other significant factors. The presence of an endotracheal tube also elevated her blood pressure, as did the pain she experienced when she was extubated and awake.

Hypotension. McGovern defines hypotension as a fall in systolic blood pressure to less than 90 mm Hg, or a 50 mm Hg fall in an individual whose blood pressure was elevated above the normal range (McGovern & Tillen, 1980). Depending on blood volume, hypotension can be a direct complication of the operative procedure itself. Surgical blood loss can result in hypovolemia, hemorrhage, or even shock, each of which may produce drastic reductions in arterial pressure.

Anesthetics, too, are responsible for the production of hypotension in the postanesthetic patient. They can decrease peripheral resistance and depress myocardial function significantly.

Decreased total peripheral resistance can be caused by vasodilation. Certain anesthetics have direct depressant and vasodilating effects on vascular smooth muscle. Such inhibition in vascular tone is dose-dependent; the higher the concentration of the agent used, the greater will be the inhibition. In his study of vascular smooth muscle and general anesthesia, Altura postulates that anesthetics could interfere with calcium mobility both at the vascular membranes and intracellularly. He also noted that the action of narcotic drugs on the peripheral circulation is very variable. Analgesics such as morphine, meperidine, and fentanyl can cause constriction, dilation, or have no effect on the peripheral circulation (Altura, 1980).

Of the inhalants, halothane has the greatest direct vasodilating properties. Barbiturates such as thiopentone also decrease peripheral resistance by causing vasodilation.

Studies have shown that general anesthetics can inhibit sympathetic nervous system activity and decrease catecholamine release. Enflurane can cause marked inhibition of epinephrine and norepinephrine secretion from the adrenal medulla (Gothert & Wendt, 1977). Halothane is also a sympathetic suppressant (Atkinson, 1982). And fentanyl can reduce cate-cholamine release as well (Benumof, 1983). Such actions can alter the stress response considerably besides creating hypotension.

Normally, the vasomotor center in the brain stimulates sympathetic nerve fibers to vasoconstrict and the adrenal medulla to secrete catecholamines. Anesthetics, however, can depress the activity of the vasomotor center. Halothane anesthesia, particularly, has been implicated in this action (Atkinson, 1982).

The baroreceptors are stretch receptors located in the heart and blood vessels which operate to stabilize blood pressure. Blood pressure rises will stimulate the baroreceptors to inhibit vasoconstrictor nerves, while falls will decrease baroreceptor activity and increase catecholamine release. The inhalants Halothane and enflurane have been shown to sensitize these structures, making blood pressure recording by them inaccurate. Conditions that can create hypotension may not activate compensatory barostatic reflexes (Price, 1967).

Spinal anesthesia is a deliberate sympathetic denervation. No arteries or arterioles become constricted following the sympathetic blockade of the spinal. Vasoconstriction can occur only in areas the spinal has not affected (Greene, 1976). Vasodilation is profound, decreasing peripheral resistance and blood pressure.

In addition to decreasing peripheral resistance, anesthetics can cause myocardial depression. Cardiac output is dependent on both stroke volume and heart rate. Unfortunately, normal cardiac function is often altered by anesthesia. Anesthetics can decrease myocardial contractility and ventricular performance, affect the electrical activity of cardiac cells, and inhibit sympathetic nervous system activity and catecholamine release. By their hypotensive, vasodilating action they can also decrease venous return to the heart. Thus, anesthetics are potent cardiac depressants, affecting stroke volume and heart rate, and decreasing myocardial function. Their ability to reduce cardiac output can result in hypotensive states.

Nursing Intervention

Obviously, the postanesthetic patient is very susceptible to the development of hypotension. The surgical procedure and the administration of anesthesia can create hypotensive conditions demanding treatment.

Nursing care of the hypotensive patient involves accurate assessment. Hypovolemia seems to be the most common cause of hypotension. Intraoperative blood loss and fluid administration should be examined. The incision site, as well as any drains or tubes, should be examined for signs of active bleeding.

Normal signs and symptoms of hypovolemia and hemorrhage may be less obvious when anesthesia has been administered. Anesthetics can produce restlessness and anxiety, cause hypotension, decrease urine output, lower body temperature, and make the patient thirsty. Such conditions are also signs and symptoms of hemorrhage and shock. Cardiac rate can be accelerated or reduced by anesthetics, in contrast to the tachycardia of hypovolemia and hemorrhage. CVP measurements and hemoglobin and hematocrit determination are thus essential.

Anesthetic-created hypotension may be self-resolving. Or it may demand active treatment with reversals or fluid administration. Supine or Trendelenburg position will temporarily increase blood pressure. The hypotension of spinal anesthesia is best resolved with the adrenergic agent ephedrine.

Case Study

Rose Dolan, a 39-year-old woman who had a simple mastectomy, became restless, hypotensive, and tachycardic shortly after admission to the PACU. The monitor revealed a sinus tachycardia of 120; BP was 90/60. Undetected by the nurse, the patient's hemovac was putting out large amounts of blood. The nurse attributed the patient's state to her anesthesia, which consisted of enflurane and fentanyl. Twenty minutes after admission, BP dropped to 70/40 and heart rate increased to 150. The anesthesiologist and the surgical service were notified and immediately came to see the patient, who was hemorrhaging.

Analysis

Anesthetics can mask the signs and symptoms of hemorrhage. The restlessness, tachycardia, and hypotension produced by anesthesia made the recognition of hemorrhage more difficult. However, proper assessment of the incision site and drain would have alerted the nurse immediately to the development of hemorrhage.

Compromised Cardiac Status

Angina and Myocardial Infarction. The delicate balance between myocardial oxygen supply and demand is usually maintained in the healthy surgical patient. Unfortunately, however, operation and anesthesia can compromise such homeostasis in the patient with preexisting cardiac disease. Oxygen supply can be reduced and demand increased, resulting in the development of angina or myocardial infarction.

Oxygen supply is dependent on both the O_2 content of arterial blood and the coronary blood flow. Hypoxemia and anemia, common states during operation, will reduce the oxygen content of the blood considerably. Hypotension can also deplete oxygen supply by compromising coronary blood flow in the diseased heart. Wynands finds that, in the heart affected by coronary artery disease, "blood flow through the myocardium is related to the degree of narrowing of the main vessels; the greater the narrowing, the more blood flow becomes pressure-dependent. When pressure falls below a critical point, blood flow will cease" (Wynands,

1978). Bradyarrhythmias, too, can decrease coronary blood flow and reduce oxygen supply. Intubation and anesthetic induction can also decrease oxygen supply.

Oxygen demands are increased by any condition that elevates blood pressure, heart rate, myocardial contractility, preload, and afterload (Wynands, 1978). Surgical stimulation, pain, anxiety, and confusion will heighten sympathetic activity and increase blood pressure and heart rate. Metabolic states such as hypothermia and hyperthermia increase myocardial oxygen demand as well. A reduction in preload due to hypovolemia, hemorrhage, or long-standing hypertension will also elevate myocardial oxygen demands, as will the increased afterload caused by valvular disease and left ventricular hypertrophy.

Upset of the critical balance between myocardial oxygen supply and demand can be detrimental to the patient with preoperative heart disease. Angina or myocardial infarction may result. In a study by Roy, ischemic ECG changes in the form of ST depression were observed in 11 of 29 patients with coronary artery disease undergoing noncardiac surgery. The incidence of perioperative infarction, occurring most commonly within the first week of surgery, has been estimated at 3 to 6.6 percent in patients with a history of cardiac disease (Goldmann & associates, 1982). Perioperative stable angina is generally not a significant operative risk, although Sapala found a history of angina and an old infarction had a perioperative mortality rate of 14 percent (Goldmann & associates, 1982). Unstable angina carries a stronger risk.

Rao and associates (1983) studied the incidence of factors related to recurrent perioperative myocardial infarction retrospectively from 1973 to 1976 (group 1) and prospectively from 1977 to 1982 (group 2). Reinfarction occurred in 28 of 364 (7.7 percent) of patients in group 1, and 14 of 733 (1.9 percent) in group 2 ($p < 0.005$). When the previous infarction was from 0 to 3 and from 4 to 6 months old, perioperative reinfarction occurred in 36 and 26 percent of group 1 patients respectively, and in only 5.7 and 2.3 percent of group 2 patients respectively ($p < 0.05$).

The two groups differed primarily in that patients in the prospective group (group 2) had the advantages of newer invasive monitoring (a Swan-Ganz catheter) in the perioperative period, which guided the titration of pharmacologic therapy to achieve the best possible physical status whenever possible; and had the benefit of new cardioactive and vasoactive drugs.

Of particular interest to nurses is the finding that although admission to the intensive care unit did not affect the incidence of reinfarction, the duration of close hemodynamic monitoring in the postoperative period may have played an important role. In group 2 patients, when the postoperative hemodynamic monitoring was done for only up to 24 hours, 8 patients out of the first 210 developed reinfarction (3.8 percent). Following this observation, 439 patients who had an infarction less than 6 months from the time of surgery, or those with associated CHF and/or undergoing upper abdominal surgery, were monitored aggressively for 72 to 96 hours postoperatively. These patients required various cardioactive and/or vasoactive drug interventions based on the hemodynamic monitoring during this period. This resulted in six reinfarctions in the 439 closely monitored and aggressively treated patients in group 2 ($p <$ 0.05).

Research has revealed that hypotension, anesthetic time, and type and timing of surgery can precipitate the development of myocardial infarction in the susceptible patient. A study by Mauney and colleagues (1970) considered a 30 percent reduction in systolic blood pressure for at least 10 minutes significant in producing infarction. The likelihood of infarction was four times greater if hypotension occurred during operation.

The choice of anesthetic technique may have little effect on cardiovascular risk. Mauney found that anesthetic time, not agent, could determine the incidence of ECG changes. Anesthetic time of 165 minutes produced no changes, while 190 minutes of anesthesia generated posterior ST and T-wave changes. Changes consistent with myocardial infarction occurred at 222 minutes of anesthesia (Mauney & associates, 1970). Interestingly, Rao and coworkers (1983) found in the prospective study that patients receiving N_2O, O_2, relaxant and narcotic anesthesia, had a higher incidence of reinfarction compared with other anesthetic drugs. The reason for this difference was not apparent.

The type and timing of surgery is also a factor in the development of ischemia and infarction. Major intraabdominal, intrathoracic, or vascular procedures are considered higher-risk procedures. Emergency surgery may also increase the incidence of infarction in patients with a history of coronary artery disease (Goldmann & associates, 1982).

Nursing Intervention

Nursing care of the postanesthetic patient with significant cardiac history consists of examining oxygen supply and demand. Conditions that affect oxygen supply, such as hypotension, hypoxemia, and anemia, should be prevented or resolved as soon as possible. Situations that increase oxygen demands, such as pain, anxiety, hypertension, hyperthermia, and hypothermia, should be treated as well.

Oxygen should always be administered to the patient who has a history of cardiac disease. Frequent vital signs and careful cardiac surveillance are also essential. ST changes are often the only reliable indicator of ischemia and infarction. The incidence of silent myocardial infarctions is increased after operation. Alterations in levels of consciousness, as well as the presence of narcotics and analgesics, may eliminate subjective complaints of infarction. Incisional pain can also mask the pain of a myocardial infarction.

If the patient does complain of chest pain, nitroglycerine or intravenous morphine administration is essential. Sedation may also prove necessary. The cardiac monitor should be closely observed for the development of arrhythmias that can occur with infarction. AV blocks, ventricular tachycardia, and ventricular fibrillation are among the most common.

In the postanesthetic patient, the diagnosis of infarction cannot be made by CPK, LDH, and SGOT levels. Surgery will elevate these enzymes. CPK isoenzymes and ECG changes are often the only reliable determinants.

Case Study

Michael Harris, a 77-year-old man who had a preoperative history of hypertension and coronary artery disease, underwent a TURP with halothane and fentanyl anesthesia. The patient was hypotensive on admission to the PACU; the monitor revealed a sinus rhythm without ectopy. Blood pressure responded to fluid administration after about 15 minutes. One hour later, ST segment changes in the form of inverted T waves were noted on the monitor. The patient was otherwise asymptomatic, denying complaints of chest pain or shortness of breath. The possibility of a silent subendocardial myocardial infarction was considered. CPK isoenzymes were obtained, and Harris was transported to the MICU for further observation.

Analysis

Because of his age and significant preoperative history, Harris was very susceptible to the development of an infarct. The prolonged hypotension, coupled with the stress of surgery, may have contributed to this state. And the presence of narcotic anesthesia may have masked normal subjective complaints of chest pain.

Case Study

Marvin Black, a 75-year-old male patient with a history of unstable angina, underwent a radical prostatectomy under spinal anesthesia. He was admitted to the PACU with a regular heart of 50 and BP of 110/70. Shortly after admission, however, the patient became severely bradycardic and hypotensive. The monitor revealed a sinus bradycardia of 30 to 35 and BP of 80/50. Atropine was administered with minimal effect. ST depression was then noted, and the patient began to complain of severe chest pain. Nitroglycerine was administered three times without relief. Morphine in 2 mg increments was then given twice, with gradual pain relief. An ECG was performed and isoenzymes obtained to rule out a myocardial infarction.

Analysis

The patient could not tolerate the bradycardia produced by spinal anesthesia. Myocardial oxygen supply was decreased, resulting in ischemia and possible infarction.

Congestive Heart Failure and Pulmonary Edema. Congestive heart failure is the result of the heart's ineffectiveness as a pump. Signs and symptoms include dyspnea, tachycardia, restlessness, anxiety, pulmonary rales, elevated central venous pressure, neck vein distention, and decreased urinary output. A variety of factors associated with operation and anesthesia can produce heart failure. Fluid and sodium overload imposed on the heart during and after surgery can cause a rapid onset of pump failure. Conditions such as fever and hemorrhage can increase the metabolic needs of the body tremendously and also decrease the heart's effectiveness as a pump. Arrhythmias, myocardial infarction, and the decreased myocardial contractility produced by anesthesia are also responsible for the development of congestive heart failure in the postanesthetic patient.

Pulmonary edema is a crisis condition that frequently results from heart failure. The capillary pressure within the lungs may become drastically elevated, and fluid pours from the circulating blood into the alveoli, bronchi, and bronchioles (Luckmann & Sorenson, 1974). Signs and symptoms of pulmonary edema include anxiety, severe dyspnea, tachycardia, pallor, cyanosis, diaphoresis, and production of large amounts of frothy pink sputum.

The presence of CHF preoperatively can be a strong risk factor. In the study by Goldman and associates (1982), a previous history of CHF increased the incidence of perioperative heart failure or pulmonary edema. Patients whose heart failure was under control at the time of surgery had a 6 percent incidence of pulmonary edema and a 5 percent incidence of cardiac death. Individuals who displayed signs and symptoms of CHF immediately prior to surgery had a 16 percent occurrence of pulmonary edema and a 21 percent occurrence of worsening CHF.

Nursing Intervention

After the diagnosis of CHF or pulmonary edema has been made, measures are taken to strengthen the heart and reduce its workload, and to relieve venous congestion. The patient should be placed in a semi-Fowler's position to ease dyspnea. Oxygen administration, cardiac monitoring, frequent vital signs, and CVP measurements are essential. Digitalization, diuretic therapy, and sedation are also vital therapeutic measures. Accurate recording of intake and output is important as well. Since diuresis can lead to hypokalemia, serum potassium levels should be obtained and potassium supplements given when necessary.

Case Study

John McHenry, a 62-year-old man with a history of severe peripheral vascular disease, underwent a left below-the-knee amputation under halothane, ketamine, and fentanyl anesthesia. Estimated blood loss was 75 cc; 900 cc of crystalloid was given intraoperatively.

The patient arrived in the PACU extubated but unstable. The monitor showed a sinus tachycardia of 120. An O_2 mask was applied at 40 percent. Level of consciousness was decreased; breathing was labored with periods of apnea. Color was dusky; skin was cool and diaphoretic. Blood-gas analysis 15 minutes later revealed a pH of 7.17, pCO_2 59, and pO_2 55. The patient was reintubated and placed on a ventilator. A chest x-ray revealed McHenry was in pulmonary edema.

Analysis
The 900 cc of crystalloid that the patient received intraoperatively resulted in fluid overload in a patient whose vascular system was compromised preoperatively. Pulmonary edema resulted. This condition was more difficult to detect, however, because of the respiratory depressant effects of fentanyl and Halothane, and the sympathetic stimulation of ketamine.

Note: Pulmonary edema in the immediate postoperative period may not be due to left ventricular failure. More than half the cases reported in the PACU are preceded by hypertension, suggesting that this problem may be related to the high pulmonary vascular pressures seen in acute postoperative hypertension. Detection is frequently made by the presence of wheezing. Elevation of the CVP and distention of the neck veins are not common findings. Treatment consists of oxygen, fluid restriction, diuresis, control of blood pressure, and mechanical ventilation if necessary.

ALTERATIONS IN URINE PRODUCTION

Decreases in Urine Output
Normally the kidneys receive 20 to 25 percent of the total cardiac output, or 1200 to 1500 ml of blood per minute (Lucas, 1976). The process of surgery and the administration of anesthesia, however, can reduce renal perfusion and subsequently decrease urine output.

Surgical procedures can reduce urine output by creating hypovolemic states. Because the patient was maintained NPO prior to surgery, intravenous fluid replacement may be inadequate. Blood loss during operation can also produce hypovolemia. And if the patient is hypovolemic and blood pressure falls, renal perfusion will be reduced. Renal vascular resistance (RVR), renin secretion, and ADH will increase, while renal blood flow (RBF) and glomerular filtration rate (GFR) will decrease. The end result is a low urine output.

The stress response to surgical stimulation can also decrease urine output significantly. According to Philbin and associates (1979), surgical stimulation results in significant elevations of vasopression (ADH) and epinephrine. Renin secretion is also increased. This results in elevations in vascular resistance and fluid retention, decreasing urine output.

Anesthetics, too, can alter renal function significantly. Their exact mechanism in doing so remains unclear, although the hypotensive, vasodilating effects of certain anesthetics may be responsible. Anesthesia has been shown to decrease RBF and GFR, and elevate RVR and ADH, resulting in decreased urine output.

Decreases in GFR and RBF of up to 50 percent have been reported with the use of halothane anesthesia (Katz & associates, 1981). A study by Deutsch and his colleagues revealed that 1.5 percent halothane anesthesia generated a 19 percent decrease in GFR and a 38 percent decrease in RBF. The use of nitrous-narcotic-muscle relaxant technique produced a 27 percent fall in GFR and a 36 percent decrease in RBF. These studies were performed in the absence of surgical stimulation. Other researchers have examined Innovar and ketamine, and found that these agents cause no change or decrease RBF only slightly (Prys-Roberts, 1980).

Spinal anesthesia itself has little effect on RBF when blood pressure remains normal. (Greene, 1981). However, urine output will decrease if blood pressure falls. According to Katz and associates (1981), "changes in renal function following spinal and epidural anesthesia tend to parallel the degree of sympathetic blockade and the amount of hypotension produced."

Nursing Intervention
Obviously, low urine outputs are common after both surgery and anesthesia. Accurate assessment is important to determine the cause of this problem. Along with decreased urine production, low CVP, cool clammy skin, rapid heart rate, and hypotension may indicate the patient is hypovolemic. Elevated CVP, dyspnea, and tachycardia may be signs of CHF. An accurate look at the fluids the patient has received intraoperatively and the estimated blood loss should be made.

If anesthesia or surgical stimulation is the cause of decreased urine output, drastic action is not necessary. Reduced renal function is only temporary.

In any event, noting the color, amount, and concentration of urine and the patient's general condition is the primary nursing measure in assessing renal function. Proper regulation of IV fluids is also important.

Alteration in Patterns of Urinary Elimination
Urination involves the coordinated action of the internal urethral sphincter, external uretheral sphincter, and the detrusor muscle of the bladder wall. Normally, when the bladder fills with urine, its walls are stretched and the individual experiences sensations of pressure. Voluntary urination then occurs by relaxing the external sphincter and the perineal muscles. (Luckmann & Sorenson, 1974). Surgical procedures and anesthetic agents can alter this normal process of urination and create difficulties in voiding.

The type of surgical procedure will affect the individual's ability to void. The necessity to lie supine after various orthopedic and neurological procedures, for example, makes voiding more difficult. Any procedure where operative handling of the bladder and associated structures is involved will alter normal urinary function. Gynecological and genitourinary surgeries may create such problems. Generalized postoperative pain and anxiety also make voiding more difficult.

Anesthesia may also create difficulties in urination by altering levels of consciousness. The somnolent patient may not realize his or her bladder is full, nor will the confused individual. And if such patients do experience sensations of bladder fullness, they may have difficulty manipulating bedpans or urinals.

Alterations in patterns of urinary elimination are especially common after spinal anesthesia. The spinal can produce difficulties in voiding by altering the basic nervous system connections with the spinal cord for bladder control. The sympathetic blockade of spinal anesthesia affects the detrusor muscle, thereby altering pressure sensations and voluntary micturition. The patient who has received a spinal may experience bladder retention or incontinence.

Nursing Intervention

Catheterization is a last resort in the care of the patient with difficulty in urination. Other measures can be performed to help the patient void independently. If the surgical procedure and the type of anesthesia permit, sitting the patient up in bed will facilitate micturition. Sleepy patients may need stimulation to keep them awake and help them void if the bladder is distended. A lack of privacy can also inhibit micturition. Privacy should be provided after assisting the patient with manipulation of bedpans or urinals. Since cold can constrict the external sphincter, warming the bedpan before placing it is a good idea.

The patient who has received spinal anesthesia should be assessed for bladder distention. If the level of the spinal remains high for a long period of time, catheterization may be necessary. Since incontinence can also occur in these patients, reassurance and explanation of why it happened can make the patient feel less upset and embarrassed.

PROBLEMS WITH INTRAVENOUS AND INTRAARTERIAL LINES

A variety of problems can develop after the introduction of intravenous lines, arterial lines, and anesthetic agents. Pain on injection, thrombophlebitis, and extravasation can make the patient's perioperative and postoperative courses uncomfortable and even hazardous. Intraarterial injection is another untoward but fortunately rare complication. Bent, broken, or clotted arterial lines are more common occurrences, demanding immediate correction.

Pain on injection is more often a problem for the patient than for the anesthetist. Kawar and Dundee (1982) found that 37 percent of the patients in their study experienced pain with injection of the intravenous agent diazepam, while thiopentone injection produced a 9 percent incidence of pain. They conclude that Valium should be injected into the larger antecubital veins to avoid this complication.

Chemical irritation of the vein wall can also lead to the development of thrombophlebitis. If small veins are used or a combination of agents is administered intravenously, the patient will be more susceptible to this condition. Such a problem most commonly occurs during the first 7 to 10 postoperative days (Atkinson, 1982). Treatment usually consists of moist heat application and rest to the affected extremity.

Extravasation of anesthetic agents is yet another complication that can make the patient's immediate postoperative course more hazardous. Besides causing pain, swelling, and redness, infiltration can prolong the action of anesthetics and make their rate of absorption unpredictable. Depending on the agent or agents administered, respiratory depression, somnia, or muscle weakness can be intermittent or sustained if extravasation has occurred.

Intraarterial injection, though infrequent, can occur in the operating room and in the PACU. The needle may be misplaced, or solutions may be inadvertently injected into the arterial line. The affected extremity will rapidly become cold and pale, and the patient will complain of severe pain. Unfortunately, intraarterial injection can lead to necrosis and eventual amputation of the limb. Sudden death has also been reported (Atkinson, 1982).

Other problems with arterial lines include bent, broken, or clotted catheters. A bent catheter should be carefully straightened and properly retaped. A broken catheter, however, presents a greater problem; surgical removal may eventually prove necessary. Repeated attempts should not be made to irrigate clotted arterial lines, as emboli may dislodge from the tip. Instead, it is best to remove the catheter.

OTHER FREQUENT COMPLICATIONS

Postspinal Headache

The incidence of headache following spinal anesthesia is surprisingly high; studies have revealed a 13 percent occurrence after intradural block (Atkinson, 1982). The cause of the postspinal headache is most probably a decrease in cerebrospinal fluid, resulting in low cerebrospinal pressure. Fluid leaks around the site of injection and alters CSF hydrodynamics. Sensitive brain structures and vessels are affected as cushioning is reduced.

Franksson estimates the average fluid loss is 10 cc per hour (Atkinson, 1982). The amount of CSF leakage can be affected by needle size and positioning. Obviously, a larger needle produces a greater dural leak from the puncture site. Sitting up in bed will also increase CSF loss. A preoperative history of headaches, as well as poor hydration, are other factors that make the individual more susceptible to the development of postspinal headache.

Nursing intervention includes prevention and treatment. The spinal injection site should first be examined. The patient should then be maintained in the supine position for the first 24 hours after spinal administration. The head of the bed may be slightly elevated, but only if necessary. If the patient complains of headache, the administration of IV and oral fluids may ease his or her pain by promoting hydration. Pain medications may also be given. Since postspinal headache is often severe, higher doses of analgesics may prove necessary.

Sore Throat

Sore throat is a common postanesthetic complaint. Intubation, the presence of oral and nasopharyngeal airways, nasogastric tubes, and the dry, irritating nature of inhalants make the individual susceptible to the development of sore throat. Frequent vomiting and coughing after surgery can also cause the patient's throat to be uncomfortably sore.

Nursing intervention consists of relieving sore throat. Mouthwashes, ice chips, and throat lozenges may temporarily alleviate the discomfort. If the patient is allowed to take oral fluids, warm beverages can be very soothing. Unfortunately, however, sore throat may remain for days or weeks after the operative procedure has been performed.

Miscellaneous Problems

A variety of untoward complications can occur because of intubation and patient positioning during operation. Corneal abrasion, tooth loss, swollen lips or tongue, and pharyngeal and laryngeal abrasions are the result of intubation. Backache and neck pain are also common complaints that arise from position during operation. With proper intubation and patient positioning, some of these complications could be avoided.

UNUSUAL COMPLICATIONS

Halothane Hepatitis

Use of the popular inhalant halothane is occasionally followed by hepatitis and even massive hepatic necrosis. This hepatotoxicity occurs in approximately one in 10,000 patients who have received this anesthetic (Bruce, 1980). Susceptibility may be increased if halothane administration is repeated within the first 30 days after operation; thus, care should be taken to use an alternate anesthetic agent.

The cause of halothane hepatitis remains uncertain. Currently, the most popular theory finds a halothane metabolite responsible for the production of hepatotoxicity (Atkinson, 1982). Prolonged intraoperative hepatic hypoxia and genetic predisposition have also been proposed as causative factors (Bruce, 1980).

Since such hepatitis does not develop in the immediate postanesthetic period, the PACU nurse has no active role in its prevention or treatment. Only later will the patient display the jaundice, pruritus, fatigue, weakness, and abdominal pain that characterize this disease.

Allergic Reactions

The incidence of developing a drug allergy in the hospital has been estimated at 1 to 4 percent, with a mortality rate of 0.005 percent (Stoelting, 1983). Anesthetic-produced allergic reactions comprise a fairly small part of this percentage. Patients at greater risk include those with a history of food or drug allergies, hay fever, and asthma, as well as those who have been repeatedly exposed to the same or similar anesthetic agent.

Agents most likely to produce allergic reactions include intravenous anesthetics (barbiturates, ketamine, and narcotics), local anesthetics, muscle relaxants (succinylcholine and nondepolarizing agents), antibiotics, and protamine (Stoelting, 1983). The fact that the patient may have received these drugs before and not experienced an allergic reaction is not always significant; repeated exposure can produce hypersensitivity.

In the susceptible individual, anesthetics can act as antigens which provoke an antibody response. Such antigen-antibodies are not beneficial to the host. The antibodies react against the foreign substance and degranulate mast cells and basophils. This inflammatory reaction leads to cell damage, and clinical manifestations are largely due to the resulting histamine release.

Allergic reactions are characterized by skin changes in the form of erythema and wheals. Edema, particularly facial edema, may also be noted. If the allergy remains unrecognized, hypotension, sinus tachycardia, bronchospasm, and hyperperistalsis can occur. Allergic reactions can even result in ventricular arrhythmias, clotting defects, leukopenia, and body temperature reduction if untreated (Stoelting, 1983).

Obviously, nursing intervention is aimed at early detection of an allergic reaction. The skin should be closely examined while nursing measures, such as taking vital signs and turning and repositioning the patient, are performed. The appearance of skin rashes and welts may signal an allergic reaction which demands immediate treatment. Antihistamines and steroids should then be administered per physician's order. These drugs are particularly effective in combatting inflammatory reactions, and can eliminate any allergic phenomena that may be in progress at the time.

If the skin is not examined and the allergic reaction progresses, hypotension, tachycardia, nausea and vomiting, and bronchospasm will result. Once again, careful patient assessment is essential. Such conditions are fairly common occurrences in the PACU, and their underlying cause may be overlooked.

Case Study

Mary Smith, age 40, was to receive an ECT in the PACU. Atropine, Pentothal, and succinylcholine were given. After succinylcholine was administered, the patient developed a rash across her chest and appeared dusky. Her color did not improve in spite of repeated attempts to ventilate her. Benadryl was given, and the patient stabilized.

Analysis

Apparently, the patient rapidly developed an allergic reaction to the depolarizing agent succinylcholine. The administration of the antihistamine Benadryl was effective in eliminating the reaction.

Toxicity of Local Anesthetics

Toxicity involves the harmful, destructive, or deadly nature of a substance. Local anesthetics have such toxic qualities, producing hypersensitivity, cytotoxicity, neurotoxicity, and even death.

Allergic reactions as a consequence of hypersensitivity are rare, but they do occur. Procaine is the most common offender, producing edema, hives, wheezing, and bronchospasm (de Jong, 1970). If the patient is sensitive to procaine, he or she will most probably develop an allergic reaction to any other ester-linked local anesthetics, such as tetracaine and chloroprocaine. Allergy to amide-linked agents such as Lidocaine, mepivacaine, and pridocaine are extremely rare (Atkinson, 1982).

Cytotoxicity involves the toxic effects local anesthetics can produce on nerve cells. Once again, such action is extremely rare in the wake of modern medicine. Metal containers and syringes of the past proved hazardous. Epinephrine-containing solutions would take up metal particles and form metallic ions, resulting in local tissue swelling and irritation. The use of glass, plastic, and stainless steel prevents such action (de Jong, 1970). However, high concentrations of local anesthetics can cause aseptic leptomeningeal irritation and damage to the parenchyma. Spinal cells and nerve roots can also be traumatized by contact with the spinal needle (Lund, 1971).

Neurotoxicity can be peripheral or central. De Jong (1970) finds that "tissue irritation could be one mechanism whereby some local anesthetics produce long-lasting nerve block, the resultant edema leading to vascular compression and diminished drug reabsorption." Once again, such consequences are uncommon but can occur.

The most obvious central sign of neurotoxicity is a generalized seizure. Both respiratory and cardiovascular performance are also compromised. The cause of such neurotoxicity is usually a high blood level of the local anesthetic produced by accidental intravascular injection, overdosage, or unusually rapid absorption of the agent (de Jong, 1970). If mortality occurs, the respiratory and cardiac depression produced by neurotoxicity are usually the cause.

Nursing Intervention

Nursing intervention for the patient with local anesthetic toxicity consists of the recognition of allergic reaction or seizure. Administration of epinephrine, steroids, and oxygen will be necessary when hypersensitivity has developed. Neurotoxicity as exemplified by seizure activity demands prompt intervention. An airway should be inserted and the patient ventilated. Rapid IV fluid administration and leg elevation should also be performed to increase blood pressure. Cardiac massage may be necessary. If time permits, siderails should be padded to protect patients from harming themselves. Diazepam administration is sometimes useful, although succinylcholine or thiopentone are often effective in controlling convulsions (Atkinson, 1982).

Case Study

Sixty-seven-year-old Robert Blake had a left inguinal herniorrhaphy performed under spinal anesthesia. On admission to the PACU he was awake and comfortable. Vital signs were stable: BP was 110/70, heart rate was 62 and regular, and respirations were 16 and deep. Sensory level was determined at T8. Twelve hours later, Blake could finally move his feet, but sensation did not return until 28 hours after the spinal was administered.

Analysis

Such prolonged insensibility and immobility were the result of the neurotoxic effects of the local anesthetic Blake had received. Edema led to vascular compression and diminished drug reabsorption.

High Spinal or Total Spinal Anesthesia

Causes of such drastic sympathetic blockade include local anesthetic overdosage, incorrect patient positioning, rapid injection speed, and variations in spinal pressure such as those with coughing or straining. Theories have suggested that dehydration or low spinal fluid pressure may also be responsible. Of interest is the observation that total spinal occurs more often in patients with large abdominal tumors or those who undergo C-section (Lund, 1971).

Phrenic nerve paralysis affecting diaphragmatic movements and respiration can occur, while block of cardiac afferent fibers from T1 to T4 can drastically reduce cardiac output. Respiratory difficulties, bradycardia, and hypotension will result.

Nursing Intervention

Nursing care of the patient with a high degree of spinal blockade involves immediate recognition and prompt intervention. First, vital signs and sensory level should be ascertained. Intubation and ventilatory assistance, rapid IV fluid administration, slight head-down position, and continuous monitoring are essential. Explanation of all procedures and emotional support is especially important if consciousness remains.

Recall

Once of the first accounts of "awareness" during apparent anesthesia appeared in 1950 (Winterbottom); since then, numerous reports and editorials have appeared in anesthesia, surgery, and medical hypnosis journals. Sia (1969) and others describe patients who were aware of events occurring in the operating room but experienced no pain. Others document patients who suffered extreme discomfort. A syndrome of traumatic neurosis following awareness has been described (Blacher, 1975). Most cases occurred during nitrous oxide relaxant anesthesia, but the complication has been reported following administration of most anesthetic agents.

Many investigators are convinced that meaningful sounds, meaningful silence, and meaningful conversation are registered and can have a profound influence upon the behavior of a patient during surgery and for many years thereafter. For this reason, the anesthesiologist—as well as the operating room nurse and PACU nurse—should treat unconscious patients with the same respect accorded patients in full possession of their senses. In recent years, the number of patients undergoing surgery under superficial chemical anesthesia has increased, and it is prudent to treat every operative patient as though he or she is capable of hearing (Bitner, 1983).

CONCLUSION

The administration of anesthesia can jeopardize the surgical patient and significantly complicate the postoperative course. Besides altering level of consciousness, anesthetics can reduce cardiovascular performance, respiration, and renal function; can eliminate effective body temperature regulation; can create gastric distress; and can even cause hepatitis.

The frequency with which serious postanesthetic complications occur can be related to age, ASA status, abdominal incision, prolonged operative procedure, preoperative intravenous antibiotic therapy, and major organ system disease (Vaughan and associates, 1981b). Many patients, however, are vulnerable to the untoward effects of anesthesia regardless of preoperative history and surgery. It is a rare individual who comes to the PACU awake, alert, oriented, mobile, comfortable, and stable.

Admittedly, most patients are far more anxious about the outcome of the surgical procedure than they are about the administration of anesthesia. But it is of vital importance for health care professionals to be cognizant of the deleterious effects of anesthetics, so that quality patient care can be delivered.

REFERENCES

Altura B et al.: Vascular smooth muscle and general anesthetics. Federation Proceedings of American Societies of Experimental Biology 39:1584–1591, April, 1980.

Atkinson R et al.: A Synopsis of Anesthesia. Littleton: John Wright & Sons, 1982.

Benumof J (Ed.): Clinical Frontiers in Anesthesiology. New York: Grune & Stratton, 1983.

Bertrand C et al.: Disturbances of cardiac rhythm during anesthesia and surgery. Journal of the American Medical Association 216:1615–1617, June, 1971.

Bitner RL: Awareness during anesthesia. In FK Orkin & LH Cooperman (Eds.), Complications in Anesthesiology. Philadelphia: Lippincott, 1983.

Blacher SS: On awakening paralyzed during surgery. Journal of the American Medical Association 234:67, 1975.

Borchardt A & Fraulini K: Hypothermia in the post-anesthetic patient. AORN Journal 36:648–661, October, 1982.

Bourke DL, Heinrich W, Rosenberg M, & Russell J: Intraoperative heat conservation using a reflective blanket. Anesthesiology 60: 151–154, Feb., 1984.

Bruce D: Functional Toxicity of Anesthesia. New York: Grune & Stratton, 1980.

Cullen D & Cullen B: Post-anesthetic complications. Surgical Clinics of North America 55:987–998, August, 1975.

de Jong R: Physiology and Pharmacology of Local Anesthesia. Springfield: Chas. C Thomas, 1970.

Donegan J: Postoperative airway management. Current Reviews for Recovery Room Nurses 3(22):1982.

Feldman S: Muscle Relaxants. Philadelphia: Saunders, 1973.

Fraulini K: Postanesthetic delirium—A conceptual approach. Current Reviews for Recovery Room Nurses 4(20):155–159, 1982.

Goldmann D et al.: Medical Care of the Surgical Patient. Philadelphia: Lippincott, 1982.

Gothert M & Wendt J: Inhibition of adrenal medullary catecholamine secretion by enflurane. Anesthesiology 46:400–403, 1977.

Greene N: The Physiology of Spinal Anesthesia. New York: Krieger, 1976.

Gronert G: Malignant hyperthermia. Anesthesiology 53:395–423, Nov., 1980.

Guyton A: Basic Human Physiology: Normal Function and Mechanisms of Disease. Philadelphia: Saunders, 1971.

Hudak C et al.: Critical Care Nursing. Philadelphia: Lippincott, 1973.

Katz J et al.: Anesthesia and Uncommon Diseases: Pathophysiologic and Clinical Correlation. Philadelphia: Saunders, 1981.

Kawar P & Dundee J W: Frequency of pain and venous sequelae following the I.V. administration of certain anesthetics and sedatives. British Journal of Anesthesiology 54:935–939, 1982.

Lucas C: The renal response to acute injury and sepsis. Surgical Clinics of North America 953–975, August, 1976.

Luckmann J & Sorenson K: Medical-Surgical Nursing: A Psychopathologic Approach. Philadelphia: Saunders, 1974.

Lund P: Principles and Practice of Spinal Anesthesia. Springfield: Chas. C Thomas, 1971.

Maclean D & Emslie-Smith D: Accidental Hypothermia. London: Blackwell Scientific Publications, 1977.

Mauney F et al.: Postoperative myocardial infarction: A study of predisposing factors, diagnosis, and mortality in a high risk group of surgical patients. Annals of Surgery 172:497–503, October, 1970.

McGovern V & Tillen D: Shock: A Clinicopathologic Correlation. New York: Masson, 1980.

Miller RD: Antagonism of neuromuscular blockade. Anesthesiology 44:318–329, 1976.

Orkin FK & Cooperman LH: Complications in Anesthesiology. Philadelphia: Lippincott, 1983.

Orlandi F: The Liver and Drugs. New York: Academic Press, 1972.

Philbin D et al.: Renin, catecholamine and vasopressin response to the stress of anesthesia and surgery. Anesthesiology 51:s121, 1979.

Price H: Circulation During Anesthesia and Operation. Springfield: Chas. C Thomas, 1967.

Price H & Ohinski S: Effects of anesthetics on the heart. Federation Proceedings of American Societies of Experimental Biology 39:1575–1579, April, 1980.

Prys-Roberts C (Ed.): The Circulation in Anesthesia. Oxford: Blackwell Scientific Publications, 1980.

Rao TLK, Jacobs HK, & El-Etr AA: Reinfarction following anesthesia in patients with myocardial infarction. Anesthesiology 59:499–505, 1983.

Rodgers R: Malignant hyperthermia: A review of the literature. Mount Sinai Journal of Medicine 50:95–98, 1983.

Sia RK: Consciousness during general anesthesia. Anesthesia and Analgesia 48:363, 1969.

Stoelting R: Allergic reactions during anesthesia. Anesthesia and Analgesia 62:341–356, 1983.

Surawicz B (Ed.): Tachycardias. Boston: Mijhoff, 1984.

Thomas J: Fighting a fatal fire. Nursing Mirror 153:48, October, 1981.

Tschirren B: Anesthetic Complications. Chicago: Year Book Med., Pub., 1980.

Vaughan MS: Shivering in the recovery room. Current Reviews for Recovery Room Nurses 3(22), 1982.

Vaughn MS: Nursing treatment of hypothermia in adult recovery room postsurgical patients. Doctoral dissertation. Tucson,: University of Arizona, 1980.

Vaughan MS et al.: Post-operative hypothermia in adults: Relationship of age, anesthesia, and shivering to rewarming. Anesthesia and Analgesia 60:746–751, October, 1981.

Vaughan R et al.: Predicting adverse outcomes during anesthesia and surgery by prospective risk assessment. Anesthesiology 59:A132, Sept., 1981b.

Walton H et al.: Ventricular cardiac arrhythmias during anesthesia: Feasibility of pre-operative recognition. Southern Medical Journal 75:27–29, Jan., 1982.

Winterbottom EH: Insufficient anesthesia. British Medical Journal 1:247, 1950.

Wynands JE: The high risk cardiac patient undergoing general surgery. The Canadian Journal of Surgery 21:475–482, 1978.

Zahorian T: Malignant hyperpyrexia: A rare anesthetic hazard. Nursing Times 77:2047–2049, Nov., 1981.

Criteria for Extubation

1. Patient not deeply anesthetized
2. Protective airway reflexes present
3. Stable cardiovascular status
4. Muscle relaxants adequately reversed
5. V_T = 3 ml/lb
6. VC = 15 ml/kg
7. Inspiratory force = -25 to -28 cm H_2O
8. $PaCO_2$ at normal level for patient when breathing spontaneously

The patient who comes to the PACU with an endotracheal tube in place should not have it removed until he or she can fulfill the above criteria for extubation. The tube should not be removed while the patient is still deeply anesthetized, as the patient's protective airway reflexes will not have returned and regurgitation or vomiting may be followed by aspiration. This is particularly important in a patient who required emergency surgery and who was anesthetized with a full stomach. In addition, the muscles of the tongue and lower jaw of a sedated individual are relaxed and the tongue may fall back into the pharynx, producing partial (snoring) or complete airway obstruction. If this occurs, it may be necessary to insert a nasopharyngeal or an oropharyngeal airway.

If the cardiovascular status is unstable, it may be unwise to impose the added stress of extubation with its possible deleterious effects on heart rate and blood pressure (e.g. tachycardia, cardiac dysrhythmias, and hypertension). These patients should remain intubated and may need ventilatory support to optimize oxygen delivery and reduce the work of breathing.

It is essential to have adequate return of respiratory muscle function prior to extubation. This can be tested by (1) assessing hand-grip strength and (2) by having the patient lift his or her head off the bed without opening the lower jaw. A nerve stimulator may be used for more exact assessment. In this case, the ability to sustain a tetanic contraction for 5 seconds or the "train-of-four" test may be used. In addition, tidal volume (V_T) and vital capacity (VC) can be measured with a respirometer and inspiratory force with a manometer attached to the endotracheal tube. It is important not only that the tidal volume be normal (3 ml/lb), but also that the VC be at least 15 ml/kg (normal 55–85 ml/kg) because this is a better measure of the patient's ability to cough and deep-breathe than is the tidal volume.

Patients who are unable to maintain an arterial carbon dioxide tension ($PaCO_2$) which is normal for them while breathing spontaneously through the endotracheal tube must remain intubated and receive mechanical ventilatory support. If allowed to breathe spontaneously, they will continue to accumulate carbon dioxide, leading eventually to carbon dioxide narcosis and death (Donegan, 1982).

APPENDIX 10–2

Arterial Blood Gases in the Operating Room and PACU

Arterial blood gases (ABG) are the only accurate way to answer the question "How well is the patient breathing?" To measure breathing is the primary use of ABGs in the OR–PACU setting. They also provide information on the acid-base status of the patient and may be drawn for this purpose only.

Normal blood-gas values are:

	Arterial	**Mixed Venous**
pH	7.40 (7.35–7.45)	7.36 (7.31–7.41)
pO_2	80–100 mm Hg	35–40 mm Hg
pCO_2	35–45 mm Hg	41–51 mm Hg
HCO_3	22–26 mEq/L	22–26 mEq/L
BE	−2–+2	−2–+2
O_2	95%	70–75%

The pO_2 (partial pressure of oxygen) is an extremely sensitive indicator of how well the lung is functioning in delivering oxygen to the blood. To correctly interpret pO_2, the FiO_2 (fractional concentration of oxygen) must be known.

FiO_2		Normal Arterial pO_2*
0.21	(room air)	80–100 mm Hg**
0.40	(mask O_2)	200–220 mm Hg
1.00	(100% O_2 by E-T Tube)	> 570 mm Hg

(*Assumes normal pCO_2 = 40.)
(**This value normally decreases with age. A pO_2 of 70 may be normal in a 70-year-old person.)

The FiO_2 may be measured directly with the Beckman O_2 meter.

A patient with a $pO_2 = 60$ on 100% O_2 ($FiO_2 = 1.0$) obviously has a much more severe problem than one with the same pO_2 on room air. Arterial pO_2 values below 50 are emergencies requiring prompt attention. Most patients will have adequate pO_2 values (over 60 mm Hg) on mask O_2. It not, a mask with a rebreathing bag will increase the FiO_2 to 0.70–0.80. If this fails, the patient should be intubated and ventilated. Five common causes of reduced arterial pO_2 are:

1. Hypoventilation
2. Reduced FiO_2 (high altitude)
3. "Diffusion-block"
4. Ventilation/perfusion (V/Q) abnormalities
5. Shunting

All will respond to increased FiO_2 except shunting. Most PACU patients have low pO_2 values secondary to V/Q abnormalities.

The pCO_2 is primarily an indicator of ventilation. Values over 40 = hypoventilation; values under 40 = hypoventilation. Common causes of ventilation abnormalities are:

Elevated pCO_2

- Depression by anesthetic agents, especially narcotics
- Airway obstruction
- Pulmonary disease
- Metabolic alkalosis
- Improperly set ventilator

Low pCO_2

- Pain
- Hypoxia
- Mechanical ventilation
- Metabolic acidosis
- Pulmonary embolus

High pCO_2 values causing low pH = respiratory acidosis. Low pCO_2 values causing high pH = respiratory alkalosis.

The pH determines the type of acid-base derangement. A pH less than 7.4 = acidosis; greater than 7.4 = alkalosis. Acid-base problems may be caused by abnormal ventilation, metabolic imbalances, or both. Acidosis is generally worse than alkalosis. Acidotic patients may have cardiac arrhythmias and hypotension.

Metabolic imbalances are determined by the base excess (BE). Negative BE (>−2) = metabolic acidosis. Postive BE (>2) = metabolic alkalosis.

The following are some examples of acid-base disturbances.

Example 1   **Normal**

pH 7.32   (7.40)
pCO_2 50   (40)
BE −2   (−2−+2)

1. Look at the pH. It is low, indicating an acidosis.
2. Look at the pCO_2. It is high, indicating a *respiratory* acidosis due to hypoventilation.
3. Look at the base excess. It is normal, indicating no metabolic component.

Example 2

pH 7.25
pCO_2 50
BE −11

1. pH = acidosis.
2. pCO_2 = respiratory acidosis—hypoventilation.
3. BE is abnormally negative, indicating an additional metabolic acidosis. Notice that the pH is lower (more acidotic) than in the first example, indicating a combined effect of both respiratory and metabolic acidosis.

Example 3

pH 7.48
pCO_2 28
BE −2

1. pH is high = alkalosis.
2. pCO_2 is low = respiratory alkalosis—hyperventilation.
3. BE is normal. This is a respiratory alkalosis without a metabolic component.

Now here's a harder one.

Example 4

pH 7.32
pCO_2 30
BE −17

1. pH = acidosis.
2. pCO_2 is low, indicating hyperventilation. This is not called a respiratory alkalosis because the pH is acid.
3. BE is negative, indicating a metabolic acidosis. This, then, is a metabolic acidosis causing hyperventilation. Note the pH is less acidotic than in the second example despite a larger BE. The effect of the acidosis on the pH has been partially compensated by the hyperventilation.

Let's try a clinical example. The patient is a 70-year-old female who was operated on for the pinning of a fractured hip. On admission to the PACU she is noted to have blue nail beds and blood pressure of 140/90. Here are the ABGs on room air:

Example 5

pH 7.35
pCO_2 44
pO_2 60
BE −2

1. pH borderline low.
2. pCO_2 borderline high.
3. BE normal.
4. The pO_2 is abnormal even for a 70-year-old. However, the physician in the PACU felt it was adequate and consistent with the postoperative state. She received 10 mg MS IV for severe pain.

After ½ hour the patient is noted to be unresponsive, with respiratory rate 12/min and BP 210/110. ABGs on room air show:

Example 6

pH 7.29
pCO_2 55
BE −2
pO_2 45

1. pH = acidosis.
2. pCO_2 = respiratory acidosis—hypoventilation.
3. BE = normal. A pure respiratory acidosis is secondary to hypoventilation.
4. pO_2 = dangerously low secondary to hypoventilation.

This lady received too much pain medication and probably needs narcan. Suppose she had an O_2 mask on. Her ABGs would now be:

Example 7

pH 7.29
pCO_2 55

BE -2
pO$_2$ 120

Note that now despite hypoventilation her pO$_2$ is fine, and her chances of developing serious problems (e.g., cardiac arrhythmias) is greatly reduced.

Could we have made this diagnosis without blood gases? The answer would seem to be obviously yes. However, what if her second set of gases showed the following (assuming she did get mask O$_2$)?

Example 8

pH 7.48
pCO$_2$ 28
BE -2
pO$_2$ 50

1. pH = alkalosis.
2. pCO$_2$ = respiratory alkalosis.
3. BE = normal metabolic status.
4. pO$_2$ = dangerously low for mask O$_2$. Some other cause for her unresponsiveness must be strongly considered; perhaps a pulmonary embolus with secondary hyperventilation.

Chapter 11

Physiologic Monitoring in the PACU

Daniel W. Gorski
Kay E. Fraulini

Progress in knowledge and technology have contributed to the advanced state of monitoring possible in a modern PACU (Fig. 11-1). A "monitor" is an instrument used to measure, display, and record (continuously or intermittently) certain physioiogic variables such as pulse, blood pressure, and respiration. Of great importance is the involvement of the person who observes the monitor, acts upon and reacts to data obtained from the monitor, and carries out any necessary treatment. This chapter begins with a look at a common monitor: arterial blood pressure. Emphasis is placed upon what, how, and when to monitor, along with complications and problems arising from the use of monitors. Monitors must be individualized, chosen by careful consideration of risk–benefit ratios, and placed and maintained by trained, competent professionals. In keeping with this, three levels of monitoring are proposed. Finally, monitoring techniques are outlined for various body systems.

It is important to emphasize that the role of the nurse in monitoring in the PACU or the intensive care unit should be clearly defined. Serving as the intermediary between physician and patient, the nurse is the monitor. In concert with electronic and communication equipment the nurse acquires, assembles, organizes, and not infrequently interprets the data to

Left ventricular pressure
Left atrial pressure
Pulmonary artery pressure
Intraventricular catheters (brain)
Central aortic pressures
CVP
Radial artery pressures
Indwelling urinary catheter
TM, Rectal, Esophageal temperature
Esophageal stethoscope
Spectrophotometric gas measurement
Nuclear cardiology
Peripheral nerve stimulator
Transcutaneous O_2 and CO_2
Three dimensional CT
Finger pulse transducer
Systolic time intervals
Doppler apparatus (and similar equipment)
Cuff BP
ECG
EEG (compressed spectral array)
RPP
Echocardiogram
Precordial stethoscope

(left vertical label) I N V A S I V E

(right vertical label) N O N I N V A S I V E

Invasive: monitor that pentrates the skin, mucosal membrane, or enters some body cavity.

Noninvasive: monitor that does not penetrate body orifice but may require a transducer.

Figure 11–1. Spectrum of monitoring devices. *(Courtesy of Blitt CD. Invasive monitoring in non-cardiac surgery. ASA Annual Refresher Course Lectures 33:(103), 1982.)*

define patient status. This latter is particularly applicable when monitoring cardiac arrhythmias, for which rapid interpretation and intervention are required. The nurse becomes the primary beneficiary of the new and sophisticated monitoring equipment available for data acquisition in the intensive care unit. Once relieved of repetitive data acquisitions and secretarial tasks, the nurse should have more time to devote to patient care and true analytical monitoring (Greenberg & Peskin, 1985).

Arterial Blood Pressure

Advances made in blood pressure monitoring mandate reading a patient's blood pressure at regular intervals and documentation of that reading on a patient's record. Consider that 100 years ago Harvey Cushing was told, "Why measure a patient's blood pressure and heart rate in the operating room; patients are there for such a short time that it is highly doubtful that any changes [in pressure] can have a significant effect on outcome [morbidity or mortality]" (Fulton, 1946). Cushing insisted on recording observations of blood pressure and heart rate on a regular basis in the operating room (Cushing, 1903); this goal is now a basic standard of care in the operating room and in the PACU during emergence from anesthesia. Records should be representative of what is happening, should be a complete measure of all physiological parameters required for a given patient, be accurate and available.

A sample of a modern PACU record is shown in Figure 11-2. The

PACU POSTOPERATIVE RECORD

TIME OF ARRIVAL _____ A.M. P.M.   DATE _____

TRANSFERRED TO ROOM _____ A.M. P.M.

LEVEL OF CONSCIOUSNESS:

		OXYGEN:	MONITOR:	AIRWAY:
	UNCONSC	VENTILATOR	EKG	ENDOTRACHEAL
	SEMICONSC	COOL/HEATED AEROSOL	CVP	ORAL
	AWAKE	CANNULA	ARTERIAL LINE	NASAL
	SPINAL	MASK	SWAN-GANZ	TRACH

TIME	B/P	PULSE	RESP.	Other Monitors ie. CVP/ SWAN-GANZ	MEDICATION, TREATMENTS AND OBSERVATIONS	PACU SCORE

I V FLUIDS GIVEN IN PACU

FLUIDS (Type)	VOLUME in PACU
1. _____	_____
2. _____	_____
3. _____	_____
4. _____	_____
Total Volume _____	
Total Blood Loss _____	
Total Urine Output	

WOUND DRAINAGE _____

PACU REMARKS:

DISCHARGE CONDITION: ☐ GOOD ☐ FAIR ☐ POOR

VITAL SIGNS: ☐ STABLE ☐ UNSTABLE

TRANSFER   TO
PER ORDER _____   ROOM _____

TIME OF D/C _____

PACU COMPLICATION: NO _____ YES _____

Figure 11–2. PACU record.

sound logic and reasoning of Cushing nearly 100 years ago is still correct today. From the cuff and mercury manometer of Riva-Rocci to sounds of Korotkoff, measurement of arterial pressure has advanced to the present state of the art, which includes arterial lines for invasive, direct monitoring of blood pressure and the Doppler monitor (Fig. 11-3A) for noninvasive, indirect monitoring. Another available method is with the Dinamap, an indirect automatic blood pressure monitor that utilizes the oscillometric principle and a microprocessor (Fig. 11-3B). Books abound on the subject of blood pressure monitoring (Daily, 1985).

Disturbances of circulation (hypotension and hypertension) are frequently seen in the PACU. Hypotension—with its clinical signs of rapid and thready pulse, cold, clammy, diaphonetic skin, pale color, disorientation, restlessness or anxiety, and possibly shallow and rapid respirations—may be blunted by the circulatory effects of residual anesthetic agents. Utilizing repeated blood pressure measurements as a guide to pressure stability, the PACU nurse should rely on these measurements more than on clinical signs.

The important questions to ask concerning monitoring are:

- What parameters do I wish to measure (in the previous example, blood pressure)?
- How should I measure that parameter (invasive versus noninvasive)?

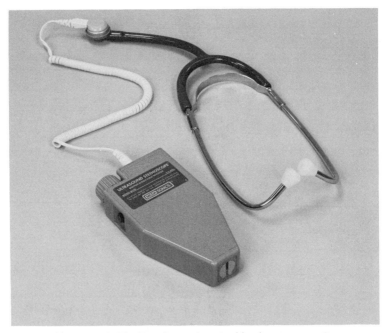

Figure 11–3A. The Doppler noninvasive blood pressure monitor.

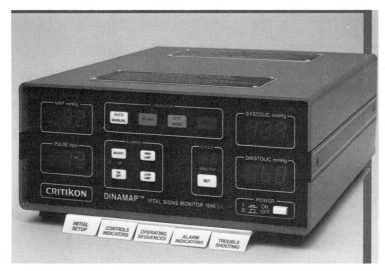

Figure 11–3B. The Dinamap noninvasive blood pressure monitor.

- When should that parameter be measured (is every 15 minutes by cuff always enough)?
- What are the appropriate, normal, physiologic limits for that parameter in a given patient?

Patients routinely have their blood pressure taken and recorded every 15 minutes in the PACU. The noninvasive, auscultatory method of blood pressure determination is commonly used, although more use of automatic noninvasive blood pressure monitoring is occurring in both the operating room and the PACU. Noninvasive monitors have the benefit of freeing the nurse's hands for other duties, but they do allow potential errors in pressure determinations due to (1) improper cuff size (arm cuff too big or small), which can cause inaccurate measurements; (2) improper deflation of cuff (too rapid cuff deflation may result in a low pressure recording); and (3) bending or kinking of the connecting tubing, which may result in recording too high a pressure. Audio and visual alarms for malfunction of the instrument are a must.

Certain patients will require arterial line placement for direct measurement of blood pressure in the operating room. Indications for and information derived from an arterial line are listed in Tables 11-1 and 11-2, respectively. The patient with an arterial line and attached monitor then enters the PACU. There are multiple problems with direct pressure measurements that the PACU nurse may face (see Table 11-3): from disconnects to improper calibration of the monitor, and from infection at the cannulation site to air embolism from a malfunctioning flush (Daily, 1985). However, a common problem noted is the following: a patient arrives in the PACU with an arterial line in place. While someone hooks

TABLE 11–1. INDICATIONS FOR ARTERIAL CANNULATION IN THE SURGICAL PATIENT

Direct Measurement of Arterial Pressure
  Cardiac surgery, especially with cardiopulmonary bypass
  Deliberate hypothermia
  Deliberate hypotension
  Intracranial operations
  Major vascular surgery—aorta, carotid, iliac, femoral arteries, vena cava
  Extensive surgery with prospect of sudden blood loss or marked shifts of body fluids
  Extensive trauma, especially with uncontrolled hemorrhage
  Thoracic or abdominal surgery with compression of the great vessels
  Noncardiac surgery in patients with significant cardiovascular disease and hemodynamic instability
  Cardiopulmonary resuscitation
  Inability to measure blood pressure indirectly (obesity, burns of the extremities)
Arterial Blood Sampling (repetitive)
  Blood gas analysis
    Pulmonary disease
    Lung surgery (one-lung ventilation)
    Major surgery (neural, cardiac, vascular, thoracic, abdominal)
  Severe metabolic derangements
    Acid–base evaluation
    Electrolyte determinations
    Glucose analysis
    Serum osmolarity measurement
  Heparin anticoagulation and protamine antagonism
    Cardiopulmonary bypass
    Arterial shunts (Gott shunt)

(From Hug C Jr.: Monitoring. In RD Miller (Ed.), Anesthesia. New York: Churchill Livingstone, 1981, p. 178.)

up the arterial line to the pressure monitor, another person records the patient's blood pressure by noninvasive methods in the opposite arm. Within minutes, the following results are noted; right arm pressure (arterial line in place) is 200/115, left arm pressure (using cuff and auscultatory method of determination) is 160/90. Which pressure should be believed? Is the right arm "normally" different from the left arm? Should the patient be treated for hypertension?

These questions are often asked and can be answered in part by understanding that, in general, indirect pressure readings are lower than direct measurements. One must understand that indirect methods of determining blood pressure measure lateral pressure on a vessel wall, while direct methods measure the onward thrust of a fluid column against the diaphragm of a recording device (Gordon, 1971). Assuming proper calibration and functioning of the pressure transducer and monitor, the direct method of pressure measurement is more accurate and subject to less variability than indirect methods. Of prime importance, no matter which method of pressure measurement is chosen, is following trends at defined time intervals. No recommendation of the superiority of one pressure measurement technique over another is made; only a plea to understand

TABLE 11–2. INFORMATION DERIVED FROM VISUAL ANALYSIS OF ARTERIAL PRESSURE

Myocardial Contractility
   The upstroke of the pulse pressure wave is dependent on left ventricular dP/dt
   A steep upstroke indicates strong left ventricular contraction
Stroke Volume
   The area under the systolic ejection phase of the pulse pressure tracing (i.e., upstroke to
     dicrotic notch) is proportional to stroke volume
Systemic Vascular Resistance
   A low dicrotic notch and a steep downstroke indicates rapid diastolic runoff and a low SVR
Hemodynamic Significance of Dysrhythmias
   The blood pressure and pulse contour following abnormal beats indicate the degree of impair-
     ment of cardiac pumping
Circulating Blood Volume
   Exaggerated beat-by-beat changes in blood pressure in relation to ventilation can indicate
     hypovolemia
   During a single cycle of ventilation:
     Positive pressure ventilation increases the stroke volume of the first beat or two and then
       decreases the stroke volume of subsequent beats
     Spontaneous ventilation decreases the stroke volume of the first beat or two and increases
       stroke volume during expiration

(From Hug C Jr.: Monitoring. In RD Miller (Ed.), Anesthesia. New York: Churchill Livingstone, 1981, p. 177.)

the differences between the techniques and to consider the indications for the measurement device (arterial line placements). A logical, systematic approach to blood pressure monitoring in the PACU (how, when, and what to monitor) will give the nurse the most reliable and accurate information about a given patient. Monitoring must be individualized, taking into account the risk–benefit ratio.

Other monitors for use in the PACU are listed in Table 11-4. This table provides indications, contraindications, normal limits, and problems specific to the monitoring device discussed.

The adage "you see what you look for" is certainly true when considering monitoring. Sophisticated equipment and techniques have taken us from the "finger on the pulse, eye on the blood, ear to the chest" day to the modern era of anesthesia monitoring. Most monitors placed in the operating room will remain in place in the PACU while the patient emerges from anesthesia. Information from these monitors will aid in diagnosis and treatment of patient problems. Table 11-5 reviews common PACU problems listed with appropriate monitors that would tell the nurse of a deviation from "normal" limits (Cullen, 1982). This list points out the fact that monitors (either invasive or noninvasive) do play an important role in patient care. To be effective, monitors should be in proper working order and checked daily by an assigned individual for problems that might cause faulty readings—and therefore faulty patient treatment—or harm to the patient such as electric shock, infection, or embolism. Table 11-4 lists common complications associated with monitors that might be used on a patient in the PACU. This list bears careful consideration, especially

TABLE 11-3. PROBLEMS ENCOUNTERED WITH ARTERIAL CATHETERS

Problem	Cause	Prevention	Treatment
Hematoma after withdrawal of needle	Bleeding or oozing at puncture site	Maintain firm pressure on site during withdrawal of catheter and for 5 to 15 minutes (as necessary) after withdrawal. Apply elastic tape (elastoplast) firmly over puncture site. For femoral arterial puncture sites, leave a sandbag on site for 1 to 2 hours to prevent oozing.	Continue to hold pressure to puncture site until oozing stops. Apply sandbag to femoral puncture site for 1 to 2 hours after removal of catheter.
Decreased or absent pulse distal to puncture site	Spasm of artery Thrombosis of artery	Introduce arterial needle cleanly, nontraumatically.	Inject lidocaine locally at insertion site and 10 mg into arterial catheter. Arteriotomy and Fogarty catheterization both distally and proximally from the puncture site result in return of pulse in more than 90% of cases if brachial or femoral artery is used.
Bleedback into tubing, dome, or transducer	Insufficient pressure on IV bag Loose connections	Maintain 300 mm Hg pressure on IV bag. Use Leur-Lok stopcocks.	Disconnect and clean transducer. Replace dome. "Fast flush" through system. Tighten all connections.
Hemorrhage	Loose connections	Keep all connecting sites visible. Observe connecting sites frequently. Use built-in alarm system. Use Luer-Lok stopcocks.	Tighten all connections.

Complication	Cause	Nursing Action	Treatment
Emboli	Clot from catheter tip into bloodstream	Always aspirate and discard before flushing. Use continuous flush device. Use 1 unit heparin/1 ml IV fluid. Gently flush 2 to 4 ml.	Remove catheter.
Local infection	Forward movement of contaminated catheter. Prolonged catheter use. Break in sterile technique	Carefully suture catheter at insertion site. Always use aseptic technique. Remove catheter after 72 to 96 hours. Inspect and care for insertion site daily, including dressing change and antibiotic or iodophor ointment.	Remove catheter. Prescribe antibiotic.
Sepsis	Break in sterile technique. Prolonged catheter use. Bacterial growth in IV fluid	Use percutaneous insertion. Always use aseptic technique. Remove catheter after 72 to 96 hours. Change in IV fluid bag, stopcocks, dome, and tubing every 24 to 48 hours. Do not use IV fluid containing glucose. Sterilize transducers before use. Use dead-ender caps on all ports of stopcocks. Carefully flush remaining blood in stopcocks after using blood sampling.	Remove catheter. Prescribe antibiotic.

TABLE 11–4. MONITORS USED IN THE PACU

Monitor	Indications	Contraindications	Normal Values	Complications and Problems
Hemodynamic/ Cardiovascular ECG	All patients post-anesthesia (general, regional, conscious sedation)		If preoperative ECG is available it should be reviewed; postanesthesia tracing should be comparable.	None
Arterial pressure Noninvasive	All patients post-anesthesia (general, regional, conscious sedation)	Inaccessibility of extremities	Within a 30% range above or below the patient's "normal" preoperative BP	Cuff not appropriate size for patient's arm, cuff too loose, kinking of connecting tube, malfunctioning of automatic BP machine, skin irritation or bruising from inappropriate application of cuff
Invasive	See Table 11-1	Inadequate collateral circulation. Infection at sites of insertion	Within a 30% range above or below the patient's "normal" preoperative BP	See Table 11-3
Central venous pressure	Lack of peripheral access. Uncertain volume status. Surgical procedure involving large blood loss/ fluid shifts/ possible air embolism. Access for Swan-Ganz catheter	Untreated pneumothorax on contralateral side	5–12 cm H_2O, unless preexisting cardiovascular disease state has altered "normal" for specific patient	Pneumothorax, infection tissue trauma

TABLE 11–4. (*Continued*)

Monitor	Indications	Contraindications	Normal Values	Complications and Problems
Swan-Ganz catheter	Patients with cardiovascular disease, causing CVP to be an unreliable indication of volume status Need for cardiac output determinations	Lack of experienced personnel Valvular heart problems Uncontrolled ventricular arrhythmias	PAP $\frac{15-28}{5-16}$ PCWP 5–16 "Normal" may be different for a patient with preexisting cardiovascular disease state	Arrhythmias, pulmonary infarction from continuous wedge, infection, tissue trauma
Monitoring of lung ventilation	All patients post-anesthesia (general, regional, conscious sedation)	None	Regular, symmetrical movement of chest wall and diaphragm with inspiration and expiration	None
Auditory	All patients post-anesthesia (general, regional, conscious sedation)	None	Clear inspiratory and expiratory breath sounds in all lung fields	None
Volume	Any patient who arrives in the PACU with an endotracheal tube in place Any patient extubated in the PACU Any patient in which there are doubts about the adequacy of volume ventilation		Tidal volume of 3–4 cc/lb body weight Negative inspiratory pressure = 20 cm H_2O Minute volume = 5–10L Vital capacity 55–85 ml/kg	No complications, may have uncooperative patient making accurate measurements difficult

(Continued)

TABLE 11–4. (*Continued*)

Monitor	Indications	Contraindica-tions	Normal Values	Complications and Problems
CO_2	Any intubated patient	None	$PaCO_2$ = 35–45	Malfunctioning of equipment
Apnea monitor	Any patient with a history of apneic spells Any patient who is excessively drowsy Any patient in which there is doubt as to the adequacy of muscle relaxant reversal	None	Respiratory rate 8–16 (adult, consider tidal volume)	Malfunctioning of equipment, "false" positive alarms
ABGs	Abnormal values obtained from any of the above Monitoring of lung ventilation	Inaccessible arterial site	pH 7.35–7.45, pCO_2 35–45, pO_2 84–104 100 − years of age/3	Hematoma, infection, emboli
CNS				
Visual reflexes	All patients post-anesthesia (general, regional, conscious sedation)	None	Extremity movement	Reflexes abnormal during emergence from anesthesia Remember to check patients who received regional anesthesia for block regression to rule out cord compression

TABLE 11–4. (Continued)

Monitor	Indications	Contraindications	Normal Values	Complications and Problems
Auditory	All patients post-anesthesia (general, regional, conscious sedation)	None	Alert, oriented to person, place, time (or status comparable to preoperative) Ability to move extremities on command	Accurate assessment cannot be made until patient almost fully recovered from anesthesia
EEG	Patients at unusual risk of CNS complications due to disease or type of surgery	None		Cost, complexity, problems of interpretation
Intracranial pressure	Patients with increased ICP due to trauma or disease and with ICP monitoring device in place	None (once device is in place)	5–15 torr	Transient changes due to coughing, straining, movement which is common in patients emerging from anesthesia Infection

Kidneys

Monitor	Indications	Contraindications	Normal Values	Complications and Problems
Urine output	Critically ill patient, elderly Extensive and/or lengthy surgery Preexisting renal disease Hypovolemia, major trauma, multiple transfusions	None (risks/benefits)	1 cc/kg/hour	Infection, tissue trauma Mechanical difficulties—obstruction of catheter

(Continued)

TABLE 11–4. (*Continued*)

Monitor	Indications	Contraindica- tions	Normal Values	Complications and Problems
Temperature				
Noninvasive Invasive	All PACU pa- tients should have some form of tem- perature monitoring to detect hypo- thermia or hyperthermia	None Inaccessibility to appropriate body cavity/ orifice	37° C ± 1°	Skin, axillary— varies with blood flow to area Rectal—varies with blood flow—fecal mass acts as insulator Esophagus—if not in lower esophagus re- flects tem- perature of respiratory gases rather than core temperature Tympanic mem- brane— membrane perforation and hemor- rhage, accu- racy very de- pendent on proper place- ment

by the physician prescribing an invasive monitoring device. The risk–benefit ratio must be considered and is an important factor in deciding what, when, and how to monitor a patient. Again, individualization of monitoring is important.

Greenberg and Peskin (1985) propose three different levels of monitoring: basic, advanced, and sophisticated.

Basic Monitoring. The set of surveillance data required daily on all patients to define degree of stability or to detect deviation constitutes basic monitoring. Surveillance is a continuous process. For those patients who reside only 24 to 48 hours in the SICU as an extension of the postoperative PACU, this is the usual level. Elderly or otherwise high-risk patients

TABLE 11–5. PROBLEMS IN THE PACU

Problem	Visual	Auditory	Mechanical	Other	Remarks
Airway obstruction	Lack of chestwall movement, nasal flaring, tracheal tug, bucking, retraction of intercostal and abdominal muscles If patient on ventilator, may see high inflation pressure Reservoir bag will not empty or refill properly	Coughing stridor Absence of breath sounds	Decreased bedside spirometer measurements (decreased TV, decreased FEV$_1$)	Signs of hypoxemia and hypercarbia	Postoperative patients during emergence from anesthesia may have airway obstruction due to lips, tongue, epiglottis, secretions, bronchospasms, and laryngospasms, sedation Anesthetic drugs + muscle relexants = beware.
Ventilation					
Hyper	Increased respiratory rate	Increased breath sounds	Increased RR/increased TV	ABG	Best way to assess ventilation is with arterial blood gas. (Look at respiratory rate and PaCO$_2$ value to determine if ventilatory rate is appropriate to keep pCO$_2$ in normal range, (5–45 mm Hg)
Hypo	Decreased respiratory rate		Decreased RR/decreased TV	ABG Apnea monitor, transcutaneous pCO$_2$ monitor, and end expired CO$_2$ monitor	

(Continued)

TABLE 11–5. (Continued)

Problem	Visual	Auditory	Mechanical	Other	Remarks
Hypoxemia	Decreased minute volume Restrictive dressings causing decreased respiratory movements Analysis of pattern of respiration	Decreased breath sounds Evidence of pulmonary edema, pneumothorax, accidental intubation of main stem bronchus with unilateral decrease in BS	Changes in lung compliance	ABG transcutaneous pO_2 monitor Chest x-ray Check vital signs	Best way to assess oxygenation is with arterial blood gas, looking at PaO_2 and FiO_2 An appropriate formula for PaO_2 for patient on room air is mean $PaO_2 = 100$ years of age $/ 3$
Pneumothorax	Decreased diaphragmatic movement on affected side Increased RR	Change in breath sounds Decrease in quantity and altered quality	Decreased TV Increased RR Sudden changes in vital signs	ABG Chest x-ray	Look for procedures in OR where incidence of pneumothorax is high: central line insertion. Surgery near diaphragm Malfunction of chest tube
Aspiration	Vomiting. May see vomitus from mouth if patient is asleep. "Silent aspiration" may occur.	Abnormal sounds in throat, wheezing, rhonchi, rales		Chest x-ray ABG	Check pH of vomitus; if below 2.0, consider need for intubation, mechanical ventilation with PEEP

Disturbance of Circulation

Hypotension	Patient is diaphoretic, color is pale. Decreased respirations	Can't auscultate blood pressure	Decreased pressure readings (palpate artery to make certain that pressure is not artificially low)	Check Hgb, Hct	Most common cause is hypovolemia. Determine amount and type of fluid replacement (crystalloid, PRBC, whole blood)
Hypertension		Patient is complaining of pain (most common cause of increased BP)			

Cardiac Instability

Dysrhythmia	ECG analysis: check lead II and lead V$_5$	Keep audio on ECG monitor	Arterial pressure monitor to determine effect of rhythm disturbance on cardiac function	Finger on pulse	Etiology of dysrhythmia must be known; e.g., PVCs must be "normal" for patient and due to pain, hypokalemia, hypoxemia, myocardial ischemia
					Etiology is different, treatment should be different
					To determine etiology of PVCs, may need ABG for PaO$_2$. Serum K+, review of EKG for signs of ischemia

(Continued)

TABLE 11–5. (Continued)

Problem	Visual	Auditory	Mechanical	Other	Remarks
Acute cardiac failure	Jugular venous distention Pulmonary edema Hypotension	S_3 noted Complaints of chest pain Dyspnea	Arterial line may show poor stroke volume Consider Swan-Ganz if event occurs in PACU		
Temperature Regulation					
Hypothermia	Shivering CNS depression ECG changes Temperature decrease	If awake, patient complains of "feeling cold" (hospital postoperative surveys show this is a very common patient complaint)	Temperature probes Temperature monitors (invasive vs. noninvasive); sites—skin, axilla, muscle, rectum, esophagus, tympanic membrane probe and Swan-Ganz monitor	Sympathetic nervous system stimulation causes increased HR, increased BP Blood glucose may be increased	Increased O_2 consumption Drug biotransformation slower Slowing of metabolic process
Hyperthermia	Sweating Temperature increase	Complaints of "feeling warm"	Body core temperature best assessed by lower esophageal probe and Swan-Ganz	Increased ventilatory work Increased respiratory rate	Always keep malignant hyperthermia in mind—may first be seen in PACU
Delayed Awakening					
Delirium (restlessness)	Inappropriate movements Altered reflexes	Inappropriate responses	None	ABG Metabolic profile Drug screen if trauma case Check intraoperative narcotic doses	Consider hypoxemia in differential diagnosis. Consider reversal agents and/or antagonists

Nausea and vomiting	Check for emesis	Patient complains (differentiate between "sharp" vs. "burning" complaints)	None	Check for abdominal/bladder distention Air in stomach, consider NG tube	Complaints of nausea following narcotic adminstration is not uncommon Increased incidence of N + V after gynecological surgery
Pain	Patient's appearance, movements	Verbal complaints	None	Question patient regarding site of pain, type of pain	Titrate narcotics, pain relief vs. respiratory depression
Renal failure	Urine output (measure with Foley for accurate output)	None	None	Check urine for pH, ketones, sugar, and blood Check specific gravity	Consider urinary bladder catheter in patients who may be hypovolemic, have major trauma, have cardiac or renal disease

(such as those with cardiac or renal failure) also benefit from this monitoring, on an elective basis.

Advanced Monitoring. This level of monitoring is indicated for patients with significantly greater deviations or greater potential for deviation as a result of their preexisting diseases, trauma, or stress. Monitoring at this level may simply require more frequent observation, not necessarily inclusion of new variables. This level of monitoring necessarily becomes more invasive. It always includes a central venous pressure line and an arterial catheter for monitoring pressures as well as easily acquiring blood samples for multiple blood-gas determinations. The majority of patients in the SICU require this level of monitoring for a period of time.

Sophisticated Monitoring. Sophisticated monitoring is reserved for patients with major traumatic or surgical stress and true multisystem disease, either acute or preexisting. These patients constitute a high-risk group and generally will not tolerate major deviations in physiology, as they are already functioning at maximal homeostatic compensation. This group of patients must have as completely uneventful and error-free a postinjury course as possible in order to recover. Thus, monitoring must be both more aggressive and more frequent. The remainder of this chapter discusses monitoring techniques for various body systems. Tables 11-6 through 11-9 utilize equations that are given in Appendix 11-1.

RESPIRATORY SYSTEM

Adequate gas exchange is essential for survival, for no other mechanism is available to provide oxygen and exchange carbon dioxide short of extracorporeal membrane oxygenation, which has not been demonstrated to be a clinically useful technique. Monitoring the respiratory system is mandatory and should include evaluation of the physical appearance of the lungs, the mechanics of respiration, and the ability to exchange gases (Table 11-6).

Impaired Oxygen Delivery

An increase in respiratory rate often reflects an increased demand for oxygen. Whether it is due to altered oxygen-carrying capacity (anemia), poor pulmonary gas exchange (adult respiratory distress syndrome), or increased oxygen consumption (sepsis), increased respiratory rate constitutes a significant early warning sign of impaired oxygen delivery. Significant increases are 20 percent between consecutive measurements. Deter-

TABLE 11–6. RESPIRATORY SYSTEM

	Mea-sured	De-rived	For-mula in Ap. 11-1.	Frequency of Observation/Recording Recommended Range in Hours		
				Basic	Advanced	Sophisticated
Chest X-ray	X			24 (12–48)	24 (12–48)	12 (6–18)
Mechanics						
Respiratory rate	X			2 (1–4)	1 (C–4)	½ (C–1)
Tidal volume	X				24 (C–24)	2 (C–6)
Minute ventilation		X	X		6 (4–12)	4 (2–6)
Vital capacity[a]	X				24	12
Inspiratory force	X				6	6
Work of breathing		X				12 (12–24)
Respiratory compliance		X	X			6
Heavy water	X					6
Gas Exchange						
Arterial blood gases[b]	X			24 (12–18)	8 (4–12)	1 (C–6)
Transcutaneous O_2	X			24 (12–48)	8 (4–12)	1 (C–6)
Transcutaneous CO_2	X			24 (12–48)	8 (4–12)	1 (C–6)
Shunt fraction		X	X		24	12 (6–24)
Alveolar-arterial gradient		X	X		24	12 (6–24)
Respiratory index		X	X			24
Cuff pressure, ET tube	X			24 (12–48)	24	24

[a]Essential for weaning from respirator; requires alert, cooperative patient.
[b]For oxygen and carbon dioxide.
C = continuous; ET = endotracheal.
(With permission of Greenburg AG & Peskin GW: Monitoring in the recovery room and surgical intensive care unit. In L Saidman & NT Smith (Eds.), Monitoring in Anesthesia (2nd ed.) Stoneham, Mass.: Butterworth, 1984.)

mination of respiratory rate along with routine chest x-ray constitutes basic monitoring for this system.

Lung Compliance

Tidal volume, minute volume, and vital capacity (available with the Wright respirometer, shown in Fig. 11-4) are useful measures of pulmonary mechanics with great prognostic significance, especially in defining the need for respiratory assistance or the ability to wean a patient from respiratory support. Inspiratory force measurements are also helpful in predicting successful weaning. A crude measure of lung compliance is obtainable by dividing peak airway pressure into volume delivered, especially if the patient is on a volume-regulated respirator. If a greater pressure is required to deliver the same volume, compliance is decreased, as might be seen in progressive adult respiratory distress syndrome. A yet more sensitive indicator of altered compliance is the measurement of lung water by the dual indicator dilution method (Tranbaugh & associates, 1980).

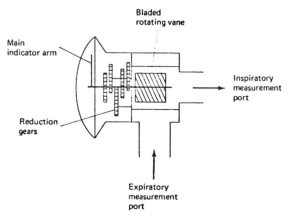

Figure 11–4. Rotating vane spirometer (Wright respirometer). *(Rarey KP & Youtsey JW: Respiratory Patient Care. Englewood Cliffs, N.J.: Prentice-Hall, 1981, p.344, with permission.)*

Work of Breathing

Perhaps the most accurate and useful measure of pulmonary mechanics is determination of the "work of breathing" (Peters & associates, 1972). Unfortunately, this requires special equipment and trained personnel. These measurements are reserved for unusual cases requiring sophisticated monitoring. Newer developments in clinical mass spectroscopy may provide a means of obtaining this variable reliably.

Arterial Blood Gases

Evaluation of pulmonary gas exchange is most easily accomplished by measurement of arterial blood gases, at least once every 24 hours for basic monitoring and more frequently for the other levels (see Appendix 10-2). Determination of shunt fraction, alveolar-arterial oxygen gradient, and respiratory index (Goldfarb & associates, 1975) are reserved for monitoring in depth, especially when there is significant pulmonary insult. Correlation to lung water measurements is also helpful here.

Recently available transcutaneous oxygen and carbon dioxide monitors, especially for neonates, may also permit close observation of these variables in a less invasive manner. If more than three blood-gas determinations are required per day, the placement of an arterial line is indicated, if only because it decreases sampling time, freeing the nurse for more critical tasks.

Transcutaneous measurements of oxygen and carbon dioxide are also seen as a system improvement, decreasing nurse involvement with sampling and perhaps decreasing patient costs. The application in adults is not yet clear and the validity of results for oxygen, especially when out of the ambient oxygen range, is questionable. This is an exciting development worth watching as it unfolds. For now it may provide trend data useful for separating circulatory from respiratory impairment in the seriously diseased patient (Tremper & Shoemaker, 1981).

In recent years, an increased awareness has developed of tracheal damage secondary to overinflation of the endotracheal tube cuff. Even with low-pressure cuffs and newer occluding devices, this remains a problem. To prevent difficulties, it is wise to monitor the endotracheal cuff pressure every 6 to 8 hours whenever the patient is intubated. Pressure should not exceed 15 to 20 cm H_2O. Ideally it should be maintained below central venous pressure to avoid venous occlusion (Fig. 11-5).

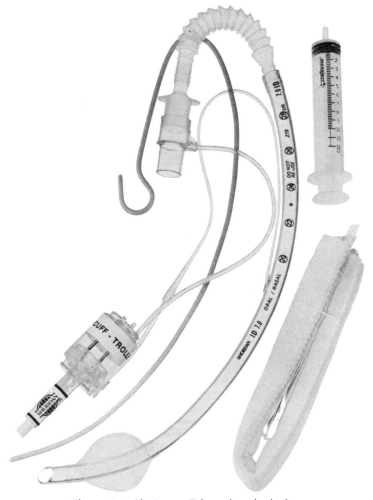

Figure 11–5. The Intensa-Tube endotracheal tube.

CARDIOVASCULAR SYSTEM

After ascertaining that an adequate oxygen supply can be taken on, delivery of that fuel to the tissues must be assessed (Table 11-7). The cardiovascular system has two major components: (1) the heart, as the pump, and (2) the vascular tree, as the delivery route. Delicate and redundant control mechanisms exist to maintain an effective interaction between components.

Monitoring arterial pressure and heart rate is synonymous with observation of vital signs. Fluctuations in these significant variables are of great prognostic value and form the basis for all monitoring efforts.

TABLE 11–7. CARDIOVASCULAR SYSTEM

	Measured	Derived	Formula in Ap. 11-1	Frequency of Observation/Recording Recommended Range in Hours		
				Basic	Advanced	Sophisticated
Arterial blood pressure (systolic, diastolic, mean)	X			2 (1–4)	1 (C–2)	$\frac{1}{4}$ (C–1)
Arterial pressure	X					
Heart rate	X			2 (1–4)	1 (C–2)	$\frac{1}{4}$ (C–1)
Pulse rate[a]	X					
ECG rhythm strip[b]						
Ectopic beats/min	X					1 (C–2)
Arrhythmias diagnosis[b]		X				
Central venous pressure	X			2 (1–4)	1 (C–2)	$\frac{1}{4}$ (C–1)
Pulmonary arterial pressure (systolic, diastolic, mean)	X				2 (C–4)	1 (C–2)
Pulmonary capillary wedge pressure	X				2 (C–4)	1 (C–2)
Left atrial pressure	X					1 (C–2)
Cardiac output	X					6 (C–24)
Left ventricular volume	X					
Cardiac index		X	X			
Total systemic resistance		X	X			
Pulmonary vascular resistance		X	X			
Cardiac work, left ventricle		X	X			
Cardiac work, right ventricle		X	X			
Stroke index		X	X			
Stroke work		X	X			
Clinical 'Starlings' curve	X					
Measurements of "contraction"						
Time-tension index		X	X			
Mean systolic ejection rate		X	X			
Central blood volume	X					

[a]As indicated on demand
[b]As indicated
C = continuous
(With permission of Greenburg AG & Peskin GW: Monitoring in the recovery room and surgical intensive care unit. In L Saidman & NT Smith (Eds.), Monitoring in Anesthesia (2nd ed.) Stoneham, Mass.: Butterworth, 1984.)

Pulmonary Artery Catheters

More recently, the flow-directed pulmonary arterial catheter has been available for obtaining data. Although the significance of variation is still being questioned, it is clear that the relationship between the left ventricular end-diastolic, left atrial, pulmonary capillary wedge (PCW), and pulmonary arterial end-diastolic pressure is legitimate in the absence of significant valvular heart disease, and thus PCW is helpful in assessing function in the left side of the heart (Shin & associates, 1975).

Flow-directed catheters are now constructed with triple lumens and integral thermistors, making them useful for determination of cardiac output when combined with cardiac output computers (Fig. 11-6). Some cardiac surgeons prefer to leave a catheter in the left atrium, through cannulation of a small pulmonary vein, for postoperative monitoring. This provides a true measure of filling pressure of the left heart, independent of the pulmonary vascular or parenchymal status.

Atrial Filling Pressure

Just as PCW challenged the accuracy of central venous pressure measurements in assessing volume and cardiac function status, newer methods of assessing the left heart—especially left ventricular volume—have raised some questions about the accuracy of PCW. Under most circumstances, left atrial filling pressure reflects the left ventricular volume and thus can be used to construct a "clinical Starling curve," a plot of cardiac output against filling pressure. However, using a variety of invasive (implanted crystals) and noninvasive (cineangiography) techniques, it appears that left ventricular volume, especially when the left ventricular wall loses compliance, does not correlate well with PCW pressure (Calvin & associates, 1981). This observation does not negate the use of the Swan-Ganz catheter but rather implies there will be situations in which it provides less than sufficient data.

Cardiac Output

It is thus possible to selectively monitor systemic perfusion pressures, filling pressures in the right and left sides of the heart, and pulmonary vascular dynamics, as indicated by patient risk evaluation. At more advanced monitoring levels, a measure of blood flow—cardiac output—is not only a useful variable by itself but, more importantly, is a factor in many equations for derived variables. The pressure/flow relationship is usually expressed as vascular resistance, and reflects the vascular tone as well as the size of the perfusion bed. Total systemic resistance and pulmonary vascular resistance can be calculated and are helpful in establishing degree of functional impairment. Manipulation of these variables pharmacologically for certain states can only be accomplished if they are in fact observed.

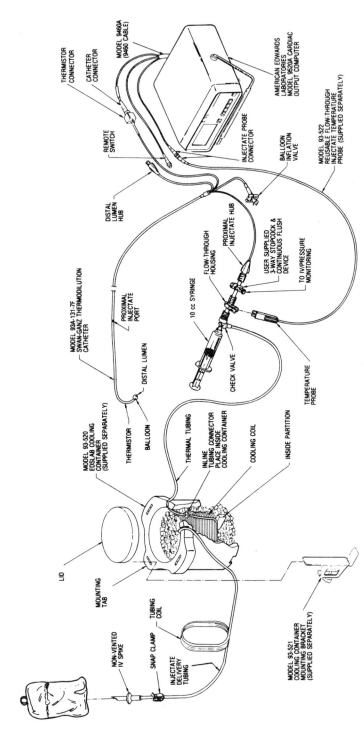

Figure 11–6. CO-Set, closed injectate delivery system, Cold injectate. (*Courtesy of American Edwards Laboratories.*)

Indexes

A variety of indexes can be calculated (such as cardiac index or stroke index, which measures left ventricular ejection volume), and by normalization to body surface area, values can be compared with normal or expected reference population data. Further derivation of right or left ventricular stroke work or minute work is possible. Calculation of these variables as part of the monitoring effort is reserved for the most sophisticated level.

Cardiac Contractility

Measurement of cardiac contractility has also been proposed as a means for evaluating cardiac function. Both mean systolic ejection rate and time–tension index have been evaluated. Unfortunately, they have little prognostic value, and their physiologic implication, apart from reflecting the effects of cardiotonic pharmacologic agents, awaits further elucidation.

For now, pressures, flow, and resistance are the most clearly understood and useful data in the monitoring effort. Determination of cardiac output is part of the sophisticated monitoring level and should also be used when a patient with significant cardiac disease is monitored at the advanced level.

HEMATOLOGIC/COAGULATION SYSTEM

The values in this system provide information about hemoglobin, clotting factors, and blood elements which may signal systemic disease, inability to respond to stress, or a major bleeding diathesis, independent of cause. These variables are commonly known and routinely used, and all except for red cell indexes are measured directly. Table 11-8 relates them to monitoring levels.

Fluids and Electrolytes

The internal environmental composition of the body is reflected in the status of the fluid and electrolyte system (Table 11-9). Maintaining stability and correcting deficits in fluid and electrolytes must be given high priority in monitoring and therapy.

MONITORS

A major contribution to the current practice of medicine is made by the galaxy of monitoring equipment and techniques developed in the past two decades. They have played a vital role in improving our ability to prevent, recognize, and treat many conditions that previously contributed to morbidity and mortality.

TABLE 11–8. HEMATOLOGIC/COAGULATION SYSTEM

	Mea-sured	Frequency of Observation/Recording Recommended Range in Hours		
		Basic	Advanced	Sophisticated
Hemoglobin	X	24	24	12
Hematocrit	X			12 (4–12)
Red cell count	X			24
Red cell indices	X			
White cell count[a]	X			(8–24)
Differential count	X			
Platelets	X			
Prothrombin time	X	Only if indicated	Only if indicated	
Partial thromboplastin time	X			
Fibrinogen	X			When indicated
Reticulocytes	X			
Triple P test	X			

[a]May increase if sepsis suspected.
(With permission of Greenburg AG & Peskin GW: Monitoring in the recovery room and surgical intensive care unit. In L Saidman & NT Smith (Eds.), Monitoring in Anesthesia (2nd ed.) Stoneham, Mass.: Butterworth, 1984.)

Securing the Swan-Ganz

The Swan-Ganz thermodilution catheter is a triple-lumen catheter inserted into the right heart to measure cardiac output, central venous pressure, pulmonary artery pressure, and pulmonary wedge pressure (Fig. 11-7). One port contains a thermistor tip to which the cardiac output monitor is connected.

The patient who needs Swan-Ganz monitoring should have intensive nursing care (Table 11-10).

Before insertion, explain the procedure to the patient. Record the patient's vital signs. Check the position of ECG electrodes and clarity of the oscilloscope signal. Have lidocaine and a defibrillator handy. Set up equipment at bedside. Position the patient comfortably, preferably supine, with arm extended at an angle of 60 to 90 degrees to the body and externally rotated upward. If the external jugular approach is to be used, place the patient in the Trendelenburg position with towel rolls under the shoulders.

During insertion, watch the oscilloscope for arrhythmias. Monitor and evaluate the patient's condition and vital signs.

After insertion, monitor PAP continuously. Keep the line patent with flush solution. Anchor the transducer to the patient's arm or stationary IV pole at RA level.

To flush solution add 500 units of heparin (1:1000-unit concentration) to 500 ml bag normal saline solution and label.

TABLE 11–9. FLUID AND ELECTROLYTE SYSTEM

	Measured	Derived	Formula in Ap. 11-1	Frequency of Observation/Recording Recommended Range in Hours		
				Basic	Advanced	Sophisticated
Body weight				24	24	12 (4–24)
"Total" input				8	4	
"Total" measured output				8	4	2
Insensible loss		X	X	24	24	12
Serum electrolytes:						
Na, K, Cl, HCO_3				24	12	6 (2–8)
Mg, Ca, PO_4				48 (48–96)	24 (24–72)	24 (12–24)
Serum glucose[a]				24	24	12 (6–8)
Serum osmolality		X	X		24	24 (8–24)
Plasma volume	X					24
Red cell volume	X					24
Specific parenteral input, type, volume	X			4	2	1 (¼–1)
Specific output, site, and volume	X			4	2	1 (¼–1)
Specific output, electrolyte concentrations	X					24 (12–36)
Cumulative volume (I/O) balance		X		8	4	1 (¼–1)
Cumulative ionic concentration balance		X		8	4	24
Output, urine[b]	X			4	2	1
Output, chest tube(s)[c]	X			4	2	1 (¼–1)

[a]Diabetic acidosis/hyperglycemia more frequently.
[b]If Foley present, interval can be shortened to hourly.
[c]Depends on patient state and rate of loss.
(With permission of Greenburg AG & Peskin GW: Monitoring in the recovery room and surgical intensive care unit. In L Saidman & NT Smith (Eds.), Monitoring in Anesthesia (2nd ed.) Stoneham, Mass.: Butterworth, 1984.)

Place bag in a pressurized pump bag and inflate to a pressure of 150 mm Hg. Maintain this pressure at all times. At this pressure the intraflow will deliver 3 ml of flush solution per hour.

To inflate the balloon for PCW pressures, proceed slowly until you see a PCW tracing on the oscilloscope. Do not leave the balloon inflated any longer than it takes to record the pressures. Pulmonary infarction can occur when balloons are kept inflated or the PA line is left in the permanent wedge position.

These techniques, particularly those involving insertion of central venous pressure (CVP) monitoring lines, intraarterial catheters (A-lines), and Swan-Ganz catheters (PA lines), all carry with their application some varying degree of risk to the patient. Such risk should be minimized by outlining the anesthesiologist's position on the provision of such procedures in the delivery of anesthesia care by anesthesia care team personnel:

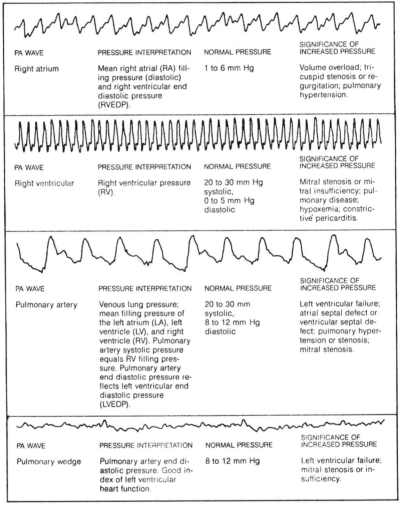

PA WAVE	PRESSURE INTERPRETATION	NORMAL PRESSURE	SIGNIFICANCE OF INCREASED PRESSURE
Right atrium	Mean right atrial (RA) filling pressure (diastolic) and right ventricular end diastolic pressure (RVEDP).	1 to 6 mm Hg	Volume overload; tricuspid stenosis or regurgitation; pulmonary hypertension.
Right ventricular	Right ventricular pressure (RV).	20 to 30 mm Hg systolic, 0 to 5 mm Hg diastolic	Mitral stenosis or mitral insufficiency; pulmonary disease; hypoxemia; constrictive pericarditis.
Pulmonary artery	Venous lung pressure; mean filling pressure of the left atrium (LA), left ventricle (LV), and right ventricle (RV). Pulmonary artery systolic pressure equals RV filling pressure. Pulmonary artery end diastolic pressure reflects left ventricular end diastolic pressure (LVEDP).	20 to 30 mm systolic, 8 to 12 mm Hg diastolic	Left ventricular failure; atrial septal defect or ventricular septal defect; pulmonary hypertension or stenosis; mitral stenosis.
Pulmonary wedge	Pulmonary artery end diastolic pressure. Good index of left ventricular heart function.	8 to 12 mm Hg	Left ventricular failure; mitral stenosis or insufficiency.

Figure 11–7. Recording pulmonary artery patterns.

1. The decision to use invasive monitoring is a medical judgment and should, therefore, be made only by a qualified physician.
2. Invasive monitoring techniques should be prescribed by a physician. Depending upon its risk, each should be applied only by a competent and trained physician or under the immediate medical direction of such a competent and responsible physician.
3. Training and awarding credentials to nonphysician members of the anesthesia care team, allowing them to perform invasive monitoring techniques, should be approved at the local medical staff level by the anesthesia department and the active medical staff.

TABLE 11–10. SOLVING PROBLEMS WITH SWAN-GANZ CATHETER

The Problem	If the Cause is . . .	The Solution is to . . .
Damped pressures	Air in system	Check intraflow, stopcock, and transducer for bubbles.
	Blood on transducer	Flush off or change transducer.
	Clot in system	Aspirate blood until no longer thickened; notify doctor.
	Catheter kinked	Cough patient or extend patient's artm to 90 degree angle from body and gently flush catheter. If problem, obtain X-ray.
	Loose connection	Check connections for security.
	Incorrect stopcock position	Correct.
Transducer imbalance	Damaged transducer	Try another transducer.
	Transducer connected to wrong amplifier	Check amplifier connection.
	Broken amplifier	Change it.
Waveform drifting	Insufficient warm-up time	Allow recommended time.
	Cable air vents kinked or coiled	Unkink or decompress.
False low reading	Damped waveform	(See section on damped pressures.)
	Transducer imbalance	Place transducer at heart level.
	Wrong calibration	Recalibrate.
False high reading	Transducer imbalance	Rebalance.
	Flush solution administered too quickly	Pour slow continual flush to 3 to 6 ml/hour.
	Air in system	Remove air from tubing/or transducer.
Configuration	Improper catheter placement	Try to wedge catheter. Obtain PCW. If problem, obtain X-ray.
	Transducer needs to be calibrated	Recalibrate.
	Transducer not at RA level	Reposition and recalibrate.
	Transducer loosely connected to catheter	Secure.
Drifting wedge pressure (with inflated balloon)	Balloon overinflation	Watch scope while inflating balloon. When waveform changes from a PA to a wedge shape, stop inflating.
PCW pressure trace unobtainable	Incorrect amount of balloon air	Deflate, start again slowly.
	Ruptured balloon	With no resistance to inflation, stop inflation. Notify doctor.

(Nursing Skillbook: Nursing Critically Ill Patients Confidently. Springhouse, Pa.: Intermed Communications, 1981, with permission.)

4. Some of the invasive monitoring tasks—namely the insertion of CVP lines placed via the upper extremity and of arterial lines (A-lines)—may be delegated to properly trained and credentialed members of an anesthesia care team. Performance, however, should be under the immediate and personal direction of the leader of the team, preferably an anesthesiologist.

5. Insertion of pulmonary artery catheters is a relatively hazardous procedure and should be done only by a properly trained physician. (American Society of Anesthesiologists, 1984).

These stipulations are appropriate and self-explanatory. As monitoring becomes more sophisticated, we should not give up "proven ways" of patient assessment, but rather increase our armamentarium of monitoring devices to see, hear, and watch more patients, especially at such a critical time as the emergence from anesthesia. To those who work in the PACU, each patient presents a challenge: what, when, and how to monitor patients so they can make a successful transition from the anesthetic state to the awake state. This goal will remain; how we will accomplish it—what methods of monitoring we will use—will change.

APPENDIX 11–1

Equations for Derived Variables in Tables 11–6 through 11–9

This appendix contains the basic equations used for the derived variables in Tables 11-6 through 11-9. The equations are organized sequentially and grouped by system.

RESPIRATORY SYSTEM

Minute ventilation:

$$\text{Tidal volume} \times \text{respiratory rate/min} = \text{ml/min}$$

Respiratory compliance:

$$\text{Tidal volume} \div \text{peak respiratory airway pressure} = \text{ml/cm } H_2O$$

Shunt fraction:

Q_s/Q_t = (alveolar O_2 content − arterial O_2 content) ÷ (alveolar O_2 content − mixed venous O_2 content)

Alveolar–arterial gradient:

$$A-aDo_2 = [(P_B - P_{H2OT})\ FiO_2 - PaCO_2] - PaO_2$$
usually when FiO_2 = 100% for consistency

Respiratory index:

$$A-aDo_2 \div PaO_2$$

CARDIOVASCULAR SYSTEM

Cardiac index:

$$CI = \text{cardiac output} \div \text{body surface area}$$

Note: For interpatient comparisons and reference standards, use of the "index" term, output normalized to body surface area, is preferred.

Total systemic resistance:

$$TSR = 79.9\ (\text{mean aortic pressure} - \text{mean central venous pressure} \div CI$$
(Requires expression of CVP as mm Hg)

Pulmonary vascular resistance:

$$PVR = 79.9\ (\text{mean pulmonary arterial pressure} - \text{PA wedge}) \div CI$$

Left ventricular or cardiac work:

$$LVCW = CI \times \text{mean aortic pressure} \times 0.0136$$

Right ventricular or cardiac work:

$$RVCW = CI \times \text{mean pulmonary arterial pressure} \times 0.0136$$

Stroke index:

$$SI = \text{cardiac index} \div \text{heart rate}$$

Stroke work, left ventricle:

$$SI \times \text{mean aortic pressure} \times 0.1135$$

Time-tension index:

$$TTI = \text{mean aortic pressure} \times \text{heart rate} \times \text{duration of systole}$$

Mean systolic ejection rate:

$$SER = SI \div \text{duration of systole (in ml/sec/m}^2)$$

Central blood volume:

$$CBV = CI \times 16.7 \times \text{mean transit time (in ml/m}^2)$$

(Calculation of mean transit time requires an indicator–dilution curve using a dye; the thermal device will not yield this number.)

OXYGEN TRANSPORT

Arteriovenous O_2 difference:

a-vDo_2 = arterial O_2 content − mixed venous O_2 content (in ml/100 ml)

Oxygen extraction ratio:

$$O_2 \text{ ER} = \text{arteriovenous } O_2 \text{ difference} \div \text{arterial } O_2 \text{ content}$$

Oxygen consumption:

$$Vo_2 = \text{arteriovenous } O_2 \text{ difference} \times CI \times 10 \text{ (in ml/min/m}^2)$$

Oxygen availability:

$$O_2 \text{ availability} = \text{arterial } O_2 \text{ content} \times CI \times 10 \text{ (in ml/min/m}^2)$$

FLUID AND ELECTROLYTES

Insensible loss:

$$[\text{Today's weight (kg)} + \text{total output (ml) last 24 hours}] - [\text{yesterday's weight (kg)} + \text{total input}]$$

Serum osmolality:

$$1.86(\text{Na}) + \text{BUN}/2.8 + \text{gluc}/18 + 19$$
(This represents the best estimate based on current data)

Miscellaneous

Free water clearance:

Urine volume − [(osmolality urine ÷ osmolality plasma) × urine volume]

Creatinine clearance, estimated:

$$[(140 - \text{age})(\text{weight kg})] \div (72 \times \text{serum creatinine})$$
(Take 85% of value for females.)

(With permission of Greenburg AG & Peskin GW: Monitoring in the recovery room and surgical intensive care unit. In L Saidman & NT Smith (Eds.), Monitoring in Anesthesia (2nd ed.) Stoneham, Mass.: Butterworth, 1984.)

REFERENCES

American Society of Anesthesiologists: Statement on invasive monitoring in anesthesiology. New Orleans: ASA, Oct., 1984.

Blitt CD: Invasive monitoring in non-cardiac surgery. ASA Annual Refresher Course Lectures 33:103, 1982.

Calvin JE, Driedger AD & Sibbald WJ: The hemodynamic effect of rapid fluid infusion in critically ill patients. Surgery 90(61), 1981.

Cullen DJ: The recovery room. Seminars in Anesthesia 1(4):333–339, 1982.

Cushing H: On routine determinations of arterial tension in operating room or clinic. Boston Medical and Surgical Journal 148 (250), 1903.

Daily EK & Schroeder JS: Techniques in bedside hemodynamic monitoring. St. Louis: C.V. Mosby, 1985.

Fulton JF: Harvey Cushing: A biography. Springfield, Ill.: Chas. C Thomas, 1946.

Goldfarb MA, Ciurej TF, McAslan TC, et al.: Tracking respiratory therapy in the trauma patient. American Journal of Surgery 129:255, 1975.

Gordon AS: Practical aspects of blood flow measurements. Oxnard, Calif.: Statham Instruments, 1971.

Greenburg AG & Peskin GW: Monitoring in the recovery room and surgical intensive care unit. In L Saidman & NT Smith (Eds.), Monitoring in anesthesia (2nd ed.). Stoneham. Mass.: Butterworth, 1985, pp 405–436.

Hug CC Jr: Monitoring. In RD Miller (Ed.), Anesthesia. New York: Churchill Livingstone, 1981, pp. 157–201.

Peters RM, Hilberman M, Hogan JS, et al.: Objective indications for respiratory therapy in post-trauma and postoperative patients. American Journal of Surgery 124:267, 1972.

Shin B, McAslaw TC & Avella R: Problems with measurement using the Swan-Ganz catheter. Anesthesiology 43:474, 1975.

Tranbaugh RF, Lewis FR, Christensen JH, & Elings VB: Lung water changes after thermal injury. The effects of crystalloid resuscitation and sepsis. American Journal of Surgery 192:479, 1980.

Chapter 12

Later Postanesthetic Problems: The First 48 Hours

Kay E. Fraulini

We now know that many patient responses to anesthesia are much more delayed or prolonged than was once supposed. For this reason, it is important that PACU nurses and nurses who assume responsibility for patients beyond the PACU be well-informed regarding later postanesthetic occurrences. For the sake of order, these will be examined according to body system.

RESPIRATORY COMPLICATIONS

The type of anesthetic and the site of operation influence the reduction in arterial oxygen tension (PaO_2) seen following anesthesia and surgery (Fig. 12-1). Abdominal operations are associated with the most prolonged reductions in PaO_2. Although the PaO_2 may be normal in the immediate postoperative period, some investigators believe that abdominal operations under regional anesthesia are associated with the greatest reduction in $PaCO_2$ after 24 hours.

Hypoventilation is defined as inadequate alveolar ventilation resulting in an increase in the arterial carbon dioxide tension ($PaCO_2$). In the postoperative period, hypoventilation occurs as a result of poor respira-

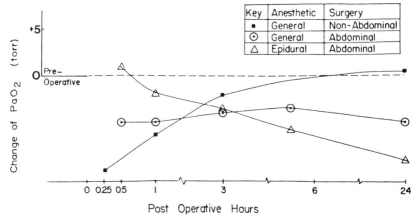

Figure 12–1. Reduction in arterial oxygen tension by type of anesthetic and site of surgery. *(From Marshall BE & Wyche MQ: Hypoxemia during and after anesthesia. Anesthesiology 37:178, 1972.)*

tory drive, poor muscle function, a high production rate of CO_2, or as the direct result of acute or chronic lung disease.

Central respiratory depression is seen with any anesthetic, but according to some authors is more common following intravenous than inhaled anesthetics. Narcotic anesthetics produce a respiratory depression that is detectable by a shift of the CO_2 response curve downward and to the right. Neurolept and narcotic anesthetic techniques can produce a biphasic respiratory depression with respiratory depression intraoperatively, which dissipates with arrival in the PACU only to be followed by a second period of respiratory depression (Fig. 12-2). Narcotic-induced respiratory depression can be reversed by use of narcotic antagonists. When

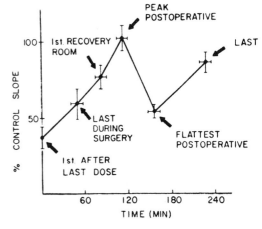

Figure 12–2. Biphasic respiratory depression exhibited by patients receiving neurolept agents supplementary to N_2O anesthesia. *(From Becker LD, Paulson BA, Miller RD, et al.: Biphasic respiratory depression after fentanyl-droperidol or fentanyl alone used to supplement nitrous oxide anesthesia. Anesthesiology 44:291, 1976.)*

small doses are used, these agents can reverse the narcotic-induced respiratory depression without altering pain relief; however, the duration of action of currently available antagonists is shorter than that of most narcotics, and the dose has to be repeated at least once. Larger doses of these agents reverse the analgesic effects of the narcotics and result in a patient in severe pain who often develops tachycardia and hypertension. This increase in rate pressure product (HR × systolic blood pressure) results in large increases in myocardial oxygen consumption and possibly ischemia in patients with coronary artery disease. An inadequate central respiratory drive can also be seen with certain neurosurgical procedures such as cervical cordotomy.

Poor respiratory muscular function occurs following surgery and often contributes to hyperventilation. The site of the incision affects the ability to take a large breath as measured by vital capacity (VC). Nearly all patients have reduction in VC, showing as much as a 60 percent reduction on the day of surgery (Fig. 12-3).

A vital capacity in excess of 15 ml/kg should transiently provide an adequate postoperative ventilatory reserve and allow for adequate deep breathing and coughing. The observation that VC is reduced by 50 to 75 percent within 24 hours following thoracic or abdominal surgery was first reported in 1927 (Shapiro, 1980). This observation has been reconfirmed numerous times and has proven to be extremely consistent. Since the normal adult vital capacity ranges between 55 and 85 ml/kg of normal body weight, any acute decrease in VC of up to 75 percent would leave most normal individuals with a VC greater than 15 ml/kg.

The postoperative VC reduction occurs gradually over 12 to 18 hours following the surgical procedure. This means that the patient's ventilatory

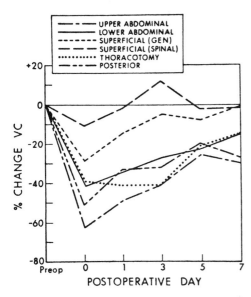

Figure 12–3. Change in vital capacity following surgical procedures at various sites. *(From Ali J, Weisel RD, Laung AB, et al.: Consequences of postoperative alterations in respiratory mechanics. American Journal of Surgery 128:376, 1974.)*

reserve will usually be significantly less 12 hours postoperatively than immediately following the surgical procedure. A clinical axiom of respiratory evaluation in the postsurgical patient is that the VC is maximally reduced 12 to 18 hours postoperative, and then gradually improves unless complications intervene. Most patients with an uncomplicated course approach their preoperative vital capacity levels by the third or fourth postoperative day. Some studies indicate that it is actually a slower process (Figs. 12-4A and 12-4B).

Clinical Guidelines

The reproducibility of surgically induced vital capacity reduction has allowed the following clinical guidelines to be developed and proved reliable beyond any reasonable doubt (Shapiro, 1980):

1. Elective upper abdominal procedures or thoracic procedures involving splitting of the sternum will, within 24 hours, result in a 60 to 75 percent decrease in the preoperative vital capacity.
2. Elective lower abdominal or thoracic procedures will, within 24 hours, result in a 30 to 50 percent decrease in the preoperative vital capacity.
3. Elective nonthoracoabdominal procedures will usually result in little postoperative vital capacity reduction; however, reductions resulting from anesthesia and narcotics are variable.

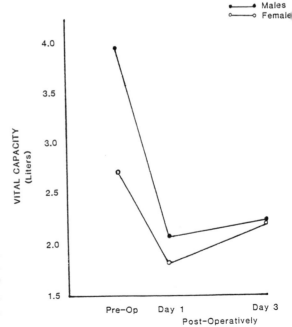

Figure 12–4A. Reduction in vital capacity by surgery. *(Fraulini KE: Effect of hand and pillow methods of incisional splinting for postoperative deep breathing and coughing on vital capacity and inspiratory pressure in cholecystectomized patients. Unpublished master's thesis. Loyola University of Chicago, 1980.)*

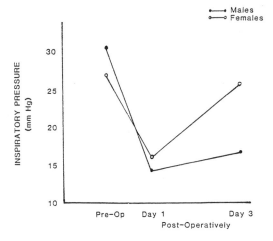

●———● Males
○———○ Females

Figure 12–4B. Postoperative effects on negative inspiratory pressure in cholecystectomized patients. *(Fraulini KE: Effect of hand and pillow methods of incisional splinting for postoperative deep breathing and coughing on vital capacity and inspiratory pressure in cholecystectomized patients. Unpublished master's thesis. Loyola University of Chicago, 1980.)*

Routine Monitoring

The simplest means of clinically monitoring the postoperative severity of vital capacity reduction is to serially observe the respiratory rate. Acute decreases in VC usually result in rapid and shallow ventilatory patterns. When an adult postoperative patient's rate becomes progressively faster in the first 12 hours and approaches 30 per minute, it usually reflects significant loss of ventilatory reserve unless significant pain is present. In such circumstances it is advisable to serially measure VC, tidal volume, and arterial blood gases in addition to making frequent clinical chest examinations (Shapiro, 1980).

Pulmonary Complications of Surgical Intervention

Most patients survive the acute restrictive pulmonary insult of elective thoracic and abdominal surgery with few detectable clinical problems. However, cardiopulmonary homeostasis is significantly stressed in many patients and results in complications. These postoperative pulmonary complications may be separated into two general categories: acute ventilatory failure and atelectasis/pneumonia. Although they are often difficult to clinically differentiate, it is convenient to separate them for purposes of discussion. For simplicity and clarity, variables such as cardiovascular, hepatorenal, and CNS function, as well as surgical technique and general medical care, are not emphasized in the following discussion; however, these variables must always be considered in an actual clinical evaluation.

Acute Ventilatory Failure. Acute ventilatory failure is defined as the sudden inability of the pulmonary system to adequately meet the metabolic demands of the body in reference to carbon dioxide hemeostasis. Through blood gas measurements this condition is clinically detectable by an arterial pCO_2 of greater than 50 mm Hg in conjunction with a pH below 7.30.

This may occur secondary to the significant increase in the energy required for adequate physiologic ventilation in the first 24 postoperative hours, especially when vital capacity becomes less than 10 ml/kg for a significant period of time. In addition, any increase in airway resistance will increase the work of breathing while any cardiovascular, hepatorenal, or CNS abnormality will decrease the patient's ability to meet increased energy requirements for ventilation.

A general guideline and reference point for estimating the probability of ventilatory failure in the first 24 hours is as follows. For an upper abdominal procedure in a patient with a normal cardiovascular, hepatorenal, and central nervous system:

> If percent FVC + percent FEV_1/FVC is less than 100, there is a 50 percent chance of that patient experiencing acute ventilatory failure in the first 24 hours.

This rule of thumb reflects the fact that if the patient is normal in all systems except pulmonary, and that pulmonary disease significantly limits ventilatory reserve, the chances of ventilatory failure caused by the surgical insult are great. Of course, significant disease in any other organ system will increase the chances of ventilatory failure.

Hypoxemia. Mild hypoxemia (PaO_2 70–90 mm Hg breathing room air) is expected for 48 hours in patients with normal, uncomplicated recovery. Moderate hypoxemia (PaO_2 50–70 mm Hg breathing room air) is common in patients with preexisting pulmonary disease and pulmonary complications. This hypoxemia is usually due to shunt effect and is correctable with 30 to 40 percent oxygen supplementation.

Atelectasis/Pneumonia. A decrease in FRC, decreased vital capacity, and the absence of periodic deep inflation are believed the main factors contributing to retained secretions and stasis pneumonia. It stands to reason that any intrinsic lung abnormality would tend to exaggerate the process.

The incidence of atelectasis and pneumonia after abdominal and thoracic surgery has been reported at rates varying from 12 to 80 percent. The disparity is probably explained by such variables as (1) the surgical procedure undertaken, (2) surgical technique, (3) preoperative condition of the patient, (4) preoperative and postoperative care, (5) retrospective versus prospective investigation, and (6) criteria used for diagnosing atelectasis and pneumonia. The single most useful clinical factor for delineating the high risk postoperative patient for atelectasis and pneumonia is the abnormal expiratory spirogram. This simple, inexpensive, and noninvasive bedside measurement has proven to be an effective means of delineating the patient at risk for postoperative pulmonary complications.

Preoperative Evaluation

The anticipated abdominal or thoracic surgical procedure must be clearly identified. Past medical history of preexistent lung disease, smoking, sputum production, exercise tolerance, and restrictive and obstructive phenomena must be examined. Preexistent cardiovascular disease (dyspnea on exertion, orthopnea, paroxysmal nocturnal dyspnea, dependent edema), evidence of congestive heart failure, angina, and myocardial infarctions must be elicited. The evaluation of preexistent renal disease and metabolic disease must be noted. Physical examination as to body weight, state of nutrition, color and temperature of the skin, chest configuration, skeletal abnormalities, pattern of ventilation, and auscultatory findings of the chest, including heart tones and murmurs, are essential. General laboratory studies, including electrocardiogram and chest x-ray, must be evaluated. At a minimum, a forced expiratory spirogram must be obtained and, if indicated, complete pulmonary function studies accomplished. Also if indicated, a blood gas measurement to further evaluate the pulmonary gas exchange should be accomplished.

A reliable system for generally arriving at a risk category for pulmonary complication in the patient undergoing abdominal or thoracic surgery is put forth in Table 12-1. Each of the five categories is evaluated and the patient ascribed a total score from 0 to 7. (Only one category is assigned for each variable, making 7 the highest score possible.)

Low Risk (0 points). When the patient receives no points, there should be little expectation that he or she will have pulmonary complications postoperatively. Incentive spirometry may prove useful, but above all the patient must be encouraged to frequently cough and deep-breathe. Oxygen therapy is usually not necessary after discharge from the PACU.

Moderate Risk (1 or 2 points). These patients have a significant incidence of postoperative complications—that is, atelectasis, pneumonia, decreased basilar breath sounds, fever of unknown origin, or mild hypoxemia. However, if properly treated these entities should not prove life threatening. Incentive spirometry is definitely indicated as a prophylactic measure and therapeutic measures (aerosol, IPPB, CPT) should be instituted when indicated. Serious consideration should be given to daily vital capacity measurements and arterial blood gas measurements to aid the physician in a pulmonary evaluation. Oxygen therapy is often indicated for several postoperative days.

High Risk (3 or more points). These patients should be seriously considered for remaining in an intensive care area for 24 to 48 hours postoperatively. Serial evaluation of cardiopulmonary reserve is indicated as well as evaluation for aggressive bronchial hygiene therapy.

A preoperative FVC of less than 20 ml/kg places the patient at high

TABLE 12–1. CLASSIFICATION SYSTEM FOR RISK OF PULMONARY COMPLICATION FOLLOWING THORACIC AND ABDOMINAL PROCEDURES

		Points
I.	**Expiratory Spirogram**	
	A. Normal (%FVC + %FEV$_1$/FVC 150)	0
	B. %FVC + %FEV$_1$/FVC = 100–150)	1
	C. %FVC + %FEV$_1$FVC 100	2
	D. Preoperative FVC 25 ml/kg	3
	E. Postbronchodilator FEV$_1$/FVC 50%	3
II.	**Cardiovascular System**	
	A. Normal	0
	B. Controlled hypertension, MI without sequelae for more than two years	0
	C. Dyspnea on exertion, orthopnea, PND, dependent edema, congestive heart failure, angina	1
III.	**Nervous System**	
	A. Normal	0
	B. Confusion, obtundation, agitation, spasticity, discoordination, bulbar malfunction	1
	C. Significant muscular weakness	1
IV.	**Arterial Blood Gas Measurement**	
	A. Acceptable	0
	B. PaCO$_2$ above 50 mm Hg or PaO$_2$ below 60 mm Hg on room air	1
	C. Metabolic pH abnormality above 7.50 or below 7.30	2
V.	A. Expected ambulation (at minimum sitting at bedside) within 36 hours	0
	B. Expected complete bed confinement for at least 36 hours	1

0 points = Low risk
1–2 points = Moderate risk
3 points = High risk
(From Shapiro B. Evaluation of respiratory function in the perioperative period. ASA Annual Refresher Course Lectures, 1980.)

risk for acute ventilatory failure in the postoperative period. These patients deserve careful evaluation and may be candidates for elective ventilator support.

Significant preoperative irreversible airway obstruction will significantly increase the postoperative work of breathing and diminish bronchial hygiene capability. In our experience, a patient free of pulmonary infection who manifests a postbronchodilator percent FEV$_1$/FVC of less than 50 percent should be considered at high risk for postoperative pulmonary complications.

Once again, careful preoperative evaluation will allow the practitioner to develop a plan of care that will cover the patient in the critical postanesthetic period, extending as it does beyond the PACU stay.

Other Respiratory Variables

Failure to antagonize neuromuscular blocking agents may result in inadequate respiratory muscle function postoperatively. This can be due to inadequate excretion of the drug, as in renal failure, or to the presence of other drugs that attenuate neuromuscular blockade, such as gentamycin, neomycin, clindamycin, and furosemide. Respiratory acidosis inhibits reversal of neuromuscular blockade, as does hypokalemia. Hypermagnesemia potentiates neuromuscular blockade, as does hypothermia. Fraulini and associates (1985) found in a sample of 312 PACU adults that 71.6 percent of the patients who arrived in the PACU intubated were hypothermic. And Vaughan and associates (1981) studied 198 PACU adults and observed that 13 percent of them were hypothermic on discharge from the PACU—again, an example of a problem that may extend beyond the immediate postanesthetic period.

Body temperature is significant as a reflection of increased metabolic rate. For any given level of ventilatory function, an increased level of metabolic demand will lead to increased ventilatory demands. Elective surgery is associated with less than a 10 percent increase in metabolic rate; however, major sepsis and major accidental injury can be associated with increases up to 50 percent, while burns and thyrotoxicosis can lead to 100 percent increases. The ventilatory requirement associated with increases in body temperature is a function of the dead space.

The most significant cause of an increased metabolic rate in the PACU setting is shivering, which can cause increases up to four times the resting metabolic rate. Shivering is a function of the temperature decrease that occurs in the operating room, the age of the patient, and the anesthetic used. Halothane seems to be the agent associated with the greatest degree of postoperative shivering. Patients receiving sodium nitroprusside for blood pressure control may also be especially susceptible to surface heat loss. Table 12-2 is a sample nursing care plan for the hypothermic patient. This is an example of types of nursing care plans that should be developed to address specific postanesthetic (not just surgical) complications. Postoperative patients require careful temperature monitoring beyond the PACU.

Obesity, gastric dilatation, tight dressings, and tight body casts also inhibit respiratory muscle function and can predispose to CO_2 retention. A high level of CO_2 production from sepsis or shivering can result in CO_2 retention, especially if the patient cannot increase minute ventilation.

The respiratory effect of narcotics consists of a diminution of alveolar ventilation resulting from a decrease in respiratory rate and tidal volume. In any discussion of narcotics and respiration, the underlying condition of the patient must play a major consideration. The ability of narcotics to depress ventilation is relatively greater in the older, debilitated patient, particularly if there is a significant component of CO_2 retention or cardiorespiratory disease. Pain and stimulation have been demonstrated to counteract the effect of narcotics on respiration.

The classical effect of large doses of narcotics is to reduce respiratory rate. The slow, relatively deep respirations of narcotic overdosage are so characteristic as to be of differential diagnostic value in establishing the

TABLE 12–2. NURSING CARE PLAN FOR HYPOTHERMIC PATIENTS

Nursing Diagnosis	Desired Outcomes	Time	Nursing Orders
Fluid and electrolyte resulting from:	*Maintains fluid and electrolyte balance as evidenced by:*		*Assess fluid and electrolyte imbalance*
Increased urinary output	Serum potassium of 4.0–5.4 mEq/L	Continuously with vital signs	Monitor input and output; check CVP
Decreased sodium reabsorption	Serum calcium of 9–11 mg%	Prn	Obtain serum electrolyte levels and check results
Vasoconstriction	Serum sodium of 136–142 mEq/L		
	CVP>5<15 or as ordered	Continuously	Watch for increased intravenous rates with vasodilation
	Output correlates with intake appropriately	Every hour or as ordered	Measure input–output
	Absence of apathy, seizures, confusion, arrhythmias	Continuously	Observe level of consciousness, monitor cardiac status
Hyperglycemia resulting from:	*Exhibits no sign of hyperglycemia as evidenced by:*		*Assess for signs and symptoms of hyperglycemia*
Diabetic—insulin withheld	Urine negative for sugar, stable level of consciousness	As ordered	Check urine for sugar and notify physician for 2+ or greater
Decreased insulin production	Blood glucose within normal limits	Prn with vital signs	Assess level of consciousness, obtain blood glucose levels and check results
Dehydration resulting from:	*Exhibits adequate hydration as evidenced by:*		*Assess for signs of dehydration*
Increased urinary output	Decreased viscosity of secretions	Every 1° while catheter in, otherwise with void	Measure input–output
Hypovolemia and insensible fluid loss	Moist mucous membranes		
Increased basal metabolic (BM) rate (shivering)	Elastic skin turgor	Prn	Check skin turgor and mucous membranes

TABLE 12–2. (*Continued*)

Nursing Diagnosis	Desired Outcomes	Time	Nursing Orders
	CVP>5<15 or as ordered, vital signs within normal limits	With vital signs	Check CVP
Decreased level of consciousness resulting from:	*Maintains adequate level of consciousness as evidenced by:*	*Prn*	*Assess level of consciousness*
Electrolyte imbalance, decreased metabolism of drugs	Appropriate responses to commands	Prn with vital signs	Assess patient orientation, reorient when necessary, check electrolytes
Decreased BMR	Oriented to person, able to maintain own airway	Continuously	Check for signs and symptoms of hypoxia, airway obstruction, hypoventilation
	Absence of apathy, agitation, or confusion		
Systemic hypertension resulting from:	*Maintains blood pressure within a normal range*		*Apply measures to maintain a normal blood pressure and monitor blood pressure*
Vasoconstriction, shivering, hypoxic agitation	Systolic >90<180, diastolic >50<90 or as ordered	Immediate and change prn	Apply warm blanket around head, feet and body to rewarm and vasodilate vessels
		Prn	Elevate head of bed
		Prn	Encourage deep breathing
		Prn	Insert oral/nasal airway
		Immediately	Provide O_2 therapy as ordered
		As per physician	Intravenous rate to keep vein open
Impaired peripheral perfusion resulting from:	*Maintains adequate perfusion of peripheral tissues as evidenced by:*		*Assess peripheral perfusion and apply nursing measures to improve*
Vasoconstriction	Absence of mottling, cold extremities	Immediately and prn	Apply warm blanket to aid in vasodilation of peripheral vessels

(*Continued*)

TABLE 12–2. (*Continued*)

Nursing Diagnosis	Desired Outcomes	Time	Nursing Orders
	Good capillary refill of nailbeds		
	Presence of dorsalis pedis, posterior tibial, and radial pulses		
Acidosis (metabolic) resulting from:	*Maintain arterial blood gases within normal limits for patients as evidenced by:*		*Assess for signs of acidosis*
Impaired peripheral perfusion (aner-obic)	pH 7.35–7.45 PCO_2 35–45 mm Hg TCO_2 22–28 mg/L PO_2 80–100 mm Hg O_2 saturated 95% or greater	Continuously if patient short of breath	Check for rapid, deep breathing, stupor, weakness
Increased O_2 consumption	BE -3 to $+3$, or gases that are consistent with preoperative base-line	As per physician's order	Obtain arterial gases, check results
Increased BMR (shivering)	Maintain normal electrolyte status	Prn	Monitor electrolytes
Coagulation defects resulting from:	*Exhibits no signs or symptoms of co-agulation defects as evidenced by:*	*With vital signs*	*Assess for signs and symptoms of co-agulation defects*
Increased blood viscosity	Absence of calf pain/sensation	Prn	Assess peripheral circulation until no longer hypo-thermic
Decreased platelets	Unequal leg temperature		
	$(-)$ Homan's sign	Continuously	Observe for signs and symptoms of pulmonary emboli
	Absence of sponta-neous bleeding/bruising		
	Normal coagulation test result	Per physician's order	Obtain coagulation profile and check results

(From Borchardt AC & Fraulini KE: Hypothermia in the postanesthetic patient. AORN Journal 36, Oct., 1982.)

etiology of respiratory inadequacy. Narcotics produce a small variable decrease in tidal volume. Therefore, the effect of narcotics on minute ventilation approximately parallels the effect on respiratory rate. Dripps and Comroe (1945) gave 10 to 15 mg morphine intravenously and witnessed a 27 percent reduction in respiratory rate within 7 to 9 minutes. With routine small intramuscular doses, the effect on the arterial pCO_2 is not important, averaging a 2 to 3 torr rise. Even when the respiratory rate is only minimally affected, however, there may be a profound influence on the response to CO_2. Thus, although the resting minute ventilation may be adequate, the patient may be at risk for CO_2 retention if a challenge to respiration occurs. In the patient with marked obesity or pulmonary disease, an intrinsic respiratory challenge may be present. These patients should be carefully observed if extubated and considered for prophylactic postoperative ventilation. In general, equianalgesic doses of narcotics depress respirations equally. Nursing or medical activities may stimulate a patient and transiently antagonize narcotic-induced respiratory depression. When these stimuli are removed, the risk of respiratory inadequacy can recur. Factors that augment the effect of narcotics are age, pulmonary disease, chest deformities, other general anesthetics, sedatives, and muscle relaxants.

The sensitivity of the respiratory center begins to return toward normal within 2 to 3 hours; however, respiratory minute volume is still considerably below normal for as long as 4 to 5 hours following therapeutic doses.

Another increasingly popular group of drugs used in the perianesthetic period is the benzodiazepines. Contrary to clinical impressions, the action of all benzodiazepines is prolonged and uncertain. The elimination half-life of diazepam is 24 to 90 hours, which is similar to that of lorazepam. With both drugs, the slow decline in plasma levels often shows a secondary "peak" at 6 to 8 hours after administration.

Diazepam is associated with a mild hypoxemia; this is not true for lorazepam. Nevertheless, lorazepam, like any other benzodiazepine, is capable of producing respiratory depression and should be used with caution in patients with pulmonary disease (Brown, 1983).

The preceding discussion of respiratory complications points to the later occurrence of many of these, after the PACU. It is essential that the surgical floor nurse or SICU nurse be well-informed regarding patient response to anesthetic agents and drugs. If these complications are anticipated and a plan of care formulated, it is reasonable to expect that unnecessary morbidity and mortality can be avoided.

Postoperative Pain Management as it Relates to Respiration

Only with careful assessment and very judicious titration of drugs (especially narcotics and tranquilizers) can the nurse ensure the respiratory integrity of the postanesthetic patient. The question which follows, of course, is how does the nurse in the PACU and beyond manage the patient's postoperative pain. The following pages will attempt to answer that question. A guiding principle should be the individualization of pain management.

The rather routine postoperative orders for intramuscular narcotic and sedative, or tranquilizer, for all patients does not represent an enlightened approach to postanesthetic pain management. Chapter 10 offers some guidelines regarding pain management in the PACU. The following discussion examines pain management as it extends beyond the PACU.

The first question to ask is what is the incidence of postoperative pain? The wide variation in patient response to surgical procedures is evident in studies reporting on postoperative drug use. Keats (1956) found that 21 percent of 104 patients having major abdominal surgery (gastrectomy or colectomy) received either one dose or no pain medication during the postoperative period. Papper and associates (1952) found that 44 percent of 237 patients received little or no pain-alleviating narcotics while recovering from surgery; Jaggard and coworkers (1950) found the same for 36 percent of 1005 postoperative patients. Papper's study also included 108 patients with intrabdominal or intrathoracic procedures, of which 27 percent recovered from surgery without complaints of postoperative pain and without receiving any medication. Parkhouse and associates sought to determine correlations between types of surgical procedures and the proportions of patients requiring postoperative analgesia. Data obtained from approximately 1000 patients demonstrated the following results: cholecystectomy and gastric surgery, 95 percent; upper abdominal surgery, 82 percent; inguinal herniorrhaphy surgeries, 48 percent; neck and head (superficial) surgical procedures, 55 percent; and minor procedures of the chest wall and scrotal areas, 20 percent. Similar results regarding associations between sites of surgical procedures and postoperative analgesia have been reported by Loan and Dundee (1967) and Keats (1956).

Results of these early studies are reinforced by later ones. Keats has combined data from several sources. All categories of postoperative patients are included and the data obtained present an interesting summary of the variation in reports of postoperative pain experienced by patients. According to Keats, approximately 40 percent of all postoperative patients never complain of pain; an additional 20 percent are relieved of pain by receiving morphine doses of 10 mg or less; slightly more than 10 percent require more than 10 mg of morphine for relief of pain; and the remaining patients (slightly less than 10 percent) never achieve pain relief even with the administration of narcotics. Bonica supports these findings, and comments that in general about one-third of all surgical patients do not experience postoperative pain, as evidenced either by a lack of complaint or by not actively seeking medication. He states that placebos are effective in alleviating pain in one-third to one-half of postoperative pain complaints.

Epidural Morphine Infusion. Epidural analgesia to prevent postoperative pain has proven a valuable technique for patients who have undergone thoracic and major abdominal surgery.

Epidural injection of narcotics produces analgesia by diffusion across the dura into the subarachnoid space and subsequent absorption into the spinal cord. Narcotics enter the CSF at a rate that is dependent on physio-chemical characteristics such as oil–water solubility, acid–base strength of the morphine, and the pH of the intercellular fluid. When the narcotic reaches the CSF, penetration from the water phase of the CSF to the lipid phase of the CNS occurs at the speed determined by the relative aqueous and lipid solubilities of the drug (Bromage & associates, 1982).

Morphine has a strong receptor-binding characteristic and a low lipid solubility. It acts at spinal cord levels to inhibit the synaptic transmission of pain impulses. It can bypass the blood–brain barrier in high concentration by entering the CSF directly and then diffuse by passing from the aqueous phase to the lipid phase in the spinal cord tissues. Since morphine has a low lipid solubility and is not tightly bound, it remains in the aqueous phase of the CSF for prolonged periods of time. This extends the duration of the drug (Bailey & associates, 1984).

Catheter Insertion. Bailey and associates (1984) propose that epidural catheter insertion be performed under sterile conditions in either the holding area of the operating room or the operating suite. The OR nurse supports the patient in the lateral decubitus or upright sitting position. The patient's neck and back are flexed to provide maximum opening of the interlaminal spaces. It is beneficial for the nurse to stand in front of the patient both to support and maintain proper position.

The nurse monitors the patient's vital signs, level of consciousness, pupil size and reaction to light, and motor and sensory response in extremities, and records the data. The anesthesiologist selects the proper lumbar interspace, and the area is prepared aseptically. In the midline of the lumbar region, the skin and ligaments are infiltrated with a local anesthetic. A 17-gauge, 9-cm needle is placed through the skin wheal to make a hole, and a 17-gauge Touhy needle with a Huber point is inserted into the epidural space with the curved bevel pointing in the direction of the patient's head. The safest point of entry into the epidural space is in the midline, midlumbar region L_1 to L_4. The distance between the epidural space and the skin is approximately 4 to 6 cm, although in obese patients the distance may be greater than 8 cm.

A catheter with a wire stylet is inserted through the needle. The markings on the catheter (11, 12, 13, 14, 15, 16 cm) indicate the distance from the tip. Withdrawal of the epidural catheter should be avoided while the introducing needle is still in place or else the tip of the catheter may be sheared off. Catheters may become hard and brittle and break off after being left in place several days; also the laminal or spinal ligaments of osteoarthritic patients may grip the catheter and break it.

Catheters may also become knotted if too much catheter is inserted. Inadvertent cannulation of an epidural vein, subarachnoid cannulation resulting in total spinal anesthesia, and perforation of the dura, which may give the patient a spinal headache, are rare possibilities. Most complications are due to insertion of too much catheter. A length of 4 cm is sufficient, but short enough to avoid serious problems (Bromage, 1978).

When the catheter has passed the needle point into the epidural space, the Touhy needle is removed from the patient's back over the catheter and stylet. This is followed by withdrawal of the wire stylet. A needle adapter is connected in the free end of the catheter. To prevent dislocation, the nurse tapes the catheter along the midline of the back and around the shoulder (Snow, 1982). The nurse also checks the site for bleeding and drainage.

Once the solution is injected, it spreads horizontally and longitudinally. It also spreads posteriorly to the region of the dorsal root, subsequently entering the cerebral spinal fluid. Anesthesia is obtained when the lumbar and thoracic spinal nerves in the epidural space are blocked. Motor paralysis is only partial. Surface landmarks will indicate segmental blockade. The nurse must know these landmarks to assess the progression and recession of anesthesia.

The patient may arrive in the PACU with the epidural morphine infusing via infusion pump, or the infusion may be started in the PACU. The epidural infusate is usually preservative-free morphine SO_4, 10 mg diluted in 100 cc 0.9 normal saline IV bag. It is infused at a rate of 0.1 mg per hour. This dosage may be increased by order of the anesthesiologist if the patient experiences pain. Supplemental systemic narcotics may also be administered.

The epidural catheter is normally left in place for 72 hours to provide analgesia. Once again, it is important that the floor and ICU nurses become knowledgeable regarding this mode of pain therapy, since patients usually have this catheter in place after leaving the PACU.

Nursing Care. The nurse must be aware of morphine's potential side effects and complications. The patient may experience apprehension due to lack of knowledge about hospitals and procedures, fear of inadequate pain relief, and misconceptions regarding the epidural catheter. The nurse should encourage the patient to verbalize concerns about surgery and pain. Usually, good preoperative teaching can alleviate the patient's fears. Teaching should include instruction regarding the surgical procedure, plans for postoperative pain management, the catheter insertion technique, and the infusion pump.

In addition to observing the patient postoperatively for complications, the nurse should be aware of potential side effects secondary to the epidural morphine infusion. Due to hypalgesia (decrease in pain and sensation), nonrespiratory side effects occur first. Itching, nausea, and vomiting occur first due to absorption of morphine from the dura into the spinal cord. Morphine, a poorly lipid-soluble agent, tends to stay in the water phase of the CSF and is carried wherever the CSF bulk flows. Side effects are dose-dependent. Pruritis can occur in 2 to 3 hours when morphine reaches the mid to upper thoracic segments. There may be no signs of urticaria, it may be generalized, or it may affect only the trunk, extremities, face, or genital region. An antihistamine such as diphenhydramine HCl (Benadryl) may be given. Nausea and vomiting can develop in 4 to 6 hours when hypalgesia extends to the upper cervical area, causing stimulation of the emetic trigger zone. An antiemetic, such as trimetholienzamide HCl (Tigan) or prochlorperazine (Compazine) may be given. Naloxone (Narcan) can also be administered to relieve the pruritis, nausea, and vomiting, but other problems may occur (see below).

Hypotension may be caused by vascular disturbances. Rapid infusion of fluids and administration of vasopressors may be required to counteract the hypotension, as well as frequent monitoring of vital signs and neurologic assessment, including levels of consciousness, pupil size and reaction to light, and motor and sensory response in extremities. Frequency of routine monitoring of vital signs depends on the institution. Often patients are monitored every 15 minutes until stable, and then every 2 to 4 hours.

Decreased muscle tone and sensation, with IV hydration, can quickly create urinary retention. It may persist for up to 20 hours in the young and even longer in the elderly.

The nurse must maintain an accurate intake and output record. Repeated doses of naloxone may be given to reverse urinary retention and could be an alternative to a Foley catheter. The need for a Foley catheter could be a serious consideration in orthopedic prosthetic operations, where the risk of urinary infections and bacteremia can have disastrous consequences for survival of the prosthesis.

Respiratory depression is another potential side effect. Meiosis, which occurs between the 6th and 9th hour, is an early sign of respiratory depression. This may be a significant problem in patients with severe chronic obstructive pulmonary disease.

Late respiratory depression is related to lipid–water solubility of the narcotic and to cerebral spinal fluid flow within the subarachnoid and ventricular systems. It is the most serious side effect and may be life threatening hours after surgery. It is important to assess the signs and symptoms of respiratory depression including quality of breathing (deep or shallow), compliance pattern (regular or irregular), and rate of respirations (below, above, or within normal range). Respiratory depression is more likely to occur if intraspinal or parenteral narcotics are combined. Respiratory parameters such as tidal volume and minute volume can be measured. Arterial blood gases may also be obtained.

Naloxone corrects respiratory depression. Its action is not completely understood, but it is thought to compete with narcotics for the same receptor sites. Two problems may arise with naloxone. Respiratory depression will be corrected, but there will be a loss of analgesia, and the patient may experience increased pain. Secondly, respiratory depression may recur when naloxone wears off. The half-life of naloxone is approximately 30 minutes. Naloxone should be taped to the head of the bed at all times and should be administered if the respiratory rate is below 8 per minute. The average dose of naloxone is 0.4 mg intravenously or intramuscularly, but it may also be given as a continuous infusion. There is disagreement regarding the need for a cardiac or apnea monitor during the first 24 hours; but there is general agreement that an infusion rate of 0.4 mg per hour or more requires a monitor. The maximum dose is 0.6 mg per hour.

Epidural catheters should be left in place no longer than 72 hours. Local tissue reaction around the tip tends to seal off the catheter in a fibrin pocket and further infusion of medication becomes painful and ineffective after this time.

Infection of the epidural space and the catheter site are rare. The nurse must assess the site for redness, tenderness, warmth, and any drainage. The infusion tubing should be replaced only when the morphine solution bag is changed. The dressing (a small occlusive dressing with clear tape) should not be changed.

A number of factors have been responsible for decreased epidural infections. Catheter design is better and the physical size is smaller than first attempts. Multidose vials of local anesthetics have been replaced by single-dose ampules, decreasing chance for contamination. Micropore bacterial filters have added an extra line of defense against contamination in continuous epidural techniques.

Epidural morphine infusion is an effective and relatively safe route for postoperative analgesia. Lanz and associates (1982) performed research supporting the use of epidural morphine. Following lumbar epidural anesthesia for orthopedic operations, 174 patients underwent the following study. At the end of surgery under double-blind conditions, 57 patients in group 1 received 0.1 mg/kg of morphine in 15 ml of normal saline epidurally and normal saline 0.01 ml/kg intramuscularly. Patients in group 2 (57 patients) received intramuscular morphine 0.1 mg/kg and normal saline 15 ml epidurally. Patients in group 3 (60 patients) received normal saline 15 ml epidurally and normal saline 0.01 ml/kg intramuscularly.

Postoperative pain was less frequent, of shorter duration, and less severe following epidural morphine (group 1). Sympathetic block was only partial; patients still noticed pressure due to a dressing or cast. There was no motor blockade and active mobilization occurred earlier. Following epidural morphine, alertness was heightened, patients were more cooperative, and respiratory depression and postoperative pneumonia were less than after systemic administration of narcotics. Additional need for analgesia and sedation was also significantly less following the use of epidural morphine.

Tests with terminal cancer and low back pain patients have been inconclusive. In obstetrics, epidural morphine infusion is effective in some patients. In one study of only eight patients conducted by Crawford, 2 to 6 mg of morphine injected epidurally was ineffective in relieving labor pain. In yet another study, 60 patients undergoing cesarean sections had only modestly diminished postoperative pain and required other forms of analgesia.

Although it is a relatively new technique in postoperative pain relief and some studies are inconclusive, epidural morphine appears to be an effective and safe means of postoperative analgesia. Researchers continue to study its effectiveness. In the future, epidural morphine may be the preferred analgesia for continuous pain relief.

Techniques of regional anesthesia have been used for the relief of postoperative pain in order to avoid narcotic-induced respiratory depression. Intercostal nerve blocks, when used to relieve pain of cholecystectomy, result in less fluctuation in arterial blood gases, earlier ambulation, and earlier hospital discharge than does use of narcotics (Bridenbaugh & associates, 1973). The availability of longer-acting local anesthetics makes this a possible method for managing postoperative pain; however, the placement and repetition of the block does take time and there is always the risk of pneumothorax. Nevertheless, these blocks can be effective and probably desirable in patients with severe lung disease in whom narcotic analgesics may provide too little analgesia and too much respiratory depression. The reader is referred to Chapter 6 for further discussion of nerve blocks.

Opiate Receptor Pharmacology. Further insights into opiate receptor properties (Table 12-3) may lead to more selective analgesic molecules. Currently, development of opiates for clinical use faces two major obstacles: (1) the receptor agonists carry the stigma and real clinical liabilities of respiratory depression as well as addiction or abuse potential, or both; and (2) sigma receptor agonists (and to a lesser extent, kappa agonists) tend to include psychotomimetic dysphoric effects often accompanied by autonomic stimulation.

The use of high dose narcotic anesthesia techniques for certain high risk patients has focused more attention on pharmacology of new paren-

TABLE 12–3. OPIATE RECEPTOR SUBGROUPS

Opiate Receptor Subgroup	Agonists	Antagonists	Effects	Anatomic Location
Mu (μ)	Morphine Morphiceptin Buprenorphine (?)Nalbuphine(?)	Naloxone Naltrex- one Nalor- phine	Analgesia Euphoria Physical dependence Respiratory depression Hypothermia Bradycardia Miosis	Hypothalamus Thalamus Guinea pig ileum Brain stem Spinal cord
Kappa (κ)	Ketocyclazocine Ethylketocyclazocine Pentazocine Butorphanol (?)Nalbuphine(?) Bremazocine	Naloxone *weakly* MR 2266	Analgesia Sedation Miosis (?)Respiratory depres- sion(?)	Hypothalamus Thalamus Cortex
Sigma (σ)	SKF 10,047 (N-allylnormetazo- cine) Cyclazocine Nalorphine Phencyclidine	Naloxone *partially*	Tachycardia Hypertonia Tachypnea Mydriasis Dysphoria Hallucinations Mania	Striatum Brain stem Spinal cord
Delta (δ)	Enkephalin	Naloxone	Inhibits mouse vas deferens Autonomic effects Analgesia (?)Microcirculation(?)	Mouse vas def- erens CNS ANA
Epsilon (ε)	β-endorphin	Naloxone	Inhibits rat vas deferens Autonomic effects Analgesia (?)Microcirculation(?)	Rat vas defer- ens CNS ANS

teral analgesics by anesthesiologists. An outgrowth of experimental work with the endogenous opioid polypeptides has been development of new analgesics that are classified as agonist–antagonist narcotics. The hallmark of this group of drugs, totally distinguishing them from the true opiates and synthetic opiates, is the low addiction liability they apparently possess. This class of drugs, the forerunner of which was pentazocine (Talwin), has never acquired much clinical popularity for use during balanced anesthesia techniques, or even for postoperative pain relief. The reasons are manifold but may revolve about a degree of nonpredictability and fear of the psychic problems of dysphoria and hallucinations (sigma receptor stimulation). Butorphanol (Stadol) has been accepted for balanced anesthesia and postoperative analgesia in several centers, however. Its hallucinogenic effects seem to be less than with pentazocine.

Nalbuphine (Nubain) is structurally similar to naloxone and oxymorphone, and was originally thought to produce analgesia primarily by acting at mu receptors with actions, effects, onset, duration, and potency similar to morphine. Subsequent studies, however, demonstrated that nalbuphine reached a limit in respiratory depression and contribution to anesthesia (0.22 MAC), and prevented further effects of morphine (Sederberg, 1981). These results were interpreted to suggest that nalbuphine binds as an agonist to kappa receptors, and binds with no effect to mu receptors. Ceilings for respiratory depression and anesthesia correspond to about 30 mg in adults.

The therapeutic importance of ceiling respiratory depression does not relate to the usual therapeutic use of nalbuphine, because respiratory depression at single doses recommended for analgesia are associated with the same respiratory depression as an equivalent analgesia dose of morphine (Romagnoli & Keats, 1980).

Patient-controlled analgesia (PCA), or demand analgesia, is a fairly recently developed dosing technique that has gained recognition as an efficacious mode for the administration of parenteral analgesics. The technique permits self-administration of boluses of analgesic drugs into an in-dwelling intravenous line using a device developed especially for this purpose. "Lock-out intervals" imposed by the system are designed to prevent redosing prior to attainment of peak pharmacological effect from previous boluses. Reports on the technique have been uniformly favorable.

Transcutaneous electric stimulation (TENS) seems to alleviate the appreciation of pain (Melzack & Wall, 1965). The stimulators are small battery-powered portable units that can be worn via flat, rubber electrodes. This form of therapy has the major advantage of having virtually no side effects, and it is therefore to be highly recommended as a treatment form for the chronic pain patient. As with other forms of stimulation-produced analgesia (acupuncture, massage, and so on), the TENS electrodes are usually placed in the painful area surrounding an incision. The patient then adjusts the dial settings for frequency and strength of stimulus. The stimulators provide a low intensity stimulus of some 5 to 200 Hz, which produces a tingling or vibration sensation. The mechanism by which the pain is relieved is believed to be suppression of the pain stimulus by a nonpain sensation, whether at spinal cord levels or higher centers. A gating mechanism has been invoked as an explanation. (Melzack, 1975).

Clearly, a TENS unit is best suited to an awake, alert patient who can manage the psychomotor skill of adjusting the dial.

Parenteral Narcotics. The most common therapy of pain management postoperatively today is parenteral narcotics. It is generally agreed that in the PACU, pain can be managed by small intravenous doses of narcotics. The use of small IV doses allows the anesthesiologist and nurse to titrate the dose needed for adequate pain relief while carefully monitoring the respiratory and circulatory depressant effects. Maximal respiratory depression occurs 7 to 10 minutes following a small dose of morphine (1–3 mg) given intravenously. However, maximal narcosis does not occur for 30 minutes. Careful titration of narcotics intravenously often results in analgesia sooner than does larger intramuscular doses.

Once the patient leaves the PACU it is usually not acceptable nursing policy to administer IV narcotics. Intramuscular narcotics are most often ordered; the nurse is confronted with the problem of narcotic-induced respiratory depression. There are several ways the nurse on the floor can avoid this:

1. The nurse should be aware of the drugs administered in the perianesthetic period, including preoperative, intraoperative, and drugs given in the PACU. With this knowledge of drug action and interaction, the nurse is able to make informed decisions regarding when to administer narcotics and how much to give. Careful assessment of the patient's complaint is also indicated—is he or she really having pain or is it anxiety, fear, or disorientation? It is important to treat the source of the complaint, not just give patients something to quiet them down.

2. It would be most helpful to begin interdisciplinary conferences to discuss management of postoperative pain. The fact that the surgeon is the one who orders postoperative pain medication is based solely on custom. It seems much more appropriate that the anesthesiologist order pain therapy and that it be individualized to meet the needs of the patient. Nurses could be instrumental in bringing about changes in practice toward the more logical procedure of pursuing a creative course uniquely designed for each postoperative patient. A major goal of this approach is prevention of serious postoperative respiratory depression.

3. A nurse who has any question about administering a postoperative narcotic should consult the physician. The nurse may be able to negotiate for a smaller dose or a placebo. Also, the nurse should become sophisticated regarding alternate modes of pain therapy. Viable alternatives, as previously mentioned, include nerve blocks, epidural infusions, and TENS.

4. As more and more nursing units are conducting clinical investigation, postoperative pain should rank high as a concept that deserves nursing study. Only as we design studies and collect data can we adequately answer the question of how to best manage postoperative pain without creating significant respiratory depression.

Perhaps the agonist–antagonist group of drugs is a step in the direction of how to best manage postoperative pain without creating significant respiratory depression. But once again, we will not have the answers until we have much broader experience with them.

CARDIOVASCULAR COMPLICATIONS

It is the goal of postanesthesia care units to resolve circulatory problems before returning the patient to his or her room. However, there is always the possibility that some of these problems may linger or recur in the later postanesthetic period. The present section gives an overview of those variables that may affect circulation.

Some drugs used in modern therapeutics can affect the course of anesthesia unfavorably. Although drugs with this potential do not invariably cause hypotension, it is important to be aware of possible interactions. Of chief concern are the adrenal steroids, the antihypertensives, the beta-adrenergic blockers and the tranquilizers, drugs that may merely potentiate the moderate reduction in blood pressure often seen with general anesthetics. On occasion a patient may develop profound hypotension during or following anesthesia under these circumstances. The possibility of drug interactions as a cause of hypotension should be added to the nurse's assessment. Implicit in this is the expectation that the surgical floor nurse reads the anesthesia and PACU record and has a working knowledge of the drugs and agents administered in the perianesthetic period.

The commonest cardiovascular complications of anesthesia are dysrhythmias and hypotension (see Chapter 10). Hypotension is never far away under general anesthesia, as most anesthetic agents tend to produce some degree of depression of the heart and peripheral vasomotor tone either directly or by their depressant action on the brain.

Predisposing Factors

Preexisting Cardiovascular Disease. The patient with cardiovascular disease is susceptible to complications during anesthesia. It is wise in this context to regard no elderly patient as having a completely healthy cardiovascular system.

Anesthetic Agents. Some volatile anesthetic agents—especially Halothane have the propensity for producing dysrhythmias, some of them potentially hazardous. Halothane is particularly likely to produce hypotension.

Increased Catecholamine Levels. Serious ventricular dysrhythmias are likely to occur in the presence of high circulating levels of catecholamines. These catecholamines, of which adrenaline is the most likely to produce dysrhythmias, may be exogenous (injected) or endogenous (produced within the body). Other intraoperative factors include hypoxia and hypercarbia and direct or reflex stimulation.

Excessive Premedication. The tendency of the opioids to lower arterial blood pressure is well known. Several pharmacologic actions contribute to this, including depression of the vasomotor center, reduction in skeletal muscle tone, depression of respiration, and dilation of peripheral blood vessels owing to a direct action or secondary to release of histamine. Circulatory depression often takes the form of postural hypotension, an intolerance to the upright position. Passive tilt to the 50 or 60 degree head-up position is used experimentally to demonstrate derangement of circulation induced by drugs. The inference is that the opioids will reduce the ability to compensate for circulatory stress such as hemorrhages, trauma, or change in position. Although this can clearly be demonstrated with tilt after administration of morphine or meperedine to the healthy patient, it is of interest that morphine and other opioids in large doses are used as analgesics in poor-risk patients for operation.

This is not to suggest that the circulatory response to tilt is unimportant or that opioids in the elderly or very ill are not without risk, but rather to point out that advantage is taken of these analgesics under highly controlled conditions in which intraarterial pressure is monitored continuously and vasopressor drugs and fluids are immediately available. However, opioids administered intravenously during routine anesthesia or postoperatively before patients recover completely from general anesthesia may be followed by hypotension. For this reason, it is best to reduce the dose of opioid (2.5 mg of morphine or 25 mg of meperidine), to give incremental doses, and to observe the blood pressure response. These are cardinal rules (algorithms) not only for the PACU nurse but for the SICU or surgical floor nurse as well.

Several of the barbituric acid derivatives—secobarbital and pentobarbital, for example—disturb the circulation least when given in 50 to 150 mg doses intravenously or intramuscularly before anesthesia. However, large doses may depress the circulation at several levels. Similarly, diazepam—more commonly used for premedication—rarely causes hypotension in the usual therapeutic doses. The incidence of complication rises sharply when opioids are combined with either barbiturates or diazepam. Although it is sometimes difficult to judge accurately the amount of premedication that will produce the desired tranquility to reaction, it is safer to err on the side of smaller doses than to seek marked sedation at the risk of arterial hypotension.

Vascular Absorption of Local Anesthetics. Operating room, PACU, and floor nurses should also be alerted to the consequences of vascular absorption of local anesthetics. Rapid absorption of local anesthetics from mucous membranes or other highly vascular tissues may cause marked hypotension. Probable causes of lowered blood pressure include depression of the myocardium and vasomotor centers as well as dilatation of peripheral vessels as a result of direct action. Prior administration of barbiturate does not protect against these effects and, indeed, may heighten circulatory depression.

It is not wise to leave critically ill or elderly patients scheduled for local anesthesia unattended during an operative procedure.

Hypotension can be minimized by reducing the total quantity of anesthetic injected per unit of time. Use of large volumes of concentrated solutions and rapid injection are chiefly responsible for elevation of blood levels to dangerous heights.

Change in Position or Moving the Patient. Since positioning the patient in the postoperative period is usually a nursing function, a few remarks on this topic are indicated. The circulation of the anesthetized patient, particularly the critically ill, is little able to compensate for stress. Change in position to the lateral decubitus may cause a marked reduction in arterial pressure. Positional changes should be accomplished slowly and gently, and the blood pressure observed throughout.

Deep Vein Thrombosis and Pulmonary Embolism.
Pulmonary emboli arise as fragments of thrombus occurring usually in the veins of the legs or pelvis. Neither usually occurs during the anesthetic, but 3 to 14 days afterwards. Although the exact "trigger" to the formation of venous thrombi is unknown, some of the factors associated with a high incidence are known and a certain amount of prophylaxis is possible. The incidence is highest in the middle-aged and elderly, with prolonged bed rest, after major and prolonged surgery especially of the lower abdomen, pelvis and hip joint, and in patients with known coronary artery disease. Venous pooling may be prevented by elastic stockings.

Active prevention includes subcutaneous dextran-70 daily until the patient is mobile.

Hypertension
Because this is a complication most often seen acutely in the PACU, it will be discussed only briefly here.

When hypertension develops in the PACU, it is often due to pain, hypercapnea, or fluid overload. When hypertension occurs, the etiology should be investigated and treated. The presence of severe hypertension can lead to left ventricular failure, myocardial infarction, or an arrhythmia due to a sharp increase in myocardial oxygen consumption. Acute hypertension may also precipitate acute pulmonary edema or a cerebral hemorrhage.

Preexisting hypertension is present in over half of the patients who develop hypertension in the PACU. Such hypertension can be augmented if antihypertensive medications have to be abruptly withdrawn preoperatively. When hypertension does develop during recovery from anesthesia, it usually begins within 30 minutes following surgery.

Treatment. Treatment of acute hypertension involves first treating pain, hypercapnea, hypoxemia, or fluid overload. If hypertension is still present, an antihypertensive is necessary. Since postoperative hypertension usually is resolved within 4 hours of surgery, it is unnecessary to begin therapy with long-acting agents because most patients without preexisting hypertension will not need prolonged treatment (see Chapter 10 for treatment of hypertension in the PACU).

SKIN COMPLICATIONS

Ulceration of the skin over bony prominences (typically the sacrum) is always a danger in elderly or debilitated patients. This is especially true if surgery is prolonged. The floor nurse should inspect the patient's skin for pressure damage as well as burns from Bovie pads or other sources. Any complications should be shared with operating room personnel.

RENAL COMPLICATIONS

Although most postoperative renal complications are not directly related to the anesthetic (as was the case with methoxyflourane or as is the case now with some patients receiving epidural morphine infusion), there are some indirect relationships. For example, the anesthesiologist is responsible for fluid administration and replacement in the operating room. Underreplacement may lead to hypovolemia, which may lead to prerenal oliguria.

The following comments summarize knowledge regarding renal complications that the postsurgical nurse should have. Postoperative renal failure remains an important cause of death in the surgical patient. Over half of the surgical patients developing acute tubular necrosis die. Careful management in the PACU is an important aspect of preventing this complication. An in-dwelling urinary catheter is important for the early recognition of oliguria in high risk patients. Patients at high risk for renal damage are those having surgery on the heart and great vessels or major biliary surgery (especially obstructive jaundice); those requiring massive transfusion or those with prolonged hypotension; elderly patients having long procedures; and those with preexisting renal disease, major trauma, or sepsis (Mazze, 1977).

Oliguria (50 to 400 ml/day or less than 15–20 ml/hour) is the common presenting feature of most cases of postoperative renal failure. The patency of the urinary drainage system should be examined in any patient with a low or absent urinary output. Oliguric patients in whom the collecting system is patent have either a prerenal, postrenal, or renal cause for their poor urinary output. Prerenal oliguria probably is the most common form of oliguria seen in the PACU and reflects poor renal perfusion due to either hypovolemia or circulatory failure. Correction of hypovolemia usually restores the urinary output. Administration of physiologic saline, 250 to 500 ml, while monitoring the central venous pressure (CVP) should result in an increase in urine flow if hypovolemia is the problem. Patients with this degree of hypovolemia will need continued fluid administration, since it takes an extracellular fluid depletion of over 25 percent to produce oliguria. If the oliguria is not secondary to hypovolemia, cardiac failure is likely, and an inotropic agent such as dopamine (2 to 10 μg/kg/min) will increase cardiac output and increase renal blood flow. Patients with cardiac failure should have fluid therapy monitored with a pulmonary artery catheter, since central venous pressure will be an imprecise guide to left ventricular filling pressure. Diuretics such as furosemide may be beneficial in restoring urine flow in patients in whom the oliguria is due to circulatory failure; however, diuretics are extremely hazardous if given to patients who are hypovolemic. One should have an accurate idea of the ventricular filling pressure prior to the use of a diuretic in an oliguric patient.

Postrenal oliguria occurs when there is obstruction to the urinary collecting system. This comprises less than 5 percent of cases of oliguria in surgical patients, and is usually treated by surgical diversion, such as placement of nephrostomy tube. Acute tubular necrosis is the other major cause of postsurgical oliguria. Examination of the urinary electrolytes, urea nitrogen, creatinine, and osmolality in relation to the plasma values provides a guide to the diagnosis of the etiology of oliguria (Table 12-4). The urinary/plasma (U/P) osmolality ratio is the most valuable guide. Oliguric patients with a U/P ratio of 1.1:1 or less usually have acute tubular necrosis. This test is valid only if the patient has not received diuretics in the preceding 6 to 12 hours. Because of the value of this test in oliguria, the results are worth obtaining prior to the administration of a diuretic to an oliguric patient.

Following the establishment of the diagnosis of acute tubular necrosis in an oliguric postsurgical patient, fluid intake should be minimized to whatever is necessary to maintain adequate ventricular filling pressures. Dialysis is usually not needed in the first 24 hours with appropriate fluid management; however, treatment of hyperkalemia is often necessary in the PACU. Normally the serum potassium rises at a rate of 0.3 to 0.5 mEq/L/day; but after surgery this can range from 1 to 2 mEq/L/day to as

TABLE 12–4. URINARY COMPOSITION IN OLIGURIA

	Physiologic Oliguria	Prerenal Failure	Acute Tubular Necrosis
Urinary sodium	<10 mEq/L	<25 mEq/L	>25 mEq/L
Urinary specific gravity	>1.024	>1.015	1.010–1.015
Urinary/plasma osmolality	>2.5:1	>1.8:1	1.1: or less
Urinary/plasma urea	>100:1	>20:1	3:1, rarely >10:1
Urinary/plasma creatinine	>60:1	>30:1, rarely <10:1	<10:1

(From Mazze RI. Critical care of the patient with acute renal failure. Anesthesiology 47:138, 1977.)

high as 1 to 2 mEq/L/hour, the latter in patients with extensive tissue injury and sepsis. For this reason, the serum potassium should be followed closely. Hyperkalemia can be treated acutely by giving bicarbonate, calcium, and a combination of insulin and glucose. This therapy will not affect total body potassium so a slower-acting, gastrointestinal-exchange resin such as sodium polystyrene sulfonate (Kayexalate) should be given as well (Mazze, 1977).

NEUROLOGIC COMPLICATIONS

Shivering
It is important to note that shivering has two components, one neurologic and the other relating to temperature control. Pyramidal tract signs are commonly seen as the patient emerges from light planes of general anesthesia, gross clonus sometimes mimicking a convulsion. This can be controlled with methylphenidate (Ritalin) given intravenously. As previously discussed, many patients emerge from anesthesia with lowered body temperatures (Dripps & associates, 1982).

Nerve Injury
Peripheral nerves can be injured during anesthesia through stretch or compression because the anesthetized patient does not perceive pain and lacks protective muscle tone. Among the nerves commonly injured are the several divisions of the brachial plexus and the ulnar, radial, common peroneal, and facial nerves. Often it is the nurse on the surgical floor who discovers these injuries. Consequently she or he should always be alert for this complication.

To avoid brachial plexus injury, one must bear the possibility in mind and avoid extremes of position of the head and arm. When palsy develops, a careful neurologic examination should be made and recorded and measures for restoration of function immediately begun with support of the paralyzed muscles and physiotherapy. In severe injury, restitution of normal function may require as long as 6 months to a year.

The ulnar, radial, and common peroneal nerves are superficially placed; hence they are easily compressed against bone, stirrups, or the sides of an operating table, or stretched around bony eminences. Certain positions such as lithotomy or the lateral decubitus predispose to injury of these nerves. If paralysis occurs, treatment is the same as that described for brachial plexus injury.

The facial nerve may be injured by overenthusiastic attempts to elevate the jaw via pressure on the rami of the mandible or by tight application of a head strap. Weakness of the muscles about the mouth or eyes is a manifestation of this injury, usually reversible within a week or two.

Femoral nerve injury may result from faulty placement of retractors during pelvic operation (Dripps & associates, 1977).

Restlessness, Excitement, and Delirium

Because restlessness, excitement, or delirium more commonly occur on emergence from anesthesia in the PACU, the reader is referred to Chapter 10. As a reminder, Table 12-5 gives a synopsis of factors contributing to delirium.

Sensorium and Psychomotor Skills

Recovery from anesthesia has been evaluated by clinical assessment, subjective reports, physiological data, and psychophysical tests. Psychophysical tests have been used to measure perceptual proficiency, cognitive ability, and psychomotor ability, usually using rotary pursuit tests, pegboards, or track tracers. This information would be of more value to the surgical floor nurse, who has reason to expect that the patient will have these skills in order to perform certain postsurgical activities. Of course, the nurse employed in the ambulatory surgical setting should have these data before sending the patient out of the hospital. Some attempt to evaluate "street fitness" should be included in discharge preparation.

Denis and associates (1984) reported that the Bender Gestalt Track Tracer shows many characteristics of an adequate measure of recovery from anesthesia. The test is reliable, valid, objective, noninvasive, inexpensive, easily understood by patients, and of short duration (60 seconds). Moreover, it can be administered by any staff member and leaves a digitalized permanent record on paper or on microcomputer that could be used for medicolegal purposes in a day-care surgery unit.

The track tracer used by Denis and associates consists of a square and a circle that reproduce approximately Figure A of the Bender Gestalt

TABLE 12–5. FACTORS CONTRIBUTING TO DELIRIUM (Restlessness and Excitement)

Pain
Psychomotor disturbances
Fear, anxiety
Prolonged maintenance of an uncomfortable position
Distended urinary bladder
Hypoxia (after thoracic, head and neck, or upper abdominal operations)
Pneumothorax, tracheal collapse, vocal cord paralysis, respiratory depression
Arterial hypotension (cerebral hypoxia)
Scopolamine (or phenothiazines and barbiturates)
Ketamine
Water intoxication (inappropriate ADH)
Ether anesthesia
Cerebral embolism
Postcardiotomy delirium
Inhalation anesthesia

Track Tracer. The circle's diameter was 20 cm; the width of the circle's track was 5 mm in the first half and 4 mm in the second half. The side of the square was 15.5 cm and the track was 4 mm wide. The stylet was 1 mm in diameter and its tip could not be taken out of the track. A subject had to follow the track without touching the sides, starting at the junction of the circle and the square; the circle was to be completed first. The apparatus was connected to a counter that added the time the electric stylet was in contact with the edge of the track; subjects had no knowledge of their performance. The result of the test was expressed as the time the stylet was in contact with the side of the track divided by the time the subject took to complete the test. This was determined to be a reliable and valid measure of recovery from anesthesia.

This assessment of recovery from anesthesia would seem to have unlimited possibilities for nurse investigators. Since very little is really known about recovery, the potential for nurses to contribute to the body of knowledge is great. Clearly, increased use of psychophysical tests to evaluate recovery from anesthesia can only serve to safeguard the well-being of the postanesthetic patient.

SUMMARY

This chapter, which looks mainly at the later postanesthetic period (the first 48 hours), is intended not only for the PACU nurse but the medical-surgical nurse as well. The goal is to heighten awareness that the postoperative patient is not only a surgical patient but also an anesthetic patient. The review of various body system responses to anesthesia should serve to illustrate that the patient has not truly "recovered" from anesthesia when he or she leaves the PACU. For this reason, it is essential that surgical nurses have and use knowledge of anesthesia.

REFERENCES

Ali J, Weisel RD, Laung AB, et al.: Consequences of postoperative alterations in respiratory mechanics. American Journal of Surgery 128:291, 1976.

Bailey CJ, Gulczynski B, Racky D, & Vehrs K: Epidural morphine infusion—Continuous pain relief. AORN Journal 39: May, 1984.

Becker LD, Paulson BA, Miller RD, et al.: Biphasic respiratory depression after fentanyl–droperidol or fentanyl alone used to supplement nitrous oxide anesthesia. Anesthesiology. 44:291, 1976.

Borchardt AC & Fraulini KE: Hypothermia in the postanesthetic patient. AORN Journal 36: Oct., 1982.

Bromage PR: Epidural Analgesia. Philadelphia: Saunders, 1978.

Bromage PR, et al.: Nonrespiratory side effects of epidural morphine. Anesthesia and Analgesia 61:490–495, 1982.

Bromage PR, et al.: Rostral spread of epidural morphine. Anesthesiology 56:431–36, 1982.

Brown B (Ed.): New Pharmacologic Vistas in Anesthesia. Philadelphia: F.A. Davis, 1983.

Carrie LES & Simpson PJ: Understanding Anesthesia. London: Heinmann Medical Books.

Crawford JS: Experiences with epidural morphine in obstetrics. Anesthesia 36:207–209, 1981.

Cullen DJ & Cullen BL: Postanesthetic complications. Surgical Clinics of North America 55:987, 1975.

Denis R, Letourneau JE, & Londorf D: Reliability and validity of psychomotor tests as measures of recovery from isoflurane or enflurane anesthesia in a day-care surgery unit. Anesthesia and Analgesia 63:653–656, 1984.

Dripps RD & Comroe JH: Clinical studies on morphine: I. The immediate effect of morphine administered intravenously and intramuscularly upon the respiration in normal man. Anesthesiology 6:462, 1945.

Dripps RD, Eckenhoff J, & Vandam L: Introduction to Anesthesia: The Principles of Safe Practice (6th ed.). Philadelphia: Saunders, 1983.

Fogdall RP & Miller RD: Prolongation of pancuroniume induced neuromuscular blockade by clindamycin. Anesthesiology 41:407, 1974.

Foldes FF, Duncalf R & Kuwavara S: The respiratory, circulatory, and narcotic antagonist effects of of nolophine, levallophan and naloxone in anesthetized subjects. Canadian Anesthetist Society Journal 16:151, 1969.

Fraulini KE: Effect of hand and pillow methods of incisional splinting for postoperative deep breathing and coughing on vital capacity and inspiratory pressure in cholecystectomized patients. Unpublished master's thesis. Loyola University of Chicago, 1980.

Fraulini KE: Postanesthetic delirium—A conceptual approach. Current Review for Recovery Room Nurses. Lesson 20 (vol. 4) 1984, pp. 155–159.

Fraulini KE, Borchardt AC, Randall Andrews D, & Slaymaker F: Mean body temperature of recovery room adults. Anesthesia and Analgesia. Abstract 64:2, Feb., 1985, p. 213.

Goodman A & Gilman L: Pharmacologic Basis of Therapeutics (6th ed.). New York: Macmillan, 1980.

Hughes SC: New approaches to obstetric pain relief—TENS, parenterals, extradural and intrathecal narcotics.

Jacox A (Ed.): Pain: A Source Book for Nurses and Other Professionals. Boston: Little, Brown, 1977.

Jaggard RS, Zager LL, & Wilkins DS: Clinical evaluation of analgesic drugs: A comparison of NU-2206 and morphine sulfate administered to postoperative patients. Archives of Surgery 61:1073, 1950.

Keats AS: Postoperative pain: Research and treatment. Journal of Chronic Diseases 4:72, 1956.

Keats AS: Use of analgesics at the bedside. In WE Leong (Ed.), New Concepts in Pain and its Clinical Management. Philadelphia: F.A. Davis, 1967.

Lanz E, et al.: Epidural morphine for postoperative analgesia: A double blind study. Anesthesia and Analgesia 61:236–240, 1982.

Loan WB & Dundee JW: The clinical assessment of pain. Practitioner 198:759, 1967.

Longnecker DE, Grazis PA, Eggers, & Gun: Naloxone for antagonism of morphine induced respiratory depression. Anesthesia and Analgesia 52:447, 1973.

Marshall BE & Wyche MQ: Hypoxemia during and after anesthesia. Anesthesiology 44:178, 1976.

Mazze RI: Critical care of the patient with acute renal failure. Anesthesiology 47:138, 1977.

Melzack R: Prolonged relief of pain by brief intense transcutaneous somatic stimulation. Pain 1:357, 1975.

Melzack R & Wall PD: Pain mechanisms: A new theory. Science 150:971, 1965.

Miller RD (Ed.): Anesthesia (vol. 2). New York: Churchill Livingstone, 1981.

Miller RD: Antagonism of neuromuscular blockade. Anesthesiology 44:318, 1975.

Miller RD & Cullen DJ: Renal failure and postoperative respiratory failure: Recurarization? British Journal of Anesthesia 48:253, 1976.

Papper R, Brodie BB, & Rovenstein EA: Postoperative pain: Its use in the comparative evaluation of analgesics. Surgery 32:107, 1952.

Romagnoli A & Keats A: Ceiling effect for respiratory depression by nalbuphine. Clinical Pharmacology and Therapeutics, 27:478–485, 1980.

Shapiro B: Evaluation of respiratory function in the perioperative period. American Society of Anesthesiologists Annual Refresher Course Lectures, 1980.

Snow JC: Manual of Anesthesia (2nd ed.). Boston: Little, Brown, 1982.

Vaughan MS, Vaughan RW, & Cork RC: Postoperative hypothermia in adults: Relationship of age, anesthesia, and shivering to rewarming. Anesthesia and Analgesia 60:746–751, 1981.

Chapter 13

The PACU as a Special Procedures Unit

Kay E. Fraulini

This chapter describes those activities conducted in the PACU which are in addition to postanesthetic recovery of the surgical patient.

There is a trend toward performing procedures such as epidural blocks, elective cardioversion, and electroconvulsive therapy in the PACU. Presumably the expanding role of the anesthesiologist as consultant has accounted for much of this. Frost (1982) provides further rationale for this practice. Proximity to the operating room ensures that preoperative intravenous or intraarterial cannulation may be safely accomplished requiring only little additional patient transportation. In the event that serious complication or an adverse drug reaction occurs, all operative facilities and personnel are immediately available. Better utilization is made of the intensive care resources of the PACU and its staff. Diagnostic or therapeutic procedures may be efficiently carried out under sterile conditions. Advanced life support systems, including the services of both anesthesiologists and surgeons, are immediately available.

Additionally, PACU nurses are well aware of the difficulty in predicting operating times and, thus, clock-time for PACU occupancy on a daily basis. Frequently, there are periods when staffing is available but there are few if any patients in the unit. This situation occurs most predictably early in the morning before the first operative procedures are completed.

In many PACUs it has become a regular practice to schedule certain procedures to fill these anticipated gaps in occupancy.

The procedures discussed below were selected with the knowledge that some PACUs are doing even more. Therefore, this is a partial list of a growing number of special procedures being done in the PACU. Most of these are performed by an anesthesiologist with the assistance of a PACU nurse. In addition, a psychiatrist is present during electroconvulsive therapy and a cardiologist during cardioversion.

ELECTROCONVULSIVE THERAPY

Electroconvulsive therapy (ECT) is a well-established treatment for many psychiatric illnesses. Cardiovascular complications—mainly a vagotonic effect of profound bradycardia—may follow electrically induced convulsions, which may aggravate preexisting cardiovascular disease, especially in older patients. Prior to therapy, an electrocardiogram must be obtained and any cardiac arrhythmias evaluated for the need for their prior treatment to avoid serious cardiac complications. Note should also be made of osteoporosis, history of frequent fractures, back pain or intervertebral disc disease, since one of the major complications of ECT is skeletal injury caused by ECT-induced intense muscle contraction.

Emotional support of these psychiatric patients is particularly important, both because of the nature of their illness and because of their need for repeated convulsive therapy (a course of ECT usually involves eight to ten treatments over about 5 weeks).

Since these patients are frequently treated as outpatients, preoperative sedation is usually not given. The customary preanesthetic check list must be completed; this includes patient identification, consent, fasting, removal of dentures, basic laboratory tests, history, and physical examination. Dental status is particularly important because loose teeth may easily be dislodged during a seizure.

ECT should be administered in a section of the PACU that can be curtained off or isolated to provide privacy and enough space for waiting comfortably for treatment and recovery. The necessary medications to have available include atropine (total dose 1 mg), sodium pentothal (3 to 4 mg/kg body weight), and succinylcholine chloride (1 mg/kg body weight). Means to provide artificial ventilation (Ambu-bag or anesthesia machine) with enriched oxygen are also required. Oral and nasal airways, laryngoscope, and endotracheal tubes must be immediately available.

The patient is prepared and treated in bed. Blood pressure and electrocardiogram are monitored. A peripheral vein is cannulated and, after preoxygenation, atropine, the pentothal, and a short-acting muscle relaxant (usually succinylcholine) are administered. In patients with frequent premature ventricular contractions, lidocaine 1 to 2 mg/kg is given intravenously to minimize the occurrence of ventricular arrhythmias. As soon as the patient loses consciousness, ventilation must be supported. When muscle relaxation is complete, electrodes coated with sufficient paste are applied to the head. A single shock is administered, which usually induces an attenuated seizure that lasts for approximately 1 to 2 minutes.

Hypertension and tachycardia may occur about 5 minutes after the treatment. These effects are usually transient (lasting 10 to 15 minutes) and rarely require treatment. However, careful monitoring is essential. The patient should be responsive and awake within 10 minutes.

Record keeping, particularly of the amounts of medication given and the shock strength, is very important, since individual variation is particularly common in these patients because of interaction of the ECT drugs with other long-acting drugs, such as tranquilizers, sedatives, and antidepressants. Appropriate modification can then be made for managing subsequent treatments (Frost, 1982).

Schneider (1981) indicates that the patient usually experiences memory loss following ECT and may not recall the nurses, the PACU, or the previous ECT experience.

The responsibility of the nurse is to assemble the necessary equipment as prescribed by the individual institution, to confirm the NPO status of the patient, and to assist the physician during the procedure. Following the "shock," the patient is monitored in the same way as any other postintravenous anesthetic patient. Specific observations should be made for cardiac arrhythmias, respiratory distress, and airway maintenance.

CARDIOVERSION

Cardioversion is a relatively simple, safe, and effective means of converting cardiac arrhythmias to sinus rhythm. The principal indications are atrial flutter and atrial fibrillation, which are usually not life-threatening situations and may be treated electively. Other arrhythmias that respond to cardioversion include ventricular tachycardia and ventricular fibrillation, but these are emergency situations and will not be included in this context.

Elective cardioversion is usually preceeded by a trial of drug therapy; these patients are therefore generally already in the hospital. Patients with a history of atrial fibrillation are frequently maintained on anticoagulant medication, both before and after cardioversion, to avoid the hazard of postconversion embolization. Quinidine is also often given to patients for at least 24 hours prior to therapy, since approximately 10 percent of cases may be converted by this drug alone. Digitalis and beta-adrenergic blocking agents are generally discontinued on the day prior to cardioversion, since excess blood levels of these medications may render the procedure ineffective. Hypokalemia must also be corrected.

After the patient is comfortably settled in bed, essential monitoring equipment (ECG, blood pressure) is applied. Essentials for resuscitation must be at hand. A peripheral vein is cannulated. Adequate pulmonary ventilation must be maintained with an enriched oxygen supply. Light anesthesia is usually given with a small dose of sodium pentothal 2 to 3 mg/kg or diazepam (Valium) 5 mg. Deep general anesthesia is usually not required if energies of 100 msec or less are employed. The duration of shock is 2.5 msec, and pain is generally not severe. The undersedated or unanesthetized patient may complain of a sensation similar to touching an exposed electrical wire. However, repeated conversion at higher output levels in apprehensive elderly patients may require more sedation.

Prior to cardioversion, it is important to check the paddles for the presence of metallic oxide on their surfaces, which may interfere with the delivery of adequate electrical energy. Cardioversion can only be successful when a sufficient amount of a properly conductive paste is used, when the paddles are far enough apart with no bridge of gel or sweat between them, and when firm contact with the skin surface is made.

After adequate sedation and with appropriate monitoring, the paddles of the cardioverter are applied over the precordium and on the patient's back (anterolateral positions may be used, but these require slightly higher energy outputs). Initial treatment for arrhythmias of recent onset should start with low energy current (about 20 to 40 msec). If the first discharge is not successful, successive shocks of 50 to 100 msec, followed by increments of 100 wsec, are given until the arrhythmia converts. Maximal strength of safe discharge is 400 msec. There is some risk of contact electroshock to personnel, and therefore the patient is not touched when the shock is delivered.

Muscular contractions may be caused during cardioversion, but are much less severe than in ECT. However, cases have been reported of torn spinous processes, and it is therefore common practice to use small doses (0.5 mg/kg) of succinylcholine chloride and to support ventilation.

AV nodal arrhythmias may occur after shock treatment for chronic atrial fibrillation. They are usually benign and revert spontaneously. Ventricular arrhythmias may develop as a result of digitalis or quinidine overdosage, hypokalemia, hypoventilation, or metabolic acidosis. Cardiac arrest may follow cardioversion in all of these conditions, and electrical pacing may be necessary. Closed-chest massage is the emergency therapy. Hypotension may be related to multiple shocks and the high energy level delivered to the myocardium. If this condition does not promptly reverse itself, electrical pacing or intravenous catecholamines (norepinephrine, dopamine) are indicated.

Rarely, myocardial damage produced by the current may cause postconversion pulmonary edema. Therapy includes sedation, digitalis, and diuretics. Recovery is usually complete in 2 to 3 days.

Finally, the sites of application of the paddles should be inspected for any burn injury. This is more likely to happen during emergency treatment and is usually superficial, responding to conservative local treatment.

NERVE BLOCKS

Indications for performing nerve blocks in the PACU are varied. Infiltration techniques with local anesthetics are used as diagnostic, prognostic, therapeutic, and prophylactic means to manage pain. Some of the more commonly administered blocks are listed in Table 13-1.

Subarachnoid block, performed as a PACU procedure, is usually done for relief of chronic pain associated with cancer. In these patients, whose physical status is generally poor, subarachnoid alcohol block causes a chemical posterior rhizotomy. Other techniques include the use of cold, hypertonic saline injections into the subarachnoid space. Pain relief has also been reported following barbotage of cerebrospinal fluid. Injection of a local anesthetic agent combined with steroids such as methylprednisolone or dexamethasone may be effective in decreasing pain through the antiinflammatory effect. Injection should be made adjacent to the suspected site of the lesion.

Subarachnoid block is performed with sterile technique employing a commercially available spinal anesthesia kit used by anesthesiologists. A small-gauge needle (22 or 25 gauge) is inserted into the subarachnoid space at the appropriate site and a local anesthetic solution (usually tetracaine, which may be combined with epinephrine for longer action) is injected.

Epidural block is a more commonly used technique, because it may be used as a continuous therapy either for pain relief or for its sympatholytic effect. Increase in skin temperature of the lower extremities after establishment of epidural blockade diagnostically indicates the degree of benefit to be obtained by performing surgical sympathectomy. Following

TABLE 13–1. NERVE BLOCKS WHICH MAY BE CONVENIENTLY PERFORMED

Subarachnoid	Intractable pain
Epidural	Sympatholytic effect
	Pain relief
Brachial plexus	Anesthetic technique
	Intractable angina
Intercostal nerve	Postoperative pain relief
	Herpes zoster
Stellate ganglion	
Celiac plexus	

(Courtesy of Frost EAM. The recovery room as a special procedures unit. Current Review for Recovery Room Nurses 4(3):18, 1982.)

surgical reattachment of part of a limb after trauma, continuous epidural block will help to ensure maximal blood flow to the compromised area. Epidural administration of local anesthetic agents may also be used to provide continuous pain relief after upper abdominal surgery or major skin-grafting procedures, particularly in drug-addicted patients in whom avoidance of narcotic agents is preferable.

This procedure, likewise, is usually performed by the anesthesiologist using an aseptic technique. After insertion of a large-bore needle (14 to 16 gauge) into the epidural space at the appropriate site, a catheter is threaded through the needle to the desired site and the needle is withdrawn, leaving the catheter in place. Solutions of local anesthetic agents are then injected as necessary, and the block may be maintained for hours or even days.

Operations involving the hands and arms are frequently performed after local anesthetic block of the brachial plexus, which may be accomplished by either a supraclavicular or an axillary approach. Since the anesthetic technique has a relatively slow onset of action (about 20 to 30 minutes until total blockade), the procedure is frequently performed in a holding area outside the operating room or in the PACU. The technique involves placement of a small-gauge needle within the sheath of the brachial plexus and injection of 20 to 40 ml of local anesthetic solution. Brachial plexus block has also been used successfully in the therapy of angina pectoris involving pain in the left arm.

Intercostal nerve blocks are given to relieve the pain of rib fractures and to provide analgesia after abdominal surgery and thus facilitate deep breathing and coughing. Because of overlapping of the distribution of nerves, three nerves must be injected to provide complete anesthesia in one dermatome.

Stellate ganglion block is used in the treatment of vascular disease of the upper extremity. By abolishing sympathetic innervation to the upper extremity, maximal vasodilation is achieved, which is advantageous for preserving blood supply in newly anastomosed vessels or in the treatment of Raynaud's disease.

Celiac plexus block is used in the management of chronic pain, (usually cancer pain) from upper abdominal viscera. Several test blocks with local anesthetic agents are frequently undertaken initially. If they are successful, the plexus may be ablated by injection of 25 ml alcohol (50 percent).

The most frequently used local anesthetic agents are lidocaine (Xylocaine) 0.5 to 1 percent, tetracaine (Pontocaine) 1 percent, mepivacaine (Carbocaine) 1 to 2 percent, bupivacaine (Marcaine) 0.25 to 0.75 percent, and chloroprocaine (Nesacaine) 0.5 to 3 percent.

Before a nerve block is performed, an intravenous route should be secured in the patient with infusion of suitable intravenous fluid. Baseline vital signs such as blood pressure, pulse, and respiratory rate must be recorded. All measures for emergency resuscitation should be immediately available. Continuous ECG monitoring is also advisable.

Reactions or complications to local anesthetics can be separated into local and systemic categories. Local reactions include hematoma, nerve injury, and inflammation. Systemic reactions include anesthetic-induced complications such as cardiovascular collapse, seizures, and true allergy; and vasopressor responses such as tachycardia and apprehension. Local reactions are rare but may be due to direct puncture of the nerve or inadequate sterility. Systemic reactions are directly related to the concentration of the local anesthetic drugs in the blood. Injection into highly vascular areas or inadvertent intravascular injection will more rapidly result in high blood concentrations. Major complications usually involve the cardiovascular and central nervous systems. Myocardial depression, bradycardia, and severe hypotension may occur. At low blood levels, local analgesic agents may have a sedative effect on the central nervous system, but at higher levels excitation and frank seizures may develop with respiratory impairment. True allergy is extremely rare and is limited mainly to ester-type drugs such as procaine (Novocaine).

Treatment of complications includes cardiovascular and respiratory support. Sedatives such as sodium thiopental and diazepam should be available. Vasopressor infusions such as Neo-Synephrine or ephedrine may be necessary.

Severe reactions resulting from overdose of vasoconstrictor substances (usually epinephrine added to local anesthetic injections to retard absorption) include treatment with beta-adrenergic blocking drugs such as phentolamine (Regitine) and propranalol (Inderal).

The nurse is responsible for assembling the equipment necessary for the procedure. Prepared and prepackaged trays are usually used. A physician's preference card or department procedure should be developed by the staff if prepackaged trays are not being used.

The anesthesiologist or attending physician has the responsibility of explaining the procedure to the patient. The nurse assists with positioning the patient and during the procedure. Following completion of the procedure, the patient's vital signs are monitored until stable; the site of the block is observed for bleeding; and the extremity or extremities distal to the block are observed for movement, sensation, and the absence of pain.

Postural hypotension, numbness, tingling, paralysis, and pain are untoward effects one might anticipate. The patient is offered liquid refreshment and gradually ambulated if an outpatient. The patient is discharged to home in the care of a competent adult, by physician's order. An inpatient can be returned to his or her room according to the discharge policy of the PACU.

CANNULATION OF VESSELS

Anesthetic management frequently involves measurements (monitoring) from catheters inserted into veins and arteries. Establishment of these monitors can be time consuming, often favoring a decision to insert the cannulae preoperatively under the sterile conditions in the PACU rather than in the operating room. General anesthesia is not usually required. Central venous, Swan-Ganz, and arterial catheters may all be conveniently inserted in the PACU. Requirements include the necessary materials, sterile techniques, and cardiovascular monitoring equipment including suitable transducers and recording apparatus.

BLOOD PATCH

One of the complications of spinal anesthesia is headache. Although this symptom usually responds to bed rest, analgesics, and adequate hydration, occasionally the pain may persist and be incapacitating. Under these circumstances an epidural injection of normal saline (30 to 50 ml) or of the patient's own blood may be given. A catheter is inserted into the same interspace at which the subarachnoid puncture was performed and fluid injected slowly until the headache abates.

BLOOD TRANSFUSION

Occasionally, the PACU may be used as a convenient location for the chronically anemic patient to be admitted on an outpatient basis for periodic blood transfusions.

Complications of blood transfusions are listed in Table 13-2. The most serious hazards of blood transfusions include transmission of hepatitis and other infectious diseases and hemolytic transfusion reactions. Hemolytic reaction is an immediate complication of blood transfusion caused by in-

TABLE 13–2. MOST COMMON COMPLICATIONS OF BLOOD TRANSFUSION

Disease transmission (infectious and serum hepatitis, syphilis, malaria, brucellosis)
Hemolytic transfusion reaction
Circulatory overload
Bacteremia
Allergic reactions

(Courtesy of Frost EAM. The recovery room as a special procedures unit. Current Review for Recovery Room Nurses 4(3):18, 1982.)

compatibility between antibodies in the recipient's plasma and antigen in the donor erythrocytes, evidenced by general hemolysis. The most common causes of this reaction are incorrect typing or cross-matching, or errors in initial unit sampling, labeling, or administration. Symptoms and signs include shivering, apprehension, urticaria, and hypotension. Hemoglobinuria may quickly develop. The hemolytic process rapidly progresses to disseminated intravascular coagulopathy (DIC).

The major objectives in treatment are to control bleeding and to prevent renal damage (acute tubular necrosis). Treatment should generally follow these steps:

1. Discontinue the transfusion and return the blood to the bank for rechecking.
2. Support the cardiovascular system with adequate fluid replacement, vasopressors, and compatible blood as soon as it becomes available.
3. Check blood and urine for free hemoglobin.
4. Administer mannitol 0.5 G/kg intravenously and follow with furosemide 40 to 80 mg intravenously to maintain renal output of at least 100 ml/hr.
5. Treat DIC, acidosis, and hyperkalemia as necessary.
6. Sterioids may be given to modify the antigen–antibody reaction. Antihistamines may also be used.
7. Platelet counts, partial thromboplastin time, and complete blood counts should be determined hourly.
8. All steps must be carefully documented on the hospital record.

Excessive or too-rapid blood transfusion may cause circulatory overload and pulmonary edema. Respiratory difficulty may develop. Useful drugs that may be used to improve cardiac function and allow the vascular system to better tolerate expansion include calcium chloride, dopamine, and digitalis preparations. Diuretics such as furosemide may be necessary. Occasionally ventilatory support is indicated.

Pyrogens are by-products of bacteria that persist after sterilization processes. Use of disposable equipment has essentially eliminated this complication. However, errors in technique of blood collection may result in contamination, especially with gram-negative bacteria and their endotoxins. Septicemia may result and is usually fatal despite vigorous therapy. Prevention includes adequate refrigeration, dating procedures, careful biologic control, and discarding of open bottles.

Allergic reactions due to the presence in the donor blood of an antigen or antibody whose immunologic counterpart is present in the recipient occurs during about 1 percent of transfusions. The reactions, including shivering and urticaria, are usually benign, and the transfusion may be continued. Rarely, angioneurotic edema or asthma may develop and require emergency therapy with epinephrine, steroids, and respiratory support.

All blood should be warmed prior to infusion to at least close to room temperatures to decrease the incidence of cardiac arrhythmias and patient discomfort from systemic cooling. A filtration component in the administration set is also essential (platelets, however, should not be given through a blood filter). During blood transfusions, the patient should be kept warm, the ECG monitored for arrhythmias due to cold or hyperkalemia, and the infusion site should be frequently inspected for infiltration or other reactions.

RESEARCH

The PACU may also be used for monitoring patients who are participating in various anesthesia/perioperative research studies. As an example, the patient who undergoes muscle biopsy for diagnosis of malignant hyperthermia may have to remain in the PACU overnight for continuous temperature monitoring.

NURSING NEEDS

Staffing should be planned on a 1-to-1 basis for most of these procedures. Time required for electroconvulsive therapy is about 10 minutes. The patient should be completely awake and ready for discharge from the PACU within 30 minutes. A similar time frame is required for cardioversion. Depending on the indication for the administration of a nerve block, approximately 20 minutes of close patient care is indicated. Epidural saline and blood patches can usually be completed in approximately 15 minutes. However, as a catheter is frequently left in place in case further administration is necessary, these patients should be observed for 1 to 2 hours.

Blood transfusions are administered slowly, and the patient's stay in the recovery room may last several hours. After an initial observation period of about 15 minutes, critical nursing care is usually no longer essential, and monitoring of vital signs every 15 minutes is adequate.

Emotional support of all patients before, during, and after these procedures must be viewed as a major aspect of their care.

In conclusion, it must be stressed that responsibility for patient care has to be delineated. Specific policies and procedures must be developed and all staff members must be aware of them. All policies and procedures as they pertain to the PACU must be outlined in the individual hospital's manuals. The physician performing the procedure (the psychiatrist for

ECT, the anesthesiologist for blocks, the cardiologist during cardioversion) assumes medical responsibility for the patient in the PACU.

Undoubtedly the national trend to decrease in-hospital stay and improve efficiency will see greater use of PACU facilities for these kinds of therapeutic maneuvers.

BIBLIOGRAPHY

Fink M: Electroshock therapy: Myths and realities. Hospital Practice 13:77, Nov. 1978.

Frost EAM: The recovery room as a special procedures unit. Current Review for Recovery Room Nurses 4(3):18–23, 1982.

Lichtiger M & Moya F: Introduction to the Practice of Anesthesia (2nd ed.). New York: Harper & Row, 1978, Chaps. 6, 16, 17, 20, 28, 38.

Minshull D: Outpatient ECT. Nurs Mir 148:28, Feb. 1979.

Mulaik JS: Nurses questions about electroconvulsive therapy. Journal of Psychosocial Nursing and Mental Health Services 17:15, Feb. 1979.

Schneider M: The recovery room as special procedures unit. AORN Journal 34(3):490–498, Sept. 1981.

Stark DCC: Practical Points in Anesthesiology (2nd ed.). Flushing, N.Y.: Medical Exam Pub. Co., 1980, Chaps. 9, 10.

Chapter 14

Postanesthesia Care in Ambulatory Surgery

Kay E. Fraulini

INTRODUCTION

The concept of ambulatory surgery is far from new. At a meeting of the British Medical Association back in 1909, Dr. J.H. Nicoll reviewed some 7320 operations that he had performed on ambulatory patients at the Royal Glasgow Hospital for Children. In 1980 over 19 million surgical procedures were performed in community hospitals in the United States (American Hospital Association, 1981). Not too many years ago, each of these procedures would have required an overnight stay in the hospital. As a result of both significant technological advances and contemporary concerns with cost-consciousness, ambulatory surgery has gained wide acceptance and accounts for a significant portion of the surgical procedures performed in hospitals as well as in independent health facilities (Burns & Ferber, 1984).

Ambulatory surgery is defined by Burns as scheduled surgical procedures provided to patients who do not remain in the hospital overnight. Although surgery not requiring an overnight hospital stay is often performed in private physicians' offices, hospital emergency departments and freestanding, independent emergency centers, this discussion will limit itself to ambulatory surgery programs specifically designed and managed to provide hospital-scheduled surgical procedures to ambulatory patients.

An ambulatory surgery program in a hospital has one or more of the following characteristics: a separate cost center, a separate facility or specifically designated surgical suites, an independent patient registration system, and independent preoperative and postoperative settings. Surgical procedures can be performed in a variety of facilities, including the inpatient operating room suites, separate operating rooms dedicated to ambulatory surgery, a freestanding facility, or the emergency department.

Accreditation

The Joint Commission on Accreditation of Hospitals (JCAH), in its 1981 Accreditation Manual for Hospitals, specifies the following:

> When surgical services are provided in an ambulatory care setting, the policies and procedures shall be consistent with those applicable to inpatient surgery, anesthesia, and post-operative recovery, and shall address in addition to the preceeding policies and procedures, the following:
>
> Types of elective operative procedures that may be performed and the locations where they may be performed.
>
> Scope of anesthesia services that may be provided and the locations where such anesthesia services may be administered.
>
> Preoperative and postoperative transportation.
>
> An established method of intervention when the designated preoperative patient workup and preparation are incomplete. An operation shall be performed only after an appropriate history, physical examination, and any required laboratory and x-ray examinations have been completed and the preoperative diagnosis has been recorded.
>
> Postoperative care, including postanesthesia recovery patient care guidelines and the role of family members assisting in patient care. Any patient who has received other than local anesthesia shall be examined by a qualified physician before discharge and shall be accompanied home by a designated person. Written instructions for follow-up care shall be given to the patient or responsible family member, and shall include directions for obtaining appropriate physician help in the event of postoperative problems. Whenever feasible, a family member should be available to pediatric patients during the preoperative and postoperative periods.

Freestanding Versus Hospital-Based Units

Two types of ambulatory care units have been defined: freestanding and hospital based. Wolcott (1981) suggests that the emergency room is not an appropriate site for ambulatory surgery and that the physician's office can at best handle only the most trivial ambulatory surgical cases safely and well. The argument of which type of unit is best is still not settled. O'Donovan (1981) has listed nine criteria that may be used to evaluate each system (Table 14–1).

TABLE 14–1. FACTORS THAT DIFFERENTIATE AMBULATORY HOSPITAL SURGERY FROM INDEPENDENTLY OPERATED FREESTANDING FACILITIES

Criteria	In-Hospital Short-Stay Surgery	Independently Operated Freestanding Ambulatory Care Surgery Facility
Cost to patient	Probably higher, because of present hospital pricing structure, but the cost could be lower because of potentially more efficient use of capital by hospitals.	Usually lower.
Cost to community	Probably lower, but only if sufficient in-hospital surgical facilities exist in a given area.	Probably higher if it duplicates underutilized hospital surgical facilities.
Quality of care	Tends to be higher, but not in all cases.	May be very good, but peer review and other safeguards must be in effect.
Access to care		
If hospital facilities are at total capacity in the local area	Restrictive.	Would increase access by providing for much-needed additional facilities (depending on how carefully placed).
If hospital facilities are not at total capacity	Then access is not aided by duplicating services.	No increase in access.
If patients lack ability to pay	The nonprofit community hospital tends to render care based more on need of care than on ability to pay, hence access to care is increased in those instances.	Depends on individual situation.
Continuity of care	Tends to increase.	A decrease, but this is not the purpose of come-and-go surgery.
Comprehensive care	Tends to increase.	A decrease, but this is not the purpose of come-and-go surgery.
Patient satisfaction	Reduced; hospital admission policies are often bureaucratic and inefficient, but this could certainly be improved; other areas besides admission policies must also be evaluated.	Tendency toward increase, especially if admission procedures are highly streamlined and efficient.

(Continued)

TABLE 14–1. (*Continued*)

Criteria	In-Hospital Short-Stay Surgery	Independently Operated Freestanding Ambulatory Care Surgery Facility
Fragmentation of health-care delivery system	Tends to have low fragmentation.	In first-rate facility, such as the Phoenix Surgicenter, there may be consolidation because better division of labor may be provided.
Dynamics of responsiveness to changing community needs	Freestanding advocates claim that hospitals are too bureaucratic to be highly responsive; however, many hospitals may respond well because they can detect needs quickly due to their great community contact and broad range of services.	Possibly greater, depending on how well they are managed.

(*Courtesy of Thomas R. O'Donovan.*)

The actual design will depend on many factors, especially available space if it is to be an in-hospital facility. Equipment will, of course, be different in the freestanding and in-hospital units, inasmuch as the in-hospital unit will rely much more heavily on the hospital's support services—radiology, laboratory, central supply, and so on. Design will also depend on the volume of work expected and the number of operating rooms. Staff members also determine whether certain types of procedures, such as bronchoscopy, esophagoscopy, colonoscopy, thoracostomy, and cystoscopy, will be done in the unit, since this too will affect the design.

ANESTHESIA FOR AMBULATORY SURGERY

Premedication—Yes or No

The in-hospital surgical patient is usually awakened early on the morning of surgery to receive an injection to produce drowsiness and calmness before being transported to the operating room. Since ambulatory patients must transport themselves or be transported by family or friends to the outpatient surgery facility, premedicant drugs are given upon arrival there. The traditional goals of premedication are to allay anxiety, dry secretions, alleviate pain, and facilitate induction of anesthesia. These must be balanced against the goals of ambulatory surgery, one of which is rapid return home following anesthesia. Also, the need for premedication of adult patients and pediatric patients may differ.

In adults, some degree of fear and apprehension about impending anesthesia and surgery is almost universal. It has been observed that so-called psychologic premedication is consistently more efficacious than pharmacologic premedication. A friendly chat with a careful explanation of what is forthcoming is frequently more effective than a sedative-hypnotic injection. If excessive anxiety remains, a reasonable approach is to give diazepam (5–10 mg) orally with a small sip of water 60 to 90 minutes prior to induction of anesthesia.

The use of anticholinergics has been customary since the advent of diethyl ether anesthesia. Today ether is rarely used, but atropine is still frequently given preoperatively. Yet essentially all modern anesthetics can be used without drying up saliva. The only exception is ketamine; oral secretions during light ketamine anesthesia trigger hyperactive laryngeal reflexes and produce airway obstruction. Fear of bradycardia has also continued preoperative anticholinergic use. Yet slow heart rates can be treated if they develop. In general, anticholinergics are not absolutely necessary as premedication except prior to use of ketamine. Finally, few ambulatory surgery patients suffer pain; elimination of narcotics avoids potential nausea and orthostatic hypotension.

For a child an ideal premedicant would be given orally, would be rapidly absorbed, would have predictable onset and short duration of action (2 to 3 hours), and would produce a tranquil, sleepy, cooperative child without sialorrhea, bronchorrhea, nausea, vomiting, hypotension, or respiratory depression. Such a drug does not exist. And as in an adult, psychologic premedication—while not perfect—is in general better than the alternatives. Also as in the adult, the use of an anticholinergic is mandatory prior to ketamine anesthesia. The role of antacids, anticholinergics, and H_2 blockers to lower gastric volume and to increase gastric pH has not been clarified.

In general, preoperative medication is not helpful in an ambulatory patient when rapid emergence from anesthesia is desired. Preoperative medications are aimed at minimizing side effects of anesthesia.

General Anesthesia Versus Regional Anesthesia

Ambulatory surgical patients should be American Society of Anesthesiologists risk class 1 or 2 (See Table 14–2) so that either general anesthesia or certain regional techniques may be used safely. Such a choice is usually made to satisfy other requirements—namely, rapid performance of anesthesia and rapid recovery. Individual preferences are also important.

Regional anesthesia for any surgical procedure requires cooperation among the patient, anesthesiologist, and surgeon. Each must understand what the other needs and expects if the procedure is to be successful. For

TABLE 14–2. PHYSICAL STATUS CLASSIFICATION OF THE AMERICAN SOCIETY OF ANESTHESIOLOGISTS

Class 1	A normal, healthy patient.
Class 2	A patient with mild systemic disease.
Class 3	A patient with severe systemic disease that is not incapacitating.
Class 4	A patient with an incapacitating systemic disease that is a constant threat to life.
Class 5	A moribund patient who is not expected to survive for 24 hours with or without operation.
E	Emergency cases are designated by the addition of "E" to the classification number.

ambulatory surgery, even more understanding and cooperation are required. Surgery that is prolonged and involves painful manipulations is best done under general anesthesia, unless the patient has an unusually high pain threshold and is unusually stoic. Sedatives and analgesics can be given during surgery, but these may delay discharge by causing a long stay in the PACU.

General Anesthesia: Intravenous Versus Inhalational Techniques

Most general anesthetics in adults begin with induction of an ultrashort-acting barbiturate through an established intravenous infusion, which is also necessary for fluid and drug administration. Indirect blood pressure measurement with a precoidial stethoscope monitor is essential. Continuous monitoring of ECG is rapidly becoming a standard practice. Following loss of consciousness, artificial ventilation is commenced with 30 to 40 percent O_2 plus 60 to 70 percent N_2O. It is at this point that two options open: (1) anesthetic vapors (halothane or enflurane) are added to the $N_2O–O_2$ to provide anesthesia; or (2) incremental intravenous doses of narcotics, muscle relaxants, and tranquilizers are given to produce anesthesia.

The concept that a "balance" of drugs can produce the anesthetic state requires an understanding that anesthesia is actually a combination of analgesia, sleep, autonomic nervous system control, and muscle relaxation. Although historically one vapor (diethyl ether, chloroform, or cyclopropane) produced anesthesia, modern anesthesia is based on using minimal amounts of several drugs to allow surgery. This use of many drugs can degenerate into extravagant polypharmacy, but the general impression remains that using a balance of drugs provides better conditions for the surgeon and less risk for the patient. Thus, a comparison of inhalational versus intravenous techniques is really a comparison of N_2O Halothane or enflurane plus muscle relaxants, versus N_2O narcotics, muscle relaxants, and tranquilizers.

Although with inhalational anesthetics there is some hepatic metabolism with eventual renal disposition, Halothane and enflurane, with their moderate blood gas solubility and high volatility, are easily administered and easily excreted via the lungs. By contrast, intravenous drugs, once given, are irretrievable and are mainly metabolized by the liver and eliminated by the kidneys.

Administration of any general anesthetic is a process of titration to achieve reversible depression of CNS function. The proper level of general anesthesia prevents the patient from movement or autonomic hyperactivity in response to surgical stimuli. Attempts to maintain anesthesia without overdose have focused on observation of blood pressure, respiratory rate and pattern, heart rate, and eye signs to gauge depth of anesthesia. Normally, the use of intravenous techniques can provide adequate anesthesia, but there is greater fluctuation in depth of anesthesia from moment to moment. The surgeon is often unaware of this since the patient is frequently paralyzed to prevent any movement during moments of light anesthesia. The possibility that patient awareness and suffering during light anesthesia with an intravenous technique may not be recognized because of induced skeletal muscle paralysis must obviously be a concern to the anesthesiologist.

Both inhalational and intravenous agents can produce equally severe cardiorespiratory depression. In general, however, patients receiving an intravenous anesthetic show higher blood pressures and heart rates. For the "healthy" patients of the ambulatory surgery group, this would be neither advantageous nor deleterious. Cardiac arrhythmias are probably more frequent with inhalational agents but are of little consequence. However, if epinephrine is used for surgical hemostasis, an interaction with Halothane to produce ventricular extrasystoles can be so prominent as to prevent halothane use.

Anesthesia misadventures usually result from failure of pulmonary gas exchange, transport of sufficient O_2 and nutrients to vital organs, or both. Rarely do direct toxic responses occur to anesthetic drugs (either inhalational or intravenous) or their metabolites. Although a liver injury probably does occur rarely after Halothane anesthesia, this has still not been conclusively proved. Enflurane is metabolized to fluoride ion, but in insufficient amounts to produce nephrotoxicity. Nitrous oxide is an immunosuppressant, but only when given for long periods (days).

Recovery from inhalational anesthetics requires adequate alveolar ventilation and cardiac output. Even though N_2O is of low solubility and Halothane of moderate solubility, 90 percent elimination from the brain takes 3 to 5 minutes for N_2O and 15 to 20 minutes for Halothane. Recovery from an intravenous balanced anesthetic first requires excretion of N_2O. Arousal will then depend on the balance of central nervous system depression opposed by incisional pain. If narcosis remains, specific antagonists (naloxone) may be used. Ultimately, ambulatory surgery patients will tolerate and recover well from either inhalational or intravenous techniques. The choice will often depend on the anesthesiologist's personal preference and skill.

It is not always reassuring to the PACU nurse that "ultimately" the patient will recover from anesthesia. As previously discussed, the above-mentioned techniques employ drugs and agents that possess long-acting depressant effects. The anesthesiologist must be aware of this and of the problems that are presented relative to criteria for discharge from the hospital or surgicenter.

Conscious Sedation

Shane (1983) writes in *Conscious Sedation for Ambulatory Surgery* that the principal objective to be stressed is the avoidance of general anesthesia whenever possible, and the avoidance of unconsciousness, which is frequently associated with deep sedation. The present section describes conscious sedation. It is presented as a creative alternative to the more traditional modes of anesthesia, and should be of especial interest for the PACU nurse who often bears a large part of the responsibility of discharging the ambulatory surgery patient.

Conscious sedation is an art not easily learned. To be successful it requires three equally important factors. The first is the use of profound local or regional block, usually performed by the surgeon. The second factor is the use of a judicious combination of drugs that will not produce somnolence or basal narcosis but only amnesia. One must execute mature judgment in drug dosage, especially in children and in patients over 50 years of age. Errors in judgment involving overdosage will result in deep sedation, which is synonymous with general anesthesia even though general anesthetic drugs may not have been employed.

The third factor is the proper employment of a series of appropriate words and phrases to produce verbal rapport. This concept of verbal rapport, or behavioral modification, is as important as local anesthesia and the use of intravenous drugs.

The proper use of verbal rapport can actually decrease the overall dosage of both narcotics and sedative drugs, thus rendering the patient ambulatory more quickly. Verbal rapport also makes the entire approach to conscious sedation practical and logical. Without it, the concept would be eventually discarded, and once again general anesthesia would assume the ascendancy.

Verbal rapport must be established either in the patient's room or in the outpatient holding area, but not in the operating room. Once the patient enters the operating room, the environmental distraction is so overwhelming that rapport will be difficult to achieve. Fear and anxiety will so discompose the patient that, regardless of how convincing the anesthesiologist is, it will not overcome the tachycardia and apprehension caused by catecholamine release, and only half the anesthesiologist's words will be embedded in the patient's subconscious.

Verbal rapport, established before any drugs are administered, involves telling the patient the following:

1. The patient will be partially asleep or in a twilight state during the painful part of the operation.
2. The patient will be allowed to awaken toward the end of the operation and will be aware of certain sensations such as constant pressure to stop bleeding, intermittent pressure to stop bleeding, the placing of sutures to stop bleeding, application of bandages or casts, and so on.
3. When these sensations of pressure or slight discomfort become manifest, the patient is not to move, speak, cry, or protest, but is to let every muscle go limp in order to prevent an elevation of blood pressure, which could cause more bleeding.
4. If the pressure to stop bleeding is a little uncomfortable, the patient may be permitted to breathe some "sweet air" (laughing gas—not more than 30 percent nitrous oxide), which will help alleviate the pressure.

These four points, with emphasis on the control of bleeding, are basic to all approaches to ambulatory surgery under conscious sedation.

A variety of drug combinations can produce amnesia without overt respiratory or circulatory depression in both young and old patients. Shane (1983) experimented with a multitude of drug cocktails and found that two specific combinations of drugs satisfy the majority of specifications for the successful management of surgery on both outpatients and inpatients. They are, briefly, the Nisentil cocktail, consisting of Nisentil, Vistaril, atropine, and Brevital (in a separate syringe); and the Sublimaze cocktail, consisting of Sublimaze, Vistaril, atropine, Valium, and Brevital (the latter two each in separate syringes). In Shane's experience the Nisentil cocktail seems to be more predictable and dependable.

Vistaril is of prime importance in both of these amnesic cocktails. The predictability and successful management of patients under conscious sedation are highly dependent on this drug. Vistaril, without adversely affecting pulse or blood pressure:

1. Potentiates all of the other drugs in the cocktail.
2. Is a powerful antiemetic.
3. Is a powerful antigagging drug.
4. Is a powerful antinausea drug.
5. Is a bronchodilator and is useful in asthmatics.
6. Is an antisialagogue.
7. Is a dissociator (that is, it tends to dissociate the patient from

present reality without affecting normal cerebration and rational behavior).

8. Possesses an intrinsic analgesic action.

9. Is nonirritating to the cerebral cortex, whereas Valium seems to be irritating in children and in adults at higher dosages.

These drugs must be combined with intensive behavioral modification if outpatient surgery without general anesthesia is to be consistently successful.

Very often these patients return to the PACU awake and with no recall of the entire operating room experience. They can usually be discharged within 2 to 4 hours in good condition (Shane, 1983).

NURSING CARE OF THE OUTPATIENT

Whether the outpatient facility is hospital-based, hospital-affiliated, or freestanding, the standards that apply to nursing care are the same (Batstone & Van Winkle, 1983).

Many organizations now have a voice in quality control of health care. Facilities that provide for ambulatory surgical care must meet and maintain standards for accreditation set by the Association for Ambulatory Health Care, Professional Standards Review Organization; the American Society of Anesthesiologists Guidelines for Outpatient Surgery and Ad Hoc Committee on Ambulatory Surgical Care; and the Joint Commission on Accreditation of Hospitals. Nursing care in the outpatient surgical facility must be based on standards of practice as established by the nursing profession (see the appendix to Chapter 9 for the ASPAN Standards of Care Guidelines).

Preoperative Phase

The decision to have surgery as an outpatient most likely is made in the physician's office. Therefore, the office nurse may initiate the nursing intervention that the patient receives. When establishing standards of patient care in any given facility, all who provide nursing care at any time during the surgical experience should collaborate in order that roles and nursing activities may be clearly delineated. This action can serve to eliminate duplication of efforts and provide desired continuity of care with minimal professional personnel.

During the preoperative period the nurse performs two major functions: (1) collecting data from the patient to be utilized by the nurse in developing an individualized plan of care, and (2) providing information to the patient that is essential for participative patient involvement. Clearly, this is similar to the preoperative phase of the inpatient.

Patient Information Booklet

Patient information booklets are a way to communicate pertinent information to the surgical candidate. Regardless of the tool used to provide patient information, instructions to the patient must be given in writing and reinforced verbally.

Although instructions given to patients will vary somewhat depending on the policies and procedures of each facility, patients must receive specific guidelines telling them what to expect and what their responsibilities are on the night before surgery, the day of the operation, and after surgical intervention.

Instructions should be written clearly, concisely, and address specific areas of concern. The following is a list of headings to be addressed in an information booklet:

NIGHT BEFORE SURGERY

1. Meals
2. Bathing
3. Alcohol intake

DAY OF THE OPERATION

1. Makeup or fingernail polish
2. Clothing
3. Anesthesiologist, who should accompany patient to and from the hospital or surgicenter
4. Directions for family or escort
5. Average length of stay
6. Discharge
7. Instruction sheet
8. Follow-up call
9. Instructions on complications

Many outpatient facilities have found it advantageous to have the patient visit the facility 2 to 7 days before the day of surgery. Preadmission laboratory work may be done at this time, and there is opportunity for the patient and family to have a guided tour of the facility to familiarize them with the environment.

Preanesthetic assessment and interview should be similar to that described in Chapter 5. Chapter 5 also includes a detailed discussion of preoperative patient teaching. Although there are no definitive studies that support physiologic benefit from such teaching, there can be no doubt that outpatients require detailed instruction concerning their surgical (anesthetic) experience. A focus of this teaching must be on what the patient should do when he or she leaves the hospital or surgicenter.

Instructions are more likely to be followed if the patient understands why they should be followed. Information given to the patient will vary somewhat depending on the procedure, the physician, and the institution. All specific verbal instructions, especially those requiring a response from the patient, should be reinforced with written instructions.

Not to be neglected is consideration of the child patient. Teaching takes on a different perspective when the patient is a child. It is generally true that a well-prepared child is a cooperative child. The nurse must consider not only the age and level of development of the child, but the sex, previous surgical experiences of the child and parents, and the parent–child relationship. It is very important for children to know what is going to happen and how they will look and feel. The child also needs to know where the parents will be during each phase of the surgical experience. Teaching aides such as books, dolls, and puppets are helpful in conveying information to children. Having toys available for play, allowing children to bring a favorite toy or security object or their own gown, slippers, and so on, may be advantageous (Batstone & Van Winkle, 1983).

Immediate Preoperative Assessment

Assessment of patient status, physical and psychological, must continue on the day of surgery. The time that the nurse spends with the patient immediately before surgery may be brief, so it is essential that keen observation and listening skills be utilized. A thorough review of preadmission documents is essential. Patients should be accompanied to the dressing area, assigned a locker, and given appropriate attire and any necessary procedural instructions. Privacy should be ensured and the patient should be told where to go after he or she has finished changing. A preoperative checklist (Fig. 14–1) will assist in the completion of a thorough preoperative assessment in a minimal amount of time.

Postoperative Phase

Many outpatient facilities have two phases designated for the postanesthesia recovery period. Defined specific criteria must be met before discharge from either phase is permitted. If two phases are designated some facilities have found it beneficial to use a Phase 1 admission criteria for patients receiving a general anesthetic or those receiving a local or regional anesthetic with sedation. Phase 2 patients, by this criteria, are those who have received only a local or regional anesthetic without sedation, or are those patients from Phase 1 who have met Phase 1 discharge criteria—that is, they are conscious.

Phase 1. Nursing intervention in the outpatient PACU differs little from that provided for the hospitalized patients, as described in earlier chapters. Though outpatients are generally not anesthetized as deeply as those having major procedures requiring hospitalization, their altered con-

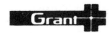

**GRANT HOSPITAL OF CHICAGO
OUTPATIENT SURGERY UNIT
PRE-OPERATIVE CHECK LIST**

(IMPRINT PATIENT INFORMATION)

Place (✓) in box to indicate item is completed and on chart.   Date: _____

Signed: ☐ Surgical and Anesthesia Consent   ☐ Patient Authorization/Statement

Physical Status: ☐ Unchanged since previous assessment on _____
                                                                  (Date)

Completed: ☐ History/Physical   ☐ Pre-op teaching/assessment sheet

Routine Testing: ☐ Hgb/Hct   ☐ Chem 24   ☐ EKG
                     ☐ CBC   ☐ Coagulation Profile   ☐ Chest X-Ray
                     ☐ Urinalysis   ☐ Other(s) _____
                     ☐ U.C.G.   ☐ R.P.R.   _____
                     ☐ Sickle Cell   ☐ Group & Rh. Factor

Removed: ☐ Valuables _____
                                                  (Specify valuables and placement)
                     ☐ Prosthesis _____
                                                  (Specify item and placement)
                     ☐ Make-up/Nail Polish/Hairpins, etc.

Wearing: ☐ Identification Band   ☐ Hospital Gown

Elimination/   am   am
  Ingestion: ☐ Voided at _____ pm   ☐ Ate/Drank at _____ pm
                     _____   ☐ Responsible Adult Present

                     T._____   P._____   R._____   B.P._____

Pre-Operative
  Medication Orders: Yes ☐   No ☐

Patient prepared and
  form completed by: _____
                                            (Signature of Nurse)

Checked in O.R. by: _____
                                            (Signature of Nurse)

Figure 14–1. Preoperative checklist. *(Courtesy of Grant Hospital of Chicago.)*

sciousness requires careful, accurate, and continuous assessment. A record similar to the one given in Chapter 4, that utilizes the REACT scoring system, can facilitate such an assessment.

Phase 2. Transfer to the second stage of recovery is generally accomplished via stretcher, and the patient is then assisted into a reclining chair. Family members are present, and together with PACU nurses encourage patients to awaken, to move about, and to get ready for ambulation. Safety measures must be implemented.

Vital signs are again checked after the transfer and recorded on a form similar to that shown in Figure 14–2; these are checked and recorded every 30 minutes during Phase 2. An overall assessment of the patient's condition should be made following the transfer. This includes checking the IV site, dressings, and so on. The recliner is first placed in the reclining position upon transfer, and adjusted gradually to a sitting position.

Grant

GRANT HOSPITAL OF CHICAGO
OUTPATIENT SURGERY UNIT

PHASE II RECOVERY ROOM RECORD
PACU

(Imprint Patient Information)

Date_____/_____/ 19_____.   Time in_____ a.m. p.m.   Time Out_____ a.m. p.m.

Operation_____

Anesthesia. General ☐.   Regional ☐.   Local w/Sedation ☐.   Local ☐.   Topical ☐.

Time	B/P	Pulse	Resp.	Medications & I.V.'s	Nurses Notes

Phase II PACU Record, Con't.

Nursing Discharge Assessment:

☐ Alert and Orientated   ☐ Vital Signs Stable   ☐ Able To Ambulate

☐ Nausea, Vomiting, Dizziness Minimal   ☐ Swallow, Cough and Gag Reflex Present

☐ Absence of Respiratory Distress   ☐ Dressings Checked.   ☐ Voided

☐ Patient Given Discharge Instruction Sheet   ☐ Take Home Medication/Prescription

☐ Responsible Adult Present To Escort Patient Home

Operative Site:_____

Follow-Up Appointment On: _____ (day)   _____ (date)   _____ (time) a.m. p.m.

Doctor's Office: Yes ☐   No ☐   Hospital: Yes ☐   No ☐

Emergency Telephone Numbers Given: Yes ☐   No ☐

Remarks & Discharge Instructions:_____

_____

_____

_____

DISCHARGE

_____ R.N.
(Signature of R.N. Discharging Patient)

Time_____ a.m. p.m.   Date_____/_____/ 19_____.

Figure 14–2. Phase II recovery record. *(Courtesy of Grant Hospital of Chicago.)*

The patient may experience nausea and vomiting following transfer to the recliner; this may be alleviated by having the patient remain quiet for a while. Soda crackers also have been found to be therapeutic, and oral fluids (if tolerated) may be offered to the patient at this time. Water, lemon-lime carbonated drinks, cola, coffee, or tea are appropriate liquids to offer. Liquids should be served at room temperature, but should be withheld if the patient is nauseated or vomiting. Solid foods, and iced or hot liquids, should not be given until clear liquids are tolerated. Babies may be given their milk or formula or the mother may be allowed to nurse if the baby is hungry.

Ambulation is accomplished when the patient's condition warrants. Some patients may need much encouragement for this first ambulation, and assistance is imperative.

Pain Management

Wetchler (1983) proposes that the role of the anesthesiologist does not end in the operating room, but carries over into management of pain, nausea and vomiting, hoarseness following extubation, and patient discharge.

Medications given in the PACU must be closely monitored and given in small, immediately effective dosages. Too much sedation, or an inappropriate route of administration, will not provide effective pain relief and may result in prolonged recovery time and possible admittance to the hospital.

Wetchler manages adult pain with fentanyl 0.25 ml IV at 5-minute intervals up to a total dose of 1 ml. This can be handled effectively by the PACU nursing staff and has been found to work satisfactorily in well over 95 percent of patients (Table 14–3). To make certain an intravenous route is always available, routine orders allow the addition of 500 ml of 5 percent dextrose and water in the PACU to any IV started during anes-

TABLE 14–3. PACU PAIN MANAGEMENT FOR ADULTS

This policy applies to patients who are at least 12 years old and weigh more than 80 lb.

1.   Fentanyl 0.25 ml IV.
2.   Repeat at 5-minute intervals as needed.
3.   Question patients as to disappearance of pain after administering each dose.
4.   Total dosage not to exceed 1 ml.
5.   Contact a member of the anesthesiology department if pain is not relieved by the above.

(Courtesy of Wetchler BV: Anesthesia in outpatients. In Mauldin BC: Ambulatory Surgery: A Guide to Perioperative Nursing Care. New York, Grune & Stratton, 1983.)

thesia. If pain persists after 1 ml of fentanyl has been administered in divided dosage, an anesthesiologist checks the patient to see if there is a reason why pain should still persist before any additional analgesia is given.

Pediatric patients also have an established fentanyl dosage based on weight (Table 14–4). For pediatric patients the initial fentanyl dosage can be repeated only once before an examination by an anesthesiologist is required. Tylenol elixir can also be used routinely. Wetchler reports great success using a combination of IV and oral pain medications in the pediatric population.

By establishing a PACU policy for pain management, the potential problem of every physician ordering different postoperative pain medications for their patients is avoided. Surgeons used to working in an inpatient environment might otherwise order morphine or meperidine in substantial intramuscular dosages for postoperative pain. One must be careful that this does not happen, because of the long-acting effects of these drugs. The operating physician should be concerned with ordering oral analgesics as take-home medications. These oral medications can also be used in the PACU once the patient has taken fluids and shown no sign of nausea or vomiting. Oral medications, particularly on an empty stomach, tend to increase nausea and vomiting. Patients are encouraged to take liquids and crackers both in the PACU and at home before taking any oral medication.

TABLE 14–4. PACU PAIN MANAGEMENT FOR INFANTS AND CHILDREN

This policy applies to patients who are less than 12 years old and weigh less than 80 lb.

The following is considered total dosage for specific patient weights:

Weight (lb)	Initial Dose μg (ml)	Total Dosage μg (ml)
20–40	5 (0.1)	10 (0.2)
41–50	7.5 (0.15)	15 (0.3)
51–60	10.0 (0.2)	20 (0.4)
61–80	12.5 (0.25)	25 (0.5)

1. Sublimaze intravenously as per above dosage/weight.
2. May repeat only once at 5-minute intervals if needed.
3. Supplement with Elixir of Tylenol.
4. Contact a member of the anesthesiology department if pain is not relieved by the above.

(Courtesy of Wetchler BV: Anesthesia in outpatients. In Mauldin BC: Ambulatory Surgery: A Guide to Perioperative Nursing Care. New York, Grune & Stratton, 1983.)

Nausea and Vomiting

A detailed account of this and other postanesthetic problems can be found in Chapter 10. Because postoperative nausea and vomiting is a major problem of outpatient anesthesia, it warrants some comments in this context.

Admittance to the hospital can result not only from uncontrolled nausea and vomiting, but also following treatment with potent antiemetics that produce prolonged somnolence. In the original droperidol studies, Janssen (1963) showed it to be 1000 times more potent an antiemetic than chlorpromazine. Although its use in ambulatory patients has been questioned because of its potential for prolonged drowsiness, droperidol has been shown to be an effective antiemetic in an outpatient setting in dosages as low as 0.25 mg (0.1 ml). When used in these low dosages, undesirable side effects are uncommon (Shelly, 1978).

Wetchler (1983) has written a policy (Table 14–5) that allows the nursing staff to institute early treatment of these symptoms without requiring specific physician's orders. Droperidol can potentiate drowsiness and, if administered during the final phases of postanesthesia care, may increase the patient's length of stay. In addition to meeting all discharge criteria, patients should be kept a minimum of 1 hour after any sedative, tranquilizing, or narcotic medications are given.

Discharge Teaching

Discharge teaching, which was initiated preoperatively, can be reviewed during Phase 2 of recovery when the patient has demonstrated that he or she can physically and mentally cope with the information and instructions needed before leaving the facility.

Discharge Criteria

Phase 2 of the recovery period is generally accomplished in approximately 1 to 1½ hours. The total recovery period (Phases 1 and 2) can last

---

TABLE 14–5. PACU POLICY FOR CONTROL OF NAUSEA AND VOMITING

Droperidol IV for persistent nausea and/or second emesis.

Patient 12 Years and Older	Children 2–12 Years	
Droperidol 0.25 ml IV.	lb	ml
If no improvement in 15 minutes,	20–25	0.1
may repeat once only.	26–50	0.15
	51–75	0.2
	76–100	0.25

A repeat dose of droperidol in pediatric patients requires examination and written order by department anesthesiologist. A department anesthesiologist should be contacted in all cases where nausea and/or vomiting persist.

(Courtesy of Wetchler BV: Anesthesia in outpatients. In Mauldin BC: Ambulatory Surgery: A Guide to Perioperative Nursing Care. New York, Grune & Stratton, 1983.)

from 2 to 4 hours (allowing time for any complications to dissipate), with an average time of approximately 2 hours.

When all criteria have been met, the patient may be prepared for discharge. Discharge criteria for Phase 2 recovery are stable vital signs; presence of swallow, cough, and gag reflexes; ability to ambulate; minimal nausea, vomiting, and dizziness; absence of respiratory distress; an alert and oriented demeanor; and a satisfactory postanesthesia score if the PACU uses a measurement system.

Tests have been developed to measure patient recovery from anesthesia (see Chapter 11). Although most of these have been found to be too involved for practical clinical usage, one that may have application in that it is simple to perform is the Trieger Psychomotor Test (Newman & associates, 1969). This test provides an objective means of measuring patient recovery by requiring the patient to draw a standard figure connected by a series of dots (Fig. 14–3). Testing is carried out preanesthesia, immediately postanesthesia, and when the patient is considered ready for discharge from the PACU. The discharge score must be equal to or lower than the preoperative score before a patient is considered eligible for discharge. Based on his studies, Trieger reached the conclusion that with the aid of his dot test, one can more objectively assess the patient's return to his or her preanesthetic state. This test might be considered a medicolegal record of the patient's discharge condition.

A study of postanesthetic morbidity in outpatients showed drowsiness to be the most common complaint during the first 24 hours (30 percent),

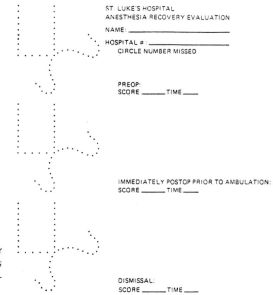

ST. LUKE'S HOSPITAL
ANESTHESIA RECOVERY EVALUATION
NAME: _____
HOSPITAL # : _____
CIRCLE NUMBER MISSED

PREOP:
SCORE _____ TIME _____

IMMEDIATELY POSTOP PRIOR TO AMBULATION:
SCORE _____ TIME _____

Figure 14–3. Trieger psychomotor test. *(Courtesy of the St. Luke's Hospital of Kansas City Ambulatory Surgery Center.)*

DISMISSAL:
SCORE _____ TIME _____

followed by headache (13 percent), anorexia and nonspecific malaise (12 percent), nausea (12 percent), dizziness (6 percent), vomiting (4 percent), and body aches (0.7 percent). The ranking order for symptoms was the same for both men and women. Women were more often affected than men, and an increase of over 20 minutes in the length of the operation was associated with both the occurrence and severity of the symptoms (Fahy & Marshall, 1969). Objective memory studies have confirmed that simple, general outpatient anesthetic techniques do affect patient memory retention in the postoperative period (Ogg & associates, 1979). Effects are maximum at 1 hour following anesthesia but return to normal limits within 3 hours (Newman & associates, 1969). This reinforces the need to give written postoperative instructions to patients.

Patients do not always follow instructions. In a survey of 100 patients who had outpatient anesthesia, it was reported that 31 went home unescorted by a responsible person; 41 patients owned their own cars and out of this number 4 drove themselves home and 30 drove within less than 24 hours from the time of surgery. A bus driver returned to his job on the same day (Ogg, 1972). It is essential that, in addition to verbal directions, patients be provided with specific written instructions to take with them for their postanesthetic and postoperative care.

Premedication and anesthetics can impair patients' psychomotor skills for varying lengths of time. Using an automobile driving simulator, Kortilla assessed recovery from anesthesia in a controlled manner (see Table 14–6), and his data can be used as a point of reference when establishing written discharge policy (Kortila, 1976, 1977). Driving simulators, reaction times, and complex psychomotor skill tests provide interesting objective information, but they are not suitable for use in everyday clinical situations.

TABLE 14–6. OUTPATIENT ANESTHESIA: RECOMMENDED MINIMAL VALUES FOR LENGTH OF STAY AND NO DRIVING

Drug	Dose	Hospital Stay (hours)	No Driving (hours)
Thiopental	6 mg/kg	3	24
Methohexital	2 mg/kg	2	24
Diazepam	10 mg IV	1	7
Meperidine	75 mg IM or IV	2–3	24
Fentanyl	0.1 mg IV	1–2	24
Fentanyl	0.2 mg IV	2	24
Droperidol	5 mg IV	4–6	24
Halothane, N_2O-O_2	(5–10 min)	2	7
Enflurane, N_2O-O_2	(5–10 min)	2	7

(Adapted from Kortila K: Minor outpatient anesthesia and driving. Modern Problems in Pharmacopsychiatry 11:91–98, 1976. With permission.)

If one utilizes a postanesthesia scoring system, it must be practical, simple, easily understandable and applicable to all postanesthesia situations. REACT, described in Chapter 4, fulfills all of these requirements (Fraulini & Murphy, 1984). A system using the numbers 1 to 10 is more easily understood when discussing a patient's postoperative condition than trying to use descriptive adjectives, and it allows physicians and nurses to communicate in a common numerical language.

In addition to using a scoring system, Wetchler's patients must meet other discharge criteria (Fig. 14–4), which are incorporated in his Phase 2 PACU record (Wetchler, 1981). When all discharge criteria have been met, an anesthesiologist checks the patient and discharges him or her. Patients who have had sedation or general anesthesia should not be allowed to leave the unit unless a responsible adult is present to take them home. Routines and policies vary among facilities, but established protocol is essential in the discharge procedure.

Follow-up Evaluation

Evaluation calls during the 24-hour period after discharge can provide effective postoperative follow-up. Questions should be asked concerning muscle aches and pains, sore throat, painful IV site, and prolonged nausea or drowsiness. If any of these problems are present, phone contact should be continued until the staff is sure of the patient's recovery. This routine is helpful not only in evaluating the status of the patient but also in giving him or her a chance to ask questions and be reassured if there have been unexpected developments (Batstone & Van Winkle, 1983).

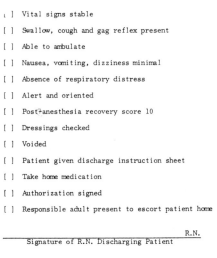

[ ]   Vital signs stable

[ ]   Swallow, cough and gag reflex present

[ ]   Able to ambulate

[ ]   Nausea, vomiting, dizziness minimal

[ ]   Absence of respiratory distress

[ ]   Alert and oriented

[ ]   Post anesthesia recovery score 10

[ ]   Dressings checked

[ ]   Voided

[ ]   Patient given discharge instruction sheet

[ ]   Take home medication

[ ]   Authorization signed

[ ]   Responsible adult present to escort patient home

_____ R.N.
Signature of R.N. Discharging Patient

Figure 14–4. Discharge criteria example. *(Courtesy of Wetchler BV. Anesthesia for outpatient surgery. AORN Journal 34:(2), 295, 1981.)*

_____ M.D.
Signature of Physician Discharging Patient

A QUALITY ASSURANCE PROGRAM

The current JCAH standard (1981) emphasizes that problems identified must be relative to the improvement of patient care. Moreover, these efforts must be coordinated and integrated into the institution's organization chart, which should show open lines of communication as well as "where the buck stops." The JCAH encourages creativity, innovation, and identification of problems, in addition to suggesting many identifying sources, such as financial data, utilization review findings, patient surveys or comments, and findings of hospital committees. For this reason the audit is no longer considered the only method of data collection. Figure 14–5 illustrates a retrospective patient care evaluation form used to document the postoperative telephone interview with the patient. Note that the form is concise and easy for the interviewer to read and mark at a glance. If the first attempt to contact the patient is unsuccessful, a second call is made.

Figure 14–6 is an explanation of positive responses and appears on the reverse side of Figure 14–5. Each "yes" response requires a specific and detailed explanation with an appropriate follow-up. Once completed, the retrospective patient care evaluation form becomes a part of the chart and thus of the formal medical record.

Buske (1984) indicates that the telephone interview provides a wealth of valid information that can be used to assess the quality and appropriateness of care delivered. Another method of retrospective interview includes asking the patient to assume the responsibility for contacting the facility. This contact can be made by telephone or by a self-addressed, postage-paid returnable questionnaire. Whichever method is used, it is incumbent on the institution to show documentation of the effort in relation to the actual impact on patient care (Redman, 1979).

Quality Assurance Based on Patient Outcomes

How can the quality of a patient's health care be properly evaluated when the length of stay is measured in hours and minutes instead of in days and weeks? Dr. Joseph Gonella believes that "patient outcomes" provide the answer, and should be the primary focus of quality assurance programs. At St. Francis Hospital in Memphis, Tennessee, 16 expected patient outcomes have been developed, and are consistent with the philosophy of the hospital in general and the Outpatient Services Department in particular (see Appendix 14–1).

An effective program should include a plan in order to provide a consistently effective quality assurance program. The JCAH suggests a written plan in which the goals and standards of care are stated. The plan, moreover, should be comprehensive enough to cover all aspects of the health care delivery mechanism in any ambulatory surgical setting. It should be flexible enough to be innovative and realistic enough to be

SAINT FRANCIS HOSPITAL, INC.
OUTPATIENT SERVICE DEPARTMENT

Pt. Name _____

1. Did patient have respiratory symptoms such as congestion, wheezing, sore throat or difficulty breathing?

   _____ General   NO   YES
   _____ Other_____   (See Reverse)

2. Did patient complain of any bleeding?

                                  NO   YES
                                                    (See Reverse)

3. Did patient experience impairment to circulation and/or nerves such as change in color,
   increased pain, numbness, swelling, tingling or coldness?

   NA   NO   YES
                                                        (See Reverse)

4. Did patient experience unusual pain at home?

                                  NO   YES
                                                    (See Reverse)

5. Did patient experience nausea and/or vomiting after discharge?

   _____ General   NO   YES
   _____ Local with sedation   (See Reverse)
   _____ Local
   _____ Block

6. Were antibiotics prescribed to be taken before surgery?

                                  NO   YES
                                                    (See Reverse)

7. Were antibiotics prescribed to be taken after surgery?

                                  NO   YES
                                                    (See Reverse)

8. Were there any signs of infection after surgery such as pus-filled or foul oder to drainage,
   pain, redness, swelling or fever?

                                  NO   YES
                                                    (See Reverse)

1st   Call—Date: _____Completed_____   2nd   Call—Date:
            _____Completed_____
                   Not Completed_____   Not Completed_____

Nurse's Signature:_____ 1st Call
Nurse's Signature: _____ 2nd Call

Figure 14–5. Retrospective patient care evaluation.

practical (Redman, 1979). The JCAH, for example, requires a review of
ambulatory surgical patients needing unplanned postoperative admission
(JCAH, 1979). Appendix 14–2 illustrates the format and results of a
review done at St. Francis Hospital on unplanned surgical admissions.
The character of the results reflects the review's ongoing nature.

1. Patient complained of respiratory symptoms including:

   _____ Congestion   _____ Sore throat   _____ Physician called
   _____ Wheezing   _____ Breathing difficulty _____ Physician seen

   Comments: _____
   _____

   Disposition _____

2. Patient complained of postoperative bleeding:

   How long did bleeding last? _____   _____ Physician called
   How much bleeding? _____   _____ Physician seen

   Comments: _____
   _____

   Disposition _____

3. Patient complained of impairment to circulation and/or nerves:

   _____ Change in color   _____ Increased pain   _____ Physician called
   _____ Tingling   _____ Coldness   _____ Physician seen
                               _____ Numbness

   Comments: _____
   _____

   Disposition _____

4. Patient complained of postoperative pain:

   _____ Mild_____ Moderate_____ Severe_____ No pain medication ordered
                       _____ Physician called   _____ Physician seen
   _____ Pain medication gave   How long did pain last before relief?_____
           tolerable relief
   _____ Pain medication did not   _____ Physician ordered pain medication after contact
           give tolerable
           relief

   Comments: _____
   _____

   Disposition _____

5. Patient complained of nausea and/or vomiting after discharge:

   How long did nausea and/or vomiting last? _____   _____ Physician called
   _____ Further treatment required   _____ Physician seen
   Comments: _____

   Disposition _____

6. Antibiotics were prescribed preoperatively:

   Name of med and dosage _____
   How long before surgery were these drugs taken?
   Comments: _____

7. Antibiotics were prescribed postoperatively:

   _____ Medication was taken as prescribed
   _____ Side effects noted
   Comments: _____
   _____

Figure 14–6. Explanation of positive responses. (*Courtesy of Buske SM. St. Francis Hospital, Memphis, Tennessee.*)

8. Patient described signs and symptoms of infection:

_____ Operative site   _____ Foul drainage and/   _____ Redness   _____ Physician
_____ Other than   or pus   _____ Swelling   called
      operative site   _____ Pain   _____ Fever   _____ Physician seen

How long after surgery did symptom appear? _____
            Med. rx'd as a result_____

Comments: _____
_____

Disposition _____

Figure 14–6. (Continued)

Problem-solving—central to the concept of quality assurance—is a cooperative effort involving clear, open lines of communication. The quality assurance plan should outline the relationship of ambulatory surgery review efforts to other departments within the institution. The plan, moreover, should indicate the mechanism by which quality assurance activities affect the vertical responsiblity within the medical staff, administration, and governing board.

REFERENCES

American Hospital Association: Hospital statistics. Chicago: AHA, 1981, p. 5.

Batstone RL & Van Winkle: Nursing care of the outpatient. In BC Mauldin: Ambulatory Surgery: A Guide to Perioperative Nursing Care. New York: Grune & Stratton, 1983.

Brown BR (Ed.): Outpatient Anesthesia: Contemporary Anesthesia Practice. Philadelphia: F.A. Davis, 1978.

Burns LA: Will multi-institutional systems serve as change agents to improve the management of ambulatory care? JACM 3:1–17, Aug. 1980.

Burns LA: Ambulatory Surgery—Developing and Managing Successful Programs. Rockville, Md.: Aspen, 1984.

Burns LA & Ferber MS: Ambulatory surgery in the United States: Trends and developments. In LA Burns: Ambulatory Surgery. Rockville, Md.: Aspen, 1984.

Buske SM: A Quality Assurance Program for Ambulatory Surgical Services in Ambulatory Surgery—Developing and Managing Successful Programs. Rockville, Md.: Aspen, 1984.

Fahy A & Marshall M: Postanesthetic morbidity in outpatients. British Journal of Anesthesia 41:433–438, 1969.

Fraulini KE & Murphy P: REACT—A new system for measuring postanesthetic recovery. Nursing 14(4):101–102, April, 1984.

Janssen PAJ: The Pharmacology of Dehydrobenzperidol. New York: Arzneim Frosch, 13:205, 1963.

Joint Commission on Accreditation of Hospitals: Accreditation manual for hospitals, 1980 edition. Chicago: JCAH, 1979, p. 69.

Joint Commission on Accreditation of Hospitals: Accreditation manual for hospitals. Chicago: JCAH, 1981, p. 66.

Mauldin BC: Ambulatory Surgery: A Guide to Perioperative Nursing Care. New York: Grune & Stratton, 1983.

Mosley T: Ambulatory surgical care. Journal of the Florida Medical Association 64:262, 1977.

Newman MG, Trieger N, Miller JC: Measuring recovery from anesthesia—A simple test. Anesthesia and Analgesia 48:136–140, 1969.

O'Donovan TP: Ambulatory Surgical Centers: Development and Management. Germantown, Md.: Aspen, 1976.

Ogg PW: An assessment of postoperative outpatient cases. British Medical Journal 4:573–575, 1972.

Ogg PW, Fischer HBJ, Bethune DW, et al.: Day case anesthesia and memory. Anesthesia 34:784–789, 1979.

Redman RR (Ed.): New JCAH quality assurance standard for hospitals. Perspective on accreditation, May–June 1979.

Shane SL: Conscious Sedation for Ambulatory Surgery. Baltimore: University Park Press, 1983.

Shelly ES & Brown HA: Antiemetic effect of ultralow dose of droperidol. ASA Annual Meeting, Chicago, 1978.

Smith CR: Patient education in ambulatory care. Nursing Clinics of North America 12:595, 1977.

Wetchler BV: Anesthesia for outpatient surgery. AORN Journal 34:2, 1981.

Wetchler BV: Anesthesia in outpatients. In BC Mauldin: Ambulatory Surgery: A Guide to Perioperative Nursing Care. New York, Grune & Stratton, 1983.

Wolcott MW: Ambulatory Surgery and the Basics of Emergency Surgical Care. Philadelphia: J.B. Lippincott, 1981.

APPENDIX 14–1

Expected Patient Outcomes, Outpatient Services Department

The patient who upon a physician's order submits to a procedure directed by the Saint Francis Hospital Outpatient Services Department can expect to be discharged from the department with the following assurances:

1. That the patient understands each form that requires a signature and why the signature or that of a responsible party is necessary.
2. That the patient understands who and how financial responsibility for the procedure will be handled and who generates the bills if other than the hospital.

3. That the patient's safety home is assured when appropriate by having a responsible person available to provide transportation.
4. That the procedures were coordinated in such a way as to provide for accuracy of scheduling as well as efficiency of time.
5. That the procedure was performed safely and accurately by qualified personnel and only according to the physician's specific instructions and plan of care.
6. That qualified personnel were available at all times to answer questions.
7. That the patient's privacy has been provided for and respected.
8. That the patient suffered no undue anxiety because the procedure was not explained.
9. That precautions to insure the patient's safety in the Outpatient Services Department have been practiced at all times.
10. That should a sudden change in the patient's condition occur requiring emergency intervention, trained personnel and necessary equipment were readily available.
11. That the patient's valuables and belongings have been kept in safekeeping until discharge.
12. That the patient understands what the prescriptions are for, when to take them and precautions to observe when taking certain drugs which affect sensory-motor function.
13. That the patient and responsible party understand exactly how to take responsibility for home care.
14. That the patient and responsible party know exactly what untoward signs and symptoms to look for after discharge which would alert them to possible problems.
15. That the patient knows who to call for help if untoward signs and/or symptoms become apparent.
16. That the patient was treated as a unique individual with the respect and dignity which is recognized as a fundamental right of every patient entering Saint Francis Hospital.

(Courtesy of Buske SM. St. Francis Hospital, Memphis, Tennessee.)

APPENDIX 14–2

Review of Unplanned Admission to the Hospital Following Surgery Done on an Ambulatory Basis

I. Concern of Study

    A. To identify the extent and causes necessitating unplanned admission to the hospital following ambulatory surgery done through the Outpatient Services Department of Saint Francis Hospital.

II. Results of Study

    A. Extent of Unplanned Admission
       1. Of the 1950 surgical cases done through the Outpatient Services Department from 1/1/80 through 12/31/80, 13 patients were admitted for further observation.
       2. This represents a 0.6 percent admission for unforeseen complications.

    B. Causes of Unplanned Admission
       1. Three patients were admitted for nausea and vomiting, one of which was also very sleepy.
       2. Two patients were admitted for unstable vital signs, particularly hypotension.
       3. Two patients were admitted due to severe pain.
       4. One patient requested admission.
       5. One patient developed a hematoma which necessitated a return to surgery and evaluation of same.
       6. One patient's physician requested 24-hour observation for bleeding after the removal of a rectal polyp.
       7. One patient was too sleepy to discharge.
       8. One patient required additional and more extensive surgery.
       9. One patient developed hoarseness, coughing and chest pain.

III. Problems Identified

    A. Seven of the 13 cases admitted appear to be the result of anesthesia-related problems, with nausea and vomiting being the most consistently repeated offenders. (Twelve of the 13 patients reviewed had been given general anesthesia.)

B. The remaining five situations requiring eventual admission appear to have no common thread of correlation other than that they could not have been anticipated preoperatively.

1. Action Recommended: Complete a study of 100 adult and 100 pediatric ambulatory surgical patients operated on under general anesthesia:

Document and compare the following:

1. age
2. weight
3. procedure
4. anesthesiologist
5. anesthesia risk
6. preoperative medications
7. anesthetics used
8. duration of anesthesia
9. length of recovery room (PACU) stay
10. medications used during recovery
11. length of outpatient observation stay
12. medications used during outpatient observations
13. incidence of anesthesia related problems during outpatient observation
14. incidence of anesthesia related problems after discharge

IV. Action Taken

A. A study of 100 adult and 100 pediatric ambulatory surgical patients undergoing general anesthesia will be completed by Sharon M. Buske, R.N., and the results submitted to the Anesthesia Medical Staff Committee for review and recommendations.

V. Follow-up Evaluation

A. Study of 100 adult and 100 pediatric patients' charts to be completed by September, 1981.

(Courtesy of Buske SM. St. Francis Hospital, Memphis, Tennessee.)

Chapter 15

The Special Patient

Kay E. Fraulini

Although the principles set forth in Chapter 9 apply to all postanesthetic patients, it becomes necessary to further elucidate certain physiologic changes that characterize "the special patient." Differences in physiology should be understood by the PACU nurse and should be appropriately worked into the nursing process and care plan. The patients described here have somewhat different needs, many times in relation to their response to anesthesia, in the postanesthesia period. Specific nursing care guidelines are not provided for each of these "special" situations, because the nurse should be able to extrapolate a plan from the physiologic data presented.

THE PEDIATRIC PATIENT

As compared with an adult, the child—especially the neonate—has unique anatomic, physiologic, and biochemical characteristics. Those people responsible for the postanesthetic care of infants and children should be familiar with these differences (Dripps & associates, 1982).

Respiratory System

The infant's upper airway is prone to obstruction because of small nares, a large tongue in relation to the size of the mandible, and abundant lymphoid tissue. The diameter of the trachea is quite small so that edema causes disproportionate narrowing of the airway.

Alveolar ventilation (V_A) of the newborn is proportionately about twice that of the adult. The high metabolic demand is met by increasing respiratory rate (f) rather than volume (Table 15–1). Dead space volume

TABLE 15–1. RESPIRATORY DATA IN THE ADULT AND NEONATE

	Adult	Neonate
Alveolar Ventilation		
V_A (ml/kg/min)	60	100–150
V_T (ml/kg)	7	6
V_D (ml/kg)	2.2	2.2
V_D/V_T	0.3	0.3
f (min)	20	40
Lung Volumes		
FRC (ml/kg)	34	30
RV (ml/kg)	17	20
FRC/TLC	0.40	0.48
RV/TLC	0.20	0.33
Respiratory Mechanics		
Total respiratory compliance	20	1
Specific respiratory compliance (compliance/L lung volume)	1	1
Total flow resistance	1	12
Specific resistance	1	1
Acid–Base Status		
$PaCO_2$ (torr)	38–40	32–35
Plasma HCO_3 (mEq/L)	24–28	17–22
pH	7.38	7.38
Alveolar–Arterial Oxygen Difference (AaD_{O2})		
Pa_{O2} (torr)	80–100	60–80
AaD_{O2} (torr)	10 (105–95)	25 (105–80)

(Courtesy of Nelson NM. Neonatal pulmonary function. Pediatric Clinics of North America 13:769, 1966.)

(V_D) is roughly the same in both the infant and adult per kilogram of body weight, and the ratio of dead space to tidal volume (V_D/V_T) remains constant (Table 15-1). However, during anesthesia it should be realized that the volume of dead space in anesthetic apparatus is more significant in the infant than in the adult owing to the smaller airway volumes of the infant.

Circulatory System
Normal neonatal systolic blood pressure is in the range of 60 to 80 torr, and pulse varies between 120 and 140 per minute. Systolic blood pressure normally rises to 100 torr and pulse rate falls to 100 per minute at about 6 years of age (Table 15–2). Accurate measurement of blood pressure in the infant and child is possible only if the proper equipment is used. Wide cuffs result in falsely low readings, whereas narrow cuffs give high values. The proper cuff covers approximately two thirds of the length of the upper arm. More sophisticated blood pressure monitoring equipment than the usual sphygmomanometer—such as the Doppler ultrasonic de-

TABLE 15–2. CARDIOVASCULAR DATA IN THE ADULT AND NEONATE

	Adult	Neonate
Stroke volume (ml)	70–80	4–5
Heart rate (min)	70	120
Cardiac output (ml/min)	4000–6000	500–600
Metabolic rate (cal/kg/hr)	1	2

Blood Pressure and Pulse		
Age	*Approximate Systolic BP (torr)*	*Approximate Pulse (rate/min)*
2 hr	60	120–160
6 days	80	120–160
6 mo	90	110–130
6 yr	100	100
10 yr	110	90
15 yr	120	80

Estimated Blood Volume	
Age	*ml/kg*
Newborn	85
Infant	80
Child	75
Adult	65

(Courtesy of Dripps, Eckenhoff, Van Dam. Introduction to Anesthesia (6th ed.). Philadelphia: Saunders, 1982.)

vice or the intraarterial catheter-transducer—is both useful and practical for complex operations in infants and children.

Heart rate is labile in infants and blood pressure is at times difficult to measure. Continuous monitoring of heart and respiratory sounds with a precordial or esophageal stethoscope is essential during pediatric anesthesia.

Temperature Control

The newborn has an incompletely developed thermoregulatory mechanism, causing it to be dependent upon the environment for maintenance of body temperature. Body surface area, especially in the premature infant, is relatively large. Neonates lack subcutaneous fat insulation, have poor peripheral vasomotor control, and inadequate sweating and shivering responses. Their main source of heat-producing energy is the brown fat (nonshivering thermogenesis) which is located largely between the shoulder blades, around the neck, and behind the sternum. Premature infants lack this brown fat.

Oxygen consumption is reduced if body temperature is kept relatively constant. Exposure of the neonate to a cold environment (< 27° C) leads to nonshivering thermogenesis, increases oxygen consumption, and induces metabolic acidosis. If body temperature falls, the cardiorespiratory system becomes depressed, especially when hypothermia occurs during anesthesia. Conservation of body heat through use of thermoregulatory blankets and other devices is important in the operative management of neonates.

Development of hyperthermia with a body temperature higher than 40° C is a dangerous complication during pediatric anesthesia. Predisposing factors are fever, dehydration, elevated ambient temperature, drugs that diminish sweating (such as atropine and scopolamine) or disturb temperature regulation (barbiturates, phenothiazines, and general anesthetics), and excessive surgical drapes. Fever increases oxygen consumption and CO_2 production, stimulates the cardiorespiratory system, and causes metabolic and respiratory acidosis. If uncorrected, convulsions, hypoxic brain damage, arterial hypotension, and cardiac arrest may occur.

Fluid Balance and Metabolism

Maintenance of fluid balance in infants and children is a special matter. The size of the body water compartments and the relative volume of circulating blood vary considerably from birth to adulthood. Renal immaturity and a high basal metabolic rate result in a greater turnover of body water and a higher daily fluid requirement in infants as compared with adults (Table 15–3). Losses of fluid are less well tolerated and result in rapid dehydration if not replaced. Investigation of operative fluid requirements in the newborn have shown that the neonatal kidney lacks the ability to retain sodium and water and that shifts of fluid and electrolytes during operation are similar to those seen in adults. The higher percentage of body mass in the form of water also necessitates a relatively higher dose of drugs—for example, succinylcholine and digoxin—per kg of body weight, owing to a larger distributional space.

Carbohydrate and fat rather than amino acids are the principal sources of metabolic fuel in the first days of life. It is therefore important to maintain glycogen stores and an adequate blood glucose level, by providing liberal quantities of glucose in intravenous fluids given during operation (10 percent glucose is recommended for premature infants).

In general, the capacity for metabolism of drugs in the neonatal period is less well established than in the infant and child. Furthermore, renal clearance rates for almost all drugs are decreased in the neonate, especially in the premature infant. Therefore, all drugs given the neonate should be administered with strict attention to dose and response (Table 15–4).

Fluid Administration

Maintenance of fluids during operation should consist of a dextrose-containing electrolyte solution. An example is 5 percent dextrose in Ringer's lactate solution (10 percent dextrose and Ringer's lactate in the neonate

TABLE 15–3. MAINTENANCE FLUIDS IN PEDIATRIC PATIENTS AND NORMAL URINE OUTPUT

Electrolytes	Daily Dose (mEq/kg)
Na	3
K	2
Cl	2

Body Weight and Age	24-Hour Fluid Requirement
Premature and full-term newborn less than 5 days old	50–70 ml/kg
Premature and full-term newborn 5 days to 1 month old	150 ml/kg
3–10 kg (over 1 month old)	100 ml/kg
10–20 kg	1000 ml + 50 ml/kg over 10 kg
20 kg to adult	1500 ml + 20 ml/kg over 20 kg

Normal Urine Output	
Age	ml/kg/hr
1–4 days	0.3–0.7
4–7 days	1.0–2.7
Over 7 days	3
Over 2 years	2
5 years to adult	1
Insensible loss	28

(Courtesy of Dripps, Eckenhoff, Van Dam. Introduction to Anesthesia (6th ed.). Philadelphia: Saunders, 1982.)

in view of the tendency toward hypoglycemia), infused at the rate of 5 to 10 ml per kg per hour, depending upon the extent of surgical dissection and estimated fluid loss from exposed viscera.

In general, blood loss should be replaced with whole blood if the loss is greater than 15 percent of the estimated blood volume (Table 15–2). Small losses are replaced with the dextrose and Ringer's solution mentioned above. Blood loss is estimated by weighing sponges and collecting suctioned blood into calibrated containers.

Nursing Care

Pang (1982) proposes that nurses must understand the pediatric patient—that is, that nurses should be pediatric nurses. They should feel comfortable dealing with infants and children and be able to recognize and immediately act upon changes in the patient's condition.

Upon admission to the PACU, oxygen should be administered to the patient. Since in response to tactile stimulation of the trigeminal area the infant usually thrashes about, oxygen can be administered by funnel

TABLE 15–4. DRUGS USEFUL IN PEDIATRIC ANESTHESIA

Drug	Dose	Remarks
Premedicants		
Atropine	0.03 mg/kg/IV or IM up to 0.6 mg	
Diazepam	0.2–0.5 mg/kg PO	
Droperidol	0.1 mg/kg/IM or IV	
Hydroxyzine	2–3 mg/kg PO	Give 45–60 min before
Morphine	0.05–0.15 mg/kg IM	procedure
Pentazocine	1–1.2 mg/kg IM	
Pentobarbital	2–3 mg/kg PO, PR, or IM	
Induction agents		
Ketamine	1–2 mg/kg IV; 5–10 mg/kg IM	
Thiopental	2–5 mg/kg IV; 20–25 mg/kg PR	2.5% solution
Methohexital	2 mg/kg IV; 15–20 mg/kg PR	10% solution
Maintenance agents		
Fentanyl	1–4 mcg/kg/hr	
Meperidine	1–1.5 mg/kg	Premedication dose
	0.5–1 mg/kg/hr	Maintenance dose
Morphine	0.05–0.2 mg/kg/hr	
Neuromuscular blockers		
Succinylcholine	2 mg/kg IV; 3–4 mg/kg IM	Newborn and infant dose
	1 mg/kg IV; 2 mg/kg IM	Child dose
D-tubocurarine	0.125–0.25 mg/kg IV initially, $\frac{1}{4}$ initial dose for maintenance	Newborn and infant dose
	0.5 mg/kg IV initially, then $\frac{1}{4}$ initial dose for maintenance	Child dose
Pancuronium	0.05–0.1 mg/kg IV initially, then $\frac{1}{4}$ initial dose for maintenance	Newborn and infant dose
	0.1 mg/kg IV initially, then $\frac{1}{4}$ initial dose for maintenance	Child dose
Metocurine	0.25 mg/kg initially, then $\frac{1}{4}$ initial dose for maintenance	
Reversal agents		
Neostigmine	0.07 mg/kg IV with atropine	Give slowly
	0.02 mg/kg IV	
Naloxone	0.005 mg/kg IM or IV	For longer lasting reversal give IM dose after IV dose
Resuscitation drugs		
NaHCO$_3$	2 mEq/kg IV, then guided by blood gases	
Calcium chloride	20 mg/kg IV slowly	10% solution
Epinephrine	0.1 ml/kg IV	1:10,000 solution
Lidocaine	1 mg (0.1 ml)/kg IV	1% solution
Atropine	0.1–0.6 mg IV	
Other drugs		
Digoxin	Premature—0.04 mg/kg PO	Oral, digitalizing dose
	Newborn—0.05 mg/kg PO	Oral, digitalizing dose
	Over 2 years—0.04 mg/kg PO	2/3 oral dose if IV, ½ of which is given initially, then $\frac{1}{4}$ dose q 6–12 h

TABLE 15–4. (*Continued*)

Drug	Dose	Remarks
Racemic epinephrine	0.25–0.5 ml in 5 ml saline	By aerosol or IPPB as needed for croup
Dexamethasone	4 mg IV	Under 2 years old
	8 mg IV	Over 2 years old
Furosemide	0.25–0.5 mg/kg IV	

(*Courtesy of Dripps, Eckenhoff, and Van Dam. Introduction to Anesthesia (6th ed.). Philadelphia: Saunders, 1982.*)

placed near the patient's nose and mouth. Vital signs—adequacy of the airway, respiratory rate, heart rate, blood pressure, and temperature—should be determined, and the color and the condition of the skin, the state of hydration, the infusion site, the drainage, and the condition of the wound and of the dressing should be assessed. The anesthesiologist should monitor the patient's airway until the nurse can devote full attention to the patient. An unreactive patient or a partially sedated patient should not be left unattended.

Assessment of Respiration

Infants are obligatory nose breathers. The tongue is almost always found to be pressed against the roof of the infant's mouth, entirely blocking any oral air exchange. Ventilation in these patients is considerably improved by the insertion of an oral airway. The oral airway should be removed as soon as laryngeal reflexes return to prevent spasm, gagging, coughing, or vomiting. In the older patient, airway obstruction may exist despite the presence of an oral airway.

Assessment of Vital Signs

Heart Rate. The average heart rate of infants and children is summarized in Table 15-2. It should be remembered that the heart rate can be influenced by atropine and by the anesthetic agents. Crying, struggling, and pain may also alter the rate.

Blood Pressure. As any PACU nurse knows, blood pressure may be one of the most difficult measurements to obtain in the pediatric patient. As previously mentioned, cuff width and length are important determinants of accuracy of blood pressure measurement. Furthermore, more reliable means of obtaining blood pressure (Doppler ultrasonic, electronic, and other devices) in infants are available.

Temperature. Rectal temperature should be obtained in all pediatric patients admitted to the PACU unless contraindicated. While the thermometer is in place, the patient should be continuously watched, since perforation of the rectum by the rigid instrument or breakage of the thermometer in the rectum are ever-present dangers. When measuring rectal temperature is contraindicated, axillary temperatures may be taken. "Normal" temperatures have been established at 99.8° F and 96.8° F rectally + 0.7° F for rectal and axillary temperatures, respectively. (MacBryde, 1957). If the patient's temperature is abnormal, attempts should be made to correct it.

There are, in general, three approaches that can be used when correcting temperature abnormalities: (1) external, (2) internal, and (3) metabolic. If the patient is only mildly hypothermic, the simpler external methods should be used. These include covering the body with warm blankets and covering the head with warm towels or a cap, using a warm water mattress, and using a radiant heat lamp. If the patient is moderately hypothermic, internal methods should be added. These methods are more limited in the postoperative period than in the intraoperative period, but can include the use of warmed parenteral fluid for intravenous infusions and ventilating the patient with warmed humidified gases. The third, metabolic, method should be used if more severe hypothermia exists, and includes the reduction of the respiratory rate.

In the hyperthermic patient, external approaches should include lowering the temperature of the room; uncovering the patient; giving tepid water baths; using a cooling mattress; and applying icebags to the head, neck, axilla, and groin. It should be remembered that direct cooling with the water mattress and icebags is uncomfortable in the conscious patient and may produce shivering. It should also be remembered that shivering increases oxygen consumption. The internal approach should include the use of cold intravenous fluids and the irrigation of the rectum with iced saline solutions. The metabolic approach should include the ventilation of the patient with unwarmed gases as well as the use of antipyretic agents such as acetaminophen and aspirin.

Emergence Delirium

In studies mainly of adult patients, belladonna alkaloids were associated with the appearance of delirium in about 20 percent of the patients (Greene, 1971). Physostigmine administered parenterally reverses the delirium induced by belladonna alkaloids. The recommended dose is twice the initial belladonna dose. Thus, a patient who has received 0.25 mg of atropine should receive 0.5 mg of physostigmine intravenously.

After the delirium is treated, the pain may be alleviated with small doses of narcotics. The preferred route of administration is the intravenous rather than the intramuscular one. This route (as described for the adult) provides for the rapid alleviation of pain by a painless technique, and allows assessment of the effect of the drug sooner than if it had been given intramuscularly.

Restraint of the Patient

In some patients, restraints are required after the emergence delirium has been treated and operative pain alleviated, to prevent self-inflicted injury or pulling on dressing, drain, or intravenous tubes. The object is to restrain without injury to the patient. When patients are too young to reason with but too active to be gently restrained, some units use padded cylinders that are long enough to cover the elbows and wide enough to fit comfortably around the arm. For smaller children, tongue depressors are taped together, while for larger children empty adhesive tape containers are used. These restraints are usually made by the nursing staff.

Postintubation Stridor

Postintubation stridor is characterized by hoarseness and by a hoarse cough. Conventional treatment has included the use of high-humidity mist therapy; oxygen enriched inspired air; corticosteroids; and if necessary, aerosolized epinepherine (Jordan & associates, 1970; Koka, 1977). The value of each of these modalities has not been clearly established.

Fluid and Electrolyte Balance

Table 15–5 summarizes the components of maintenance requirements. In the absence of sweating, insensible water loss and urine are the only significant components. These amount to about 100 ml per 100 cal expended. The item labelled as "hidden" intake is usually of no great consequence and occurs as the result of oxidation of carbohydrates and fatty acids. It becomes important, however, in cases of severe, sustained oliguria.

The usual electrolyte requirements have been derived by examining the usual oral intake, and have been determined to be approximately 2.5 mEq per 100 cal expended, of each sodium and potassium.

Hence, the usual maintenance requirements for water, electrolytes, and glucose are summarized as follows:

$$\text{Water} = 100 \text{ ml per } 100 \text{ cal}$$

$$\text{Sodium} = 2.5 \text{ mEq per } 100 \text{ cal}$$

$$\text{Potassium} = 2.5 \text{ mEq per } 100 \text{ cal}$$

$$\text{Chloride} = 5.0 \text{ mEq per } 100 \text{ cal}$$

$$\text{Glucose} = 5 \text{ gm per } 100 \text{ cal}$$

Preoperative Orientation and Parents in the PACU

Many postanesthesia nurses have developed innovative programs which include, for example, making preoperative visits to patients above the age of 2 years. If old enough, the patient along with his or her parents may be given a tour of the PACU and have an opportunity to become acquainted with the nursing routine and equipment. Although a specific preoperative

TABLE 15–5. COMPONENTS OF NORMAL MAINTENANCE WATER REQUIREMENTS.

Component	Water Required (ml/100 cal)
Output	
Insensible water loss	45
Sweat	0–25
Urine	50–75
Stool water	5–10
"Hidden" intake	12

(Modified from Winter RW (Ed.). The Body Fluids in Pediatrics. Boston: Little, Brown, 1973.)

program will not be detailed here, it is the goal of all such programs to alleviate some of the parental anxieties as well as some of the patient's problems associated with awakening in a strange environment and seeing strange faces.

Great advances have been made in hospital–parent–child relationships in recent years. However, there is still disagreement about whether all parents should be allowed free admission to the PACU. There is concern that the presence of even one parent in the PACU can produce physical and emotional interference with essential patient care. Until we have more definitive evidence from scientific studies of therapeutic benefits to the patient from the parent's presence in the PACU, it must be left to the individual hospital to establish visiting protocols.

THE PATIENT IN RENAL FAILURE

Excretion of anesthetic drugs and their metabolites by the kidney and its role in acid–base and water metabolism are essential considerations in anesthetic management and postanesthetic care. In a patient with minimal renal reserves, compounds excreted by the kidneys—the long-acting barbiturates, gallamine (Flaxedil), and succinylcholine given by constant infusion—are best avoided. Problems have been encountered in the reversal of the actions of pancuronium (Pavulon) in the presence of renal failure. Before the era of hemodialysis, which maintains the patient with renal failure in a reasonable state of biochemical balance, such patients presented a formidable array of problems: high serum potassium levels, low sodium and calcium, metabolic acidosis, and increased susceptibility to infection. Drugs used to treat these conditions added to the problems of anesthesia—antihypertensive medications, digitalis, antibiotics, and cortisone. In preparation for nephrectomy or renal transplantation, chronic dialysis returns physiologic and biochemical abnormalities toward normal values, and the risks of anesthesia and operation are consequently lessened.

But optimal conditions must be attained before operation. Starting with a borderline high serum potassium level, from 5.5 to 6.0 mEqL, several events during anesthesia may elevate potassium levels to the point of cardiac standstill or ventricular fibrillation: use of succinylcholine with attendant release of potassium; transfusion of large volumes of cold bank blood of low pH and high serum potassium; and use of sympathomimetic drugs. Hypoxia, hypercarbia, and low flow states also add to the K+ load. Low flow states with concomitant blood transfusion or release of myoglobin from traumatized tissues and the use of sympathomimetic drugs that cause renal vasoconstriction predispose to postoperative acute tubular necrosis or vasoconstrictive nephropathy (Dripps & associates, 1982).

In addition to being aware of the above physiologic abnormalities as they relate to anesthesia, the nurse must have some technical know-how related to hemodialysis, as explained in the subsequent sections.

The Shunt or A-V Fistula

Creation of an internal arteriovenous fistula, the most generally used type of bloodstream access today, is a surgical procedure in which an artery in the arm is anastomosed to a vein in a sideways or end-to-end fashion (Fig. 15–1). This creates an opening or fistula between a large artery and a large vein. The leaking of arterial blood into the venous system causes the veins to become engorged. This process takes at least 1 to 2 weeks and sometimes as long as 12 weeks to develop enough for the site to be used, making this approach inappropriate for immediate use. Peritoneal dialysis and external arteriovenous shunts may be used while the fistula is forming. Once the fistula is developed, the large veins may be punctured, using 14- or 16-gauge needles (for dialysis).

Care of the shunt site is designed to prevent clotting and infection. The shunt is usually filled with undiluted heparin. The skin at the puncture site is cleaned daily with an antiseptic solution. An antimicrobial ointment may be applied, followed by a dressing.

The site must be protected from trauma. Blood pressure readings

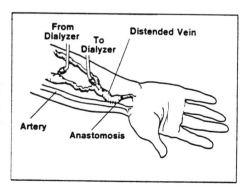

Figure 15–1. Arteriovenous fistula. (Courtesy of Welchel JD. Renal failure patients in the recovery room. Current Review for Recovery Room Nurses 2:12, 1980.)

should not be taken, nor blood specimens drawn, from the arm with the cannula. Between dialysis periods, the skin over an internal arteriovenous fistula requires only routine care with soap and water.

A good rule of thumb in all dialysis patients is to avoid any unnecessary manipulation or instrumentation of the extremity where vascular access is located (Table 15-6).

Fluids and Electrolytes

The lack of renal function in renal failure patients may severely limit the volume and type of fluid that can be safely given during and following surgery. Blood and fluid losses and administration must be monitored closely. Excessive volume replacement can produce severe hypertension, pulmonary edema, and congestive heart failure. Such stress in the presence of an already limited cardiac reserve could be catastrophic. However, inadequate volume replacement may lead to poorly tolerated hypertension. Monitoring of central venous and arterial pulse pressure, especially during and after major operative procedures, is an extremely useful guide to adequate volume management.

Maintenance fluid volume in renal failure patients varies from 1200 to 1500 cc per day. This total must include all parenteral and oral fluids received by the patient. Administration of medicines should be planned to provide for fluid conservation, because little may be left to keep intravenous lines open or for oral consumption. Except in certain situations, such as replacement of gastric drainage, saline and Ringer's solution should not be used as maintenance fluid. These fluids supply excessive sodium to the renal failure patient. The accumulation of sodium may lead to significant volume overload. One half normal saline is an excellent maintenance intravenous fluid.

The advent of routine hemodialysis has decreased but not eliminated electrolyte abnormalities. Electrolyte disturbances such as hyperkalemia remain potential hazards. Hyperkalemia can develop rapidly in the postoperative period, especially if potassium is administered with intravenous fluid replacement. Oral intake of postoperative fluids or foods with high potassium content can also contribute to hyperkalemia. As a routine precaution, serum potassium levels should be determined shortly after the patient's arrival in the PACU. Personnel managing these patients should

TABLE 15–6. MANAGEMENT OF VASCULAR ACCESS IN PACU

Do Not	Do
Apply tourniquet or cuffs	Clean daily
Obtain blood sample through	Apply protective bandage
Administer fluids or medicine through	Observe for function

(Courtesy of Whelchel JD. Renal failure patients in the recovery room. Current Review for Recovery Room Nurses 2:12, 1980.)

be familiar with the various electrocardiographic changes associated with hyperkalemia, such as peaked T waves. These changes may precede serious arrhythmias that eventually lead to cardiac arrest. The presence of serum potassium levels of 6 mEqL or greater is a medical emergency (Whelchel, 1980).

THE GERIATRIC PATIENT

The physiologic changes of aging must be considered relative to anesthetic and postanesthetic management.

Decreased Basal Metabolic Rate
Basal metabolic rate declines approximately 1 percent per year beyond age 30. Therefore, anesthetic agents will be metabolized and excreted much more slowly in elderly patients compared to younger patients. In addition, since the metabolic rate is lower in elderly patients, the requirement for anesthetic agents in this age group will likely be less.

Decreased Central Nervous System Function
Like basal metabolic rate, the function of most organs—and most importantly, that of the central nervous system (CNS)—declines during the aging process. Dementia that occurs with aging may be due to localized areas of microemboli or, more commonly, to a gradual process of decreased cerebral blood flow and decreased CNS activity (Alzheimer's disease). This very gradual process may not be distinguishable in a given patient, but the likelihood is that geriatric patients in general will have reduced requirements for anesthesia due to a gradual reduction in CNS activity. The MAC requirements for most inhalational agents gradually reduce as patients become older. This same principle is also seen with regional anesthesia, where smaller doses of local anesthetics are required to produce the same level of epidural or spinal anesthesia.

Decreased Airway Reflexes
Laryngeal, pharyngeal, and other airway reflexes are less effective in older individuals. This requires special awareness of a decreased ability to prevent pulmonary aspiration of foreign material.

Decreased Serum Protein
Protein binding is a primary determinant of the effectiveness of intravenous anesthetic agents and narcotics. Portions of administered drugs that are protein-bound remain in plasma and are ineffective in producing an effect. The unbound portions, however, are able to cross membranes into the CNS to produce an effect. As individuals age, the circulating level of serum protein, especially albumin, and the binding effectiveness of circu-

lating protein are reduced. Thus, a greater percentage of drugs is present in the geriatric patient in an unbound or effective state, and as a result, a reduced dose of intravenous anesthetic agents should be administered.

Increased Percentage of Body Fat

As individuals reach the age of 60, lean body mass (muscle) is reduced approximately 10 percent from age 20 levels. During the same time period there is also an approximate 10 percent increase in percentage body weight that is fat. Due to their high lipid solubility, anesthetic agents will be stored in the adipose tissue. Since elderly individuals have a greater percentage of body fat compared to younger patients, for the same administered dose of an anesthetic agent a greater amount of drug will be sequestered. This has the effect of delaying emergence from anesthesia since there is a protracted efflux of these agents from the lipid storage sites into the circulating plasma.

Decreased Cardiovascular Reserve

The cardiovascular changes with aging are perhaps of more importance in the perianesthetic period than any of the other age-related physiologic changes.

Cardiac index is reduced approximately 1 percent per year after age 30 (Fig. 15–2). This results in delayed induction following administration of intravenous anesthetic agents. For example, a test dose of thiopental

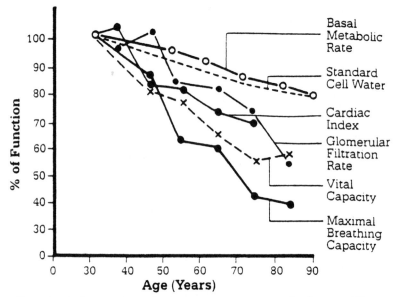

Figure 15–2. A comparison of pulmonary compartments and volumes at different ages.

may not demonstrate any effect in an elderly patient during the time frame when one expects to see a slight decrease in blood pressure or an increase in sedation in a younger patient. If adequate time is not allowed in the elderly group to permit the delayed delivery of intravenous agents to the brain and other target organs, then one may inadvertently give a repeat dose that is too large, thinking that the initial dose had no effect. On the other hand, with slower circulation times we can expect a faster onset of inhalational anesthesia. Since cardiac output is reduced, the uptake of inhalational anesthetic agents from the alveoli will also be reduced. This allows for a more rapid achievement of a high partial pressure in the alveoli, which is reflected as a high partial pressure in the blood and, in turn, in the brain—the parameter responsible for anesthetic effects.

Resting *stroke volume* remains relatively unaffected by the aging process; however, the normal response to stress may be impaired. Similarly, the maximum heart rate that may be generated by an elderly patient is considerably less than that of a younger patient. As a result, following administration of atropine or other anticholinergic drugs the resultant tachycardia will be much less in geriatric patients.

During the aging process, elastic tissue in the pulmonary perenchyma, skin, and other organs is replaced by less resilient fibrous connective tissue. *Total peripheral resistance* is increased as the rigidity of the vasculature increases and elasticity of the vasculature decreases, which explains the greater frequency of hypertension and hypertensive cardiovascular disease in geriatric patients.

Decreased Pulmonary Reserve

Pulmonary changes that occur during aging affect both the musculoskeletal supporting structure of the lung as well as the parenchyma of the lung itself. The chest becomes more kyphotic with gradual compression of the intervertebral discs. Arthritic changes occur in the ribs and costochondral junctions that reduce total lung capacity. Muscle wasting reduces the effectiveness of the diaphragm and intercostal muscles. As a result, maximum breathing capacity (Fig. 15–2), total lung capacity, and vital capacity all decline with aging (Fig. 15–3).

The age-induced parenchymal changes of the lung mimic those of emphysema. Because pulmonary reserve is reduced in the elderly patient, it is more likely that postoperative ventilation may be required. These patients may be less able to cough and clear their secretions and may require additional pulmonary toilet postoperatively.

Decreased Hepatic and Renal Function

Like most other body functions, hepatic and renal function are reduced about 1 percent per year above age 30. Most administered anesthetic agents are highly lipid soluble. These lipid-soluble drugs filtered by the glomeruli are very readily reabsorbed by renal tubules and therefore are

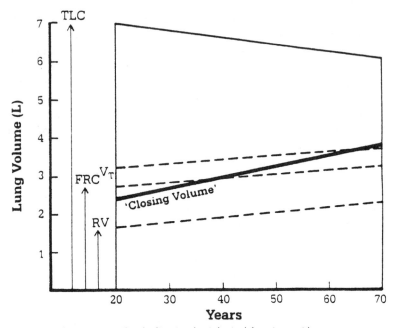

Figure 15–3. The decline in physiological functions with age.

not excreted. It is the function of the liver to convert lipid-soluble drugs by glucuronidation or other metabolic processes into water-soluble metabolites, which after filtration by the glomeruli are reabsorbed less readily by the renal tubules and excreted. During the aging process the ability of individuals to both metabolize and excrete anesthetic drugs is impaired. For example, the elimination half-life ($T_{\frac{1}{2}}$-B) of fentanyl is 265 minutes in young patients compared to 945 minutes in older patients. The reduced clearance of drugs in the aged patient also affects muscle relaxants, which suggests that muscle relaxants should be administered at less frequent intervals than in younger patients.

Choice of Anesthesia with Special Attention to Respiratory and Cardiovascular Status

The choice of anesthetic technique is clearly less important than maintenance of stable intraoperative vital signs and adequate oxygenation. Several factors, however, are worthy of review. The superiority of regional over general anesthesia in pulmonary patients is not as clear as many consultants would have us believe. There is evidence that regional anesthesia has fewer pulmonary complications in peripheral surgical procedures. However, when abdominal surgery requires a higher level of nerve block such that the abdominal musculature is paralyzed, spinal anesthesia has no advantage over general anesthesia (Tisi, 1979). Regional anesthesia for intraperitoneal surgery causes a decrease in total lung capacity (TLC), inspiratory reserve volume (IRV), and expiratory reserve volume (ERV) so that effective cough is not possible until the muscle tone returns. Rehder and associates (1975) reviewed the changes of the lung during general anesthesia. They found changes in lung volumes, ventilation perfusion (V/Q) relationships, and surfactant. In addition, general anesthesia decreases compliance of the entire respiratory system. There is decreased tone of diaphragm and intercostal muscles so that functional residual capacity (FRC) diminishes. Closing volumes tend to increase along with the decrease in FRC; therefore, airway closure takes place during tidal breathing. These changes are accentuated in the elderly patient who has decreased muscle mass and pulmonary reserves in the awake state. Hence, both regional and general anesthesia may adversely affect the patient's pulmonary status.

Another important factor that may influence the choice of specific agents may be the impact of concomittant drug therapy. Table 15–7 presents a list of drug interactions that may adversely affect the respiratory system in the perioperative period.

Likewise, the general consensus is that the particular technique (regional versus general) does not correlate with cardiac risk. Technical expertise of anesthetic administration and maintenance of stable CV parameters intraoperatively appear to be more important.

Postoperative Management

The time of emergence from general anesthesia and the immediate postoperative period are extremely strenuous and labile periods for the aged patient. There is pain, shivering, fluid shifts, and impaired oxygen exchange to upset the oxygen balance and to precipitate cardiac decompen-

TABLE 15–7. RESPIRATORY SYSTEM EFFECTS OF CONCOMITTANT DRUG THERAPY

Respiratory System Effect	Drug or Drug Interaction
Increased narcotic respiratory depression	MAOI, tricyclic antidepressants, phenothiazines, local anesthetic and inhalational agents, minor sedatives
Increased barbiturate sleep time and apnea	Phenothiazines, tricyclic antidepressants, MAOI, lithium narcotic and inhalational agents
Muscle stiffness	MAOI, anti-Parkinson agents, fentanyl
Prolonged neuromuscular blockage Nondepolarizing	Diuretics, lithium, antibiotics (mycins, Polymixin A and B, tetracycline) local anesthetic and inhalational agents
Depolarizers Lower pseudocholinesterase activity	Echothiophate, Hexafluorenium, phenelzine (MAOI), cytotoxic agents (nitrogen mustards and cyclophosphamide)

(Courtesy of Kuechel, SW. Anesthesia and the Geriatric Patient. New York: Grune & Stratton, 1983.)

sation. In addition, the administration of neuromuscular block-reversing drugs can cause dysrhythmias in patients with borderline conduction disturbances. Pain control and extubation may help prevent the tachycardia and hypertension common in the early postoperative period. Fluid administration must be adjusted to continued third-space displacement, blood loss, and urine output.

Hypotension. The occurrence of hypotension in the early postoperative period is most often the result of inadequate effective circulating volume, and its occurrence should stimulate a review of intraoperative fluid balance while a crystalloid fluid bolus is being administered. Severe hypotension warrants the use of vasopressors while the cause is being determined and treated. Additional causes of hypotension, not uncommon among the elderly, are congestive heart failure, dysrhythmias, myocardial ischemia, massive pulmonary embolism, adrenal insufficiency, myxedema, and uncontrolled diabetes. If there is no response to fluid administration or a prolonged need for large amounts of fluids or vasopressors, a PA catheter is indicated.

Hypertension. Hypertension results in an elevation of myocardial oxygen demand while decreasing the subendocardial blood flow. This may overextend the reserves of the elderly patient for myocardial oxygen supply. Pain and anxiety are likely causes of hypertension; however, before starting treatment, one must rule out hypoxemia and hypercarbia. Congestive heart failure can also present primarily as hypertension, as can myocardial infarction. Treatment should be specific if possible: pain control, supplemental oxygen, or assisted ventilation. Vasodilators will give symptomatic relief and should be used when specific therapy is slowly decreasing afterload. Detection of ischemia on an ECG is an indication for intravenous nitroglycerin to control blood pressure and ischemic changes.

Heart Failure. Postoperative congestive heart failure carries a 15 to 20 percent incidence of mortality in patients with no known heart disease and is fatal in 80 percent of patients with heart disease (Cooperman & Price, 1970). Patients suffering from chronic obstructive pulmonary disease and those with intrathoracic major vascular and upper abdominal surgery have an increased incidence of postoperative cardiac failure. In the elderly patient with limited cardiac output, congestive heart failure can be precipitated by the afterload increase of anxiety and pain, anesthetic agents, hypoxia, myocardial infarctions, pulmonary embolism, or excessive intravascular volume. Tachydysrhythmia may also result in congestive failure, especially in patients with severe coronary artery or valvular disease.

The treatment of congestive heart failure involves efforts to increase contractility while decreasing fluid excess. Combinations of diuretics, inotropes, and vasodilators are useful in these patients. Pulmonary-artery catheters may be invaluable in guiding therapy.

Dysrhythmias. Dysrhythmias are frequently encountered in the elderly postoperative patient. In addition to age, the factors that increase the incidence of postoperative rhythm disturbances include congestive heart failure; chronic lung disease; and thoracic, major vascular, and upper abdominal surgery. Tachydysrhythmias associated with severe hypotension warrant immediate cardioversion or defibrillation. Calcium channel blockers such as verapamil may be useful in treating some of these dysrhythmias (such as paroxysmal supraventricular tachycardia). Ventricular ectopic activity is probably the most common dysrhythmia seen in the elderly. This is at least in part due to the increased incidence of coronary artery disease in this population. The elderly are particularly susceptible to PVCs because of hypoxia and electrolyte disturbances frequently encountered during this period—for example, the hypokalemia associated with alkalosis secondary to overzealous controlled ventilation, particularly in those patients taking digitalis preparations.

This tendency toward dysrhythmias is only enhanced by drugs given perioperatively that increase sympathetic activity or sensitize the myocardium to catecholamines—digitalis, methylxanthines, levodopa, vasopressors, and psychotropic drugs. The treatment of choice for the suppression of PVCs in the elderly is a bolus of lidocaine followed by a constant infusion. One must be exceedingly cautious, however, when using lidocaine in the postoperative period, since the drug has anesthetic properties, can depress the myocardium, and may intensify residual neuromuscular blockade. In the elderly it is also wise to reduce the total dose because liver blood flow is significantly reduced. It may be inferred that the clearance of lidocaine will be impaired.

THE PATIENT REQUIRING ISOLATION

Since a common recommendation is that no surgery except emergency or essential surgery, such as abscess drainage, be done in patients with infectious disease, and also since it is becoming more evident that renal insufficiency can be caused by antimicrobial agents (Appel, 1977), assessment of renal function and the organ damage present from renal insufficiency should be assessed by the anesthesiologist preoperatively in the patient with infectious disease. Prophylactic antibiotics are used to prevent bloodstream seeding and sepsis from predictable bacteremic interventions. The degree of impairment of the infected organ and its effect on anesthesia should be assessed by the anesthesiologist and reported to the PACU nurse as appropriate. For instance, endocarditis merits examination of volume status; drug therapy and side effects; myocardial function; and renal, lung, neurologic, and hepatic function—those organ systems that endocarditis can affect (Roizen, 1981). With this information the nurse can do the kind of planning that may be necessary to avoid catastrophe.

Nursing Responsibilities

This patient population has long presented numerous problems in the perioperative period. Several recommendations can be made, and these should be developed into standards of care for the infected patient requiring isolation.

1. There should be specific epidemiologic guidelines as to the type of isolation required. The PACU should have more stringent guidelines for the isolation of infected cases because of the open environment and the relative host vulnerability of surgical patients.
2. In the new or renovated PACU a separate room must be constructed for the physical isolation of these patients.
3. Detailed communication from the operating room, surgeon, and anesthesiologist to the PACU is essential if target patients are to be identified and properly isolated.
4. The PACU staff must develop intelligent policies and procedures relative to the infected patient, which must be adhered to with a minimum of conflict.
5. If it is possible to anticipate these patients, nurse staffing must be provided by assignment. The entire staff should be trained in handling infectious diseases and should develop an understanding of the often critical nature of the situation that requires patient isolation (for example, multiple IV antibiotic therapy was found to be a predictor of postoperative morbidity) (Vaughan, 1982).
6. The nurse in isolation needs support from peers concerning such matters as supplies, disbursement of specimens, and communicating with physicians.

Experience has taught us that to be nonchalant about the infected patient is a mistake. These patients, especially the septic patient, are prime candidates for physiologic crises that are often precipitous in nature. The PACU nurse should therefore be prepared for the challenge of using all of her or his assessment skills and be ready to intervene quickly.

THE OBSTETRIC PATIENT

Dripps and associates (1982) remind us that anesthetic care for mothers having vaginal delivery or cesarean section entails many considerations not pertinent to surgical patients. Essentially all anesthetics given the parturient cross the placenta to affect the fetus: opioids, sedatives, tranquilizers, local and inhalation anesthetics, and to some extent neuromuscular blockers.

Unlike the usual surgical patient who comes prepared for anesthesia, the obstetric patient is rarely in optimal condition at the time. She must be suspected of having a full stomach, therefore being prone to aspiration of gastric contents, a leading cause of maternal anesthetic mortality. During labor, emergencies such as fetal distress, maternal hemorrhage, prolapsed cord, and uterine tetany demand immediate anesthesia if both mother and baby are to survive. Vaginal delivery requires the parturient to be awake and cooperative most of the time to assist the forces of labor. Common medical disorders such as diabetes mellitus, heart disease, and endocrine imbalance are aggravated by pregnancy. Others may be associated with the gravid state, such as preeclampsia/eclampsia and coagulation disorders occurring with abruptio placentae, intrauterine fetal death, and amniotic fluid embolism. For the most part, the timing of delivery is not controlled; anesthesia must be readily available at all times.

Physiologic Changes of Pregnancy and Anesthetic Implications

Respiratory Changes. Physiologic changes of pregnancy carry profound anesthetic implications. A generalized edema of the upper airway develops (thought to be a result of increased circulating levels of progesterone); thus airway obstruction is more likely to occur and the risk of trauma associated with airway insertion and laryngoscopy is increased.

The following is a summary of changes in lung function during pregnancy. Although vital capacity is unchanged, total lung volume is decreased by approximately 5 percent owing to elevation of the diaphragm. At term, alveolar ventilation is increased by approximately 40 percent, primarily a result of an increase in tidal volume. These alterations cause a 15 percent reduction in functional residual capacity, which enhances uptake of anesthetic gases. During labor without adequate pain relief, alveolar ventilation may approach three times normal, further increasing anesthetic uptake. Hyperventilation results in respiratory alkalosis, usually compensated by metabolic acidosis secondary to renal excretion of bicarbonate. At term, both basal metabolic rate and the quantity of oxygen required for physical exercise are increased by 15 percent. These alterations, combined with a decrease in functional residual capacity, increase the likelihood of maternal hypoxia. Apprehension, increased oxygen consumption, and the demands of labor are associated with maternal metabolic and lactic acidosis.

Circulatory Changes. The total blood volume at term is increased by 30 percent, an additional 1200 to 1500 ml. A larger increase in plasma volume occurs and results in a decreased hematocrit, thus explaining the relative anemia of pregnancy despite an increased red blood cell volume.

With proper dietary intake, including vitamin and iron supplementation, hematocrit rarely falls below 35 percent. About 800 ml of the increased blood volume is contained in the gravid uterus and is expressed into the peripheral circulation when the uterus contracts at delivery. Simultaneously, vascular capacity is decreased by an equal amount. This permits the healthy parturient to sustain a blood loss approaching 1500 ml without apparent difficulty. As the average blood loss in vaginal delivery and cesarean section seldom exceeds 500 and 1000 ml, respectively, transfusion with blood or colloid is rarely necessary.

Measured in the lateral decubitus position, maternal cardiac output is elevated to near maximum toward the end of the first trimester, remains elevated by about 35 percent throughout pregnancy, and does not return to normal until 2 weeks after delivery. Although blood pressure is not thereby increased, heart rate is elevated by approximately 10 to 15 beats per minute. During uterine contractions, cardiac output and blood pressure both increase; blood pressure measurement is thus accurate only in the interval between contractions. Elevation of the diaphragm causes the heart to appear enlarged on both physical examination and chest x-ray. Benign systolic heart murmurs and left axis shift may appear as pregnancy progresses.

Central Nervous System Changes. Because intraabdominal pressure increases, peridural veins become engorged and the volume of both the epidural space and the cerebrospinal fluid contained within the subarachnoid space decreases. Therefore, less local anesthetic is required for subarachnoid and epidural anesthesia. In addition, although pregnancy per se does not increase cerebrospinal fluid (CSF) pressure, painful uterine contractions and valsalva maneuvers can increase CSF pressure and markedly increase the height of an anesthetic block if local anesthetic is injected into the subarachnoid space during a contraction. The anesthetic requirement for inhaled agents is also decreased up to 40 percent during pregnancy. The central nervous system mechanism for this decrease is not completely understood but may rely on the sedative effects of increased levels of progesterone (Shnider & Levinson, 1981).

Anesthesia for Vaginal Delivery

A list of the various anesthesia techniques is presented here. Chapter 6 provides more description. The reader is also referred to obstetric anesthesia texts.

The systemic drugs administered during labor may be classified into three broad groups. Sedative tranquilizers are generally used, either alone or in combination with a narcotic, during the first stage of labor. Narcotics are used to relieve pain during the first and second stages of labor. Dissociative or amnesia-producing drugs, such as ketamine or scopolamine, are used infrequently.

Inhalational analgesia is the administration of subanesthetic concentrations of inhaled agents, either alone or as a supplement to regional or local anesthesia to provide relief of pain for the first and second stages of labor.

Regional blocks for labor and vaginal delivery are the most commonly used techniques for analgesia. Regional blocks provide pain relief while allowing the parturient to be awake and able to participate in labor and delivery. Compared with parenteral or inhalational anesthesia techniques, regional anesthesia is less likely to produce drug-induced depression in the fetus or aspiration pneumonitis in the mother. The most common forms of regional anesthesia are spinal, lumbar epidural, caudal, paracervical, pudendal, and local perineal infiltration. Each technique has a specific application and can be used to block some or all of the nerves carrying the pain impulses.

The most significant complications of regional anesthesia are severe hypotension, convulsions induced by local anesthetics, total spinal anesthesia with the resulting respiratory arrest, vasopressor-induced hypertension nerve injury, and headache secondary to dural puncture.

General anesthetic technique used for vaginal delivery is similar to that used for cesarean section. Currently Halothane and enflurane are the most popular agents for providing uterine relaxation, if necessary.

The choice of regional or general anesthesia for cesarean section depends on the reason for the operation, the degree of urgency, the desires of the patient, and the skills of the anesthesiologist.

Complicated Obstetrics
Of particular interest to the PACU nurse is the patient with obstetric complications because it is she who most often comes to the surgical PACU.

Pregnancy-Induced Hypertension. Preeclampsia and eclampsia, often referred to as toxemia of pregnancy as well as pregnancy-induced-hypertension (PIH), are among the leading causes of maternal morbidity and mortality. Preeclampsia becomes apparent after the 24th week of gestation, usually abates within 48 hours of delivery, and is characterized by the triad of maternal hypertension, proteinuria, and generalized edema. With the occurrence of grand mal convulsion, the condition is known as eclampsia, and the prognosis for both mother and fetus worsens. The cause of preeclampsia is thought to be related to a decreased placental perfusion that results in increased production of renin, angiotensin, aldosterone, and thromboplastin, and in decreased production of prostaglandin (Speroff, 1973). Immunologic factors may also be involved.

Recently investigators at Loyola University of Chicago have performed experiments that show the syndrome is associated with a microscopic organism previously unknown. The researchers have named the newly discovered wormlike organism Hydataxi Lualba. Their experiments showed the possible cause and effect relationship between the organism and the disease, as well as the fact that the organism produces disease only in the context of pregnancy. It is believed that the discovery of the organism and its association with toxemia of pregnancy is the first step in finding a cure (Lueck & associates, 1983).

The pathophysiologic changes in preeclampsia involve nearly every major organ system. There is a generalized vasoconstriction and, despite retention of sodium and water and generalized edema, the intravascular volume is usually decreased. Glomerular filtration rate, renal blood flow, renal function, and urinary output may be reduced. Fibirin deposits are present within the glomeruli and most of the small blood vessels of the body. Significant coagulopathies may occur, especially in the severely preeclamptic or eclamptic patient. Hyperreflexia and hyperexcitability of the central nervous system occur. Uteroplacental perfusion is decreased, and fetal distress is common.

Patients are usually treated with magnesium sulfate and, if necessary, drugs counteracting hypertension. Magnesium sulfate, which is used primarily to prevent convulsions, is a central nervous system depressant that also reduces hyperreflexia (Aldrete, 1974). At the neuromuscular junction, magnesium sulfate decreases the amount of acetylcholine liberated, diminishes the sensitivity of the endplate to acetylcholine, and depresses the excitability of the muscle membrane (Foldes, 1959). Thus, it increases the sensitivity of the mother to both the depolarizing and nondepolarizing skeletal muscle relaxants (Gieseche & associates, 1968; Ghoneim & Long, 1970). Therapeutic maternal blood levels of magnesium sulfate are approximately 4 to 6 mEqL (Table 15–8). Magnesium crosses the placenta and often causes the newborn to be hypotonic. High levels of magnesium in the newborn may produce respiratory depression and apnea. Intravenous administration of calcium may partially offset the neuromuscular blocking properties of magnesium in both mother and newborn.

The use of epidural, caudal, or spinal analgesia in the patient with

TABLE 15–8. EFFECTS OF INCREASING PLASMA MAGNESIUM LEVELS

Observed Condition	mEq/L
Normal plasma level	1.5–2.0
Therapeutic range	4.0–6.0
ECG changes	5.0–10
(P–Q interval prolonged, QRS complex widens)	
Loss of deep tendon reflexes	10
Sinoatrial and atrioventricular block	15
Respiratory paralysis	15
Cardiac arrest	25

(Courtesy of Shnider S & Levinson G. Obstetric anesthesia. In RD Miller (Ed.), Anesthesia (vol. 2). New York: Churchill-Livingstone, 1981.)

preeclampsia or eclampsia is controversial. Ideally, for patients with severe preeclampsia who are receiving epidural anesthesia, a central venous or pulmonary artery catheter should be placed (Strauss & associates, 1980). Before receiving the block, such patients should be hydrated with a balanced salt solution and/or plasmanate until central venous pressure is 6 to 8 cm water or until pulmonary capillary wedge pressure is 5 to 12 torr. Usually this can be accomplished with 250 ml of plasma protein fraction and 250 ml of Ringer's lactate solution. Coagulation studies should be performed before the block is given.

Emergency cesarean section may be required when the fetus is in distress. General anesthesia is indicated because of the rapidity of its effectiveness and because it minimizes the incidence of maternal hypotension. In obstetrics, the standard technique for general anesthesia is usually modified to avoid prolonged paralysis due to the interaction of magnesium with muscle relaxants, to permit the easier control of hypertension, and to avoid the use of potentially nephrotoxic or hypertensive agents. Thus, a nondepolarizing agent is not administered prior to succinylcholine. If muscle relaxants are given, their doses should be carefully titrated and their effect monitored using a nerve-muscle stimulator; low dose Halothane can be added to the nitrous oxide, and drugs such as methoxyflurane and ketamine should be avoided. If severe hypertension occurs, an intravenous antihypertensive agent such as nitroprusside (Strauss & associates, 1980), nitroglycerin (Snyder & associates, 1979), or trimethaphan can be used for short-term control of blood pressure (Shnider & Levinson, 1981).

PACU Care

In addition to the usual concerns about postanesthetic recovery care are the concerns about postpartum care. The following is a brief overview of postpartum care in the PACU.

Every 15 minutes for the first hour, the nurse should check:

- *Vital Signs.* Blood pressure should stay normal; elevation may be sign of hemorrhage. Pulse may be slow; rapid pulse may be sign of hemorrhage. Temperature is taken before transfer to postpartum room.
- *Fundus.* Tone should be firm. Boggy uterus should be massaged until firm to prevent hemorrhage. Height should be at or about one finger above or below umbilicus.
- *Lochia.* Should be moderate, and occasionally will be scant. If scant, make sure it is not collecting inside uterus; if heavy, find out cause and treat.
- *Perineum.* Unusual swelling and discoloration may be symptoms of hematoma.
- *Warmth.* Warm blanket and warm room are helpful to combat chilly feeling.

- *Bladder.* Prevent distention. A full bladder can cause bleeding by preventing the uterus from contracting; it will displace uterus upward and to the side.
- *Cleanliness.* Give perineal care and change pad as needed.

Luczun (1984) further elaborates on patient care after cesarean section. Contraction of the uterus is essential to prevent excessive blood loss or hemorrhage. After the routine PACU admission process has been completed, the fundus should be palpated (usually at the level of the umbilicus). The fundus should feel hard and firm. A uterus that cannot be felt should be massaged, a technique that facilitates the passage of blood and sometimes clots. Massaging the fundus generally restores its firm consistency, but frequent observation is necessary to ensure adequate contraction. Fluids given in an IV infusion contain oxytocin (Pitocin), usually 20 units per liter, which enhances contraction. Excessive bleeding must always be reported to the surgeon. Ergonovine maleate (Ergotrate), which produces vigorous but rhythmic contractions for approximately 3 hours following administration, is often given intravenously.

Patients who have had cesarean sections experience the pain of an abdominal incision as well as the pain of uterine contraction. Therefore, they often require some type of narcotic analgesic. Antiemetic agents may be necessary in treating the nausea and vomiting that can occur following a dose of ergonovine. The remainder of PACU care is much the same as that for abdominal surgery. Coughing and deep-breathing exercises should be performed at frequent intervals.

THE DIABETIC PATIENT

Diabetes mellitus is a long-term illness that afflicts 2 percent of Americans, occurring with greater prevalence after the age of 45. It is a chronic, hereditary disease characterized by hyperglycemia due to a relative insufficiency or a lack of insulin, which leads to abnormalities in the metabolism of carbohydrates, proteins, and fat.

There are two distinct types of diabetes: (1) growth-onset or juvenile diabetes and (2) maturity-onset or adult-onset diabetes. These forms differ not only in age of onset but in their clinical courses and complications and thus in their clinical management. People with juvenile diabetes usually lack insulin and require exogenous insulin therapy; those with maturity-onset diabetes have insulin circulating in the blood and respond more satisfactorily to oral hypoglycemic drugs such as sulfonylurea and phenformin. Both types of diabetes produce deleterious effects on the capillaries of every organ system and also on the peripheral nerves (Brunner & Suddarth, 1975).

Because diabetic patients have a 50 percent chance of undergoing an operation in their lifetime, patients suffering from this endocrine disease are frequently on the operating room schedule. Studies have shown that the diabetic patient has an increased risk for morbidity and mortality compared with the general population. This is not surprising since the diabetic patient has impaired response to infection, impaired wound healing, and increased protein breakdown (Walts, 1983).

While undergoing anesthesia for an operation, diabetic patients can show extremes in blood glucose values. Should these patients become hyperglycemic, they may have increased diuresis and severe disturbance in electrolyte balance. If this condition remains unchecked, the patients can progress to metabolic ketoacidosis, an imminent threat to life. Patients who are given insulin during an operation are potential candidates for hypoglycemia, a dangerous state that could result in brain damage. Good control of plasma glucose during anesthesia is essential.

Walts (1983) reviewed numerous articles that describe techniques of managing the diabetic during anesthesia. Generally, these papers fall into three groups.

1. Some specialists recommend that the well-managed diabetic patient not be given insulin before an operation. They reason that plasma glucose is unlikely to reach a high value if the patient is fasting. They also note that the use of insulin carries the hazard of hypoglycemia. Thus, they suggest that medication cease in the morning of the operation and be resumed when the patient returns to his or her room.
2. Most specialists recommend that a partial dose of insulin be given on the morning of the operation. They, too, recognize the danger of hypoglycemia; however, they acknowledge that the blood glucose level rises during an operation. They believe that giving a fraction of the usual dose is sufficient to prevent an excessive rise in blood glucose and yet is unlikely to produce hypoglycemia.
3. In the past decade, some physicians have recommended that insulin be administered in small doses at the time of the operation. These are primarily anesthesiologists who deal directly with the diabetic patient during the surgery.

Walts and associates (1981) undertook a study of 200 diabetic patients utilizing each of the three management techniques. Findings indicated that regardless of the management during the operation, by 10:00 P.M. on the day of the operation and at 7:00 A.M. the following morning there was no significant difference in the average blood glucose value among the three groups of insulin-taking diabetic patients. Thus, even though the titration technique seemed to be a better method of intraoperative management, the fact that careful diabetic control ceased on discharge from the PACU meant that all groups ultimately fared similarly (Table 15-9).

The recommendations of this study are that the most important principles of safe management are knowing the current plasma glucose value

TABLE 15–9. PLASMA GLUCOSE VALUES FOR DIABETICS UNDER DIFFERENT MANAGEMENT TECHNIQUES

Group	No. of Patients	Preoperative Glucose	4 Hours after Start of Operation	Evening of Operation
Insulin-taking				
Control	31	190	281	299
Partial dose	58	181	258	249
Titration	33	167	160	265
Noninsulin-taking				
Control	47	165	237	249
Titration	31	163	186	211

Average plasma glucose (mg/dl) values found at various times on day of operation.
(Courtesy of Walts LF. Managing diabetes during surgery. AORN Journal 37:5, April 1983.)

and intervening with sugar or insulin as needed. If a diabetic patient is to have optimal control, plasma glucose values must be monitored intraoperatively and postoperatively. It is of no value to learn that the intraoperative glucose was 520 mg/dl or 30 mg/dl 6 hours after the blood is drawn.

In many hospitals, the central chemistry laboratory must be mobilized to handle the stat analysis that a messenger will hand-carry. In other hospitals that already have a separate blood-gas laboratory, the technicians must be trained to provide similar service using a glucose analyzer. Once the anesthesiologist has the proper information, he or she can take appropriate action.

For general guidelines, the following recommendations can be made:

1. Obtain the plasma glucose value before anesthesia is induced. If the value is 200 mg/dl or less, repeat analysis may not be needed during the operation, provided no insulin has been given.
2. Limit the sugar infusion. Walts gives the 5 percent glucose "piggy-back" on the crystalloid (nonglucose-containing) solution. The crystalloid can be given as necessary for the patient's fluid and electrolyte needs. The glucose can be given independently at the limited rate of 125 μg/hr. This translates to 1000 ml D_5W over 8 hours.
3. If the blood glucose value reaches 250 mg/dl, give 10 units of regular insulin intravenously. Once insulin is given, plasma glucose must be measured hourly for at least 3 hours.
4. If plasma glucose falls below 80 mg/dl, the glucose rate of infusion should be doubled for at least 1 hour to check a further decline. The infusion rate may then be readjusted after the plasma glucose has been redetermined.

The Walts and associates (1981) study reveals the postoperative period as critical to the diabetic patient. The anesthesiologist can carefully control the plasma glucose of the diabetic patient in the operating room and

PACU. Unfortunately, control ceases after the patient leaves the anesthesiologist's care. Obviously, future efforts should be made in improving postoperative management. In the future it may be necessary to create an endocrine care unit where diabetic patients can remain until they can resume oral feeding. It is the responsibility of surgical personnel to provide optimal care for the patient's endocrine disease.

Nursing Responsibilities

Clearly, a priority of PACU nursing care is knowledge of the patient's blood glucose and of any insulin therapy that has been administered. This is a classic illustration of the material presented in Chapter 8—that is, information which must be reported to the PACU nurse by the anesthesiologist. In order to intelligently care for the postanesthetic diabetic patient, the nurse needs to know which regimen has been employed preoperatively and intraoperatively. It is then her or his responsibility to be able to interpret blood glucose values and correlate that with type of insulin therapy. Essential to this is an awareness of time of onset and duration of action of the specific insulin administered. Table 15–10 provides these properties of the various insulins relative to subcutaneous injection. It is important to remember that if the patient was maintained on the titration or "tight-control" method, intravenous insulin was administered intraoperatively and pharmacodynamics are altered by route of administration. Additionally, the responsibilities of the nurse postoperatively differ depending on whether the classic (nontight control) regimen or tight control regimen was employed. Table 15–11 summarizes responsibilities for patients maintained on the classic regimen. Tables 15–12 and 15–13, and Figure 15–4, provide comparable summaries for patients maintained on tight control regimens.

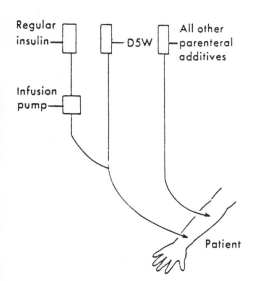

Figure 15–4. Arrangement of intravenous lines for regular insulin infusion (tight control regimen). *(Courtesy of Roizen MF. Preoperative evaluation of patients with diseases that require special preoperative evaluation and intraoperative management. In RD Miller (Ed.), Anesthesia (vol. 1). New York: Churchill Livingstone, 1981.)*

TABLE 15–10. PROPERTIES OF VARIOUS PREPARATIONS OF INSULIN

Type	Preparation	Appearance	Protein Modifier	Approximate Time of Onset* (Hours)	Approximate Duration of Action* (Hours)	Compatible Mixed with
Fast-Acting	Insulin injection, USP (regular insulin)	Clear solution	None	1	6	All preparations
	Insulin injection, USP—Insulin made from zinc-insulin crystals (regular insulin)	Clear solution	None	1	8	All preparations
	Prompt insulin, zinc suspension, USP (semilente insulin)	Cloudy suspension	None	1	14	Lente preparations
Intermediate-Acting	Isophane insulin, suspension USP (NPH insulin, isophane insulin)	Cloudy suspension	Protamine	2	24	Insulin injection
	Insulin zinc, suspension USP (lente insulin)	Cloudy suspension	None	2	24	Insulin injection semilente
	Globin zinc, insulin injection, USP	Clear solution	Globin	2	18	—
Long-Acting	Protamine zinc, insulin suspension, USP	Cloudy suspension	Protamine	7	36	Insulin injection
	Extended insulin zinc suspension, USP (ultralente insulin)	Cloudy suspension	None	7	36	Insulin injection semilente

*The figures are representative. The values may be expected to vary over a relatively wide range, depending on the dose and the individual patient.
(Courtesy of Goodman AG, Goodman, LS & Gilman A. The pharmacological basis of therapeutics (6th ed.). New York: Macmillan, 1980.)

TABLE 15–11. RESPONSIBILITIES FOR PATIENTS MAINTAINED ON CLASSIC (NONTIGHT CONTROL) REGIMEN

Aim
Avoid hypoglycemia.
Avoid ketoacidosis and hyperosmolar states.

Protocol
1. Day before surgery: NPO after midnight with a glass of orange juice at bedside for emergency use.
2. At 6 A.M. on day of surgery, institute IV fluids with plastic cannulae IV using a solution containing 5% dextrose at 125 ml/hr/70 kg.
3. After IV is instituted, give half of usual A.M. insulin dose subcutaneously.
4. Continue 5% dextrose solutions through operative period giving at least 125 ml/hr/70 kg.
5. In PACU, monitor urine sugars and acetones and blood glucose concentrations, and treat with a sliding scale.

TABLE 15–12. RESPONSIBILITIES FOR PATIENTS MAINTAINED ON TIGHT CONTROL REGIMEN 1

Aim
Keep plasma glucose between 79 and 200 mg/100 ml, which may improve wound healing and prevent wound infections.

Protocol
1. Evening before operation: obtain preprandial blood glucose level.
2. Through a plastic cannulae, begin IV infusion of 5% dextrose in water at 50 ml/hr/70 kg.
3. Piggyback to dextrose infusion an infusion of regular insulin using an infusion pump—this should be 50 units of regular insulin in 250 ml 0.9% sodium chloride; flush the line with 60 ml of infusion mixture and discard before attaching (see Fig. 15–4)—this approach is adequate to saturate insulin binding sites on tubing.
4. Set infusion rate with this equation: insulin (units/hr) = plasma glucose (mg/100 ml)/150*
5. Repeat measurements of blood glucose levels every 4 hours as needed with appropriate insulin adjustments to obtain blood glucose levels between 100 and 200 mg/100 ml.
6. Day of surgery: intraoperative fluids and electrolytes managed with nondextrose-containing solutions continued as in steps 3 and 4, above.
7. Obtain plasma glucose at start of operation and every 4 hours for the rest of the 24-hour period. Adjust insulin dosage appropriately.

Although it might not be necessary to treat hypoglycemia (blood glucose less than 50 mg/100 ml), it is important to be prepared to do so with 15 ml of 50% dextrose in water. Obviously, the insulin infusion should then be terminated.

* This denominator should be 100 if patient is taking corticosteroids (± 100 mg prednisone per day).

TABLE 15–13. RESPONSIBILITIES FOR PATIENTS MAINTAINED ON TIGHT CONTROL REGIMEN 2

Aim
Same as that of Tight Control Regimen 1.

Protocol
1.   Obtain "feedback mechanical pancreas" and set dials for desired plasma glucose regimen. Institute two appropriate IV lines.
This last regimen may well supersede all others if cost of a mechanical pancreas can be reduced and if control of hyperglycemia is shown to make a meaningful difference.

THE ONCOLOGIC PATIENT

Patients with malignancy may be essentially healthy (save for their yet to be removed malignancy) or desperately ill with nutritional, neurologic, metabolic, endocrinologic, electrolyte, cardiac, pulmonic, renal, hepatic, hematologic, or pharmacologic disability. Thus, knowledge of the other disabilities any patient with malignancy has requires search in all other systems. Many patients receive large doses of analgesics and should be kept comfortable in the perioperative period; avoidance of drug dependence is of no practical importance in terminally ill patients. More detailed information regarding specific malignancies may be found in oncologic nursing texts.

The side effects and toxicity of cancer chemotherapy relate to the agents used and dose. Table 15–14 (see pages 386–399) should be a helpful reference on chemotherapeutic agents for PACU nurses. Some of the problems seen in the PACU may be related to this therapy.

THE PATIENT RECEIVING TOTAL PARENTERAL NUTRITION

There are several metabolic problems with total parenteral nutrition. These include the syndrome of hyperosmolar hyperglycemic or nonketotic coma; dangerous hypoglycemia following unplanned discontinuation of high concentrations of intravenous glucose; hypophosphatemia; metabolic acidosis; and increased CO_2 production from metabolism of large amounts of glucose. Enhanced CO_2 formation may require initiation of artificial ventilation or may cause failure to wean the patient from long-term ventilation (Biebuyck, 1981).

It was not until the early 1970s that surgeons and anesthesiologists began to truly understand the basis of altered metabolism in the starving or undernourished patient (Cahill, 1970), and how anesthesia and trauma might interfere with "caloric homeostasis" in such a patient. Clearly, it was shown that vital tissues could use substrates other than glucose. A large proportion (19.6 percent) of basal metabolic expenditure is devoted to nourishing the central nervous systems. Investigations in humans and animals showed that the brain is able to utilize ketone bodies in addition to glucose (Owen & associates, 1967; Hawkins & Biebuyck, 1979). It also became apparent that the myocardium can utilize ketone bodies as metabolic fuel, and that both the myocardium and the liver can utilize free fatty acids. In fact, evidence accumulated to show that by raising plasma levels of free fatty acids, starvation lessened rather than enhanced the anesthetic depression of myocardial and hepatic function in experimental animals (Ko & Paradise, 1971; Biebuyck & associates, 1972). The effects of anesthetic agents on metabolic pathways, and particularly on substrate utilization by individual organs, have an important bearing on altered organ function during prolonged anesthesia.

The patient receiving TPN is considered here only from the perspective of altered metabolism of anesthetic agents and drugs. This discussion limits itself to the assessment phase of the nursing process, and is intended only to alert the nurse to possible abnormalities of anesthetic metabolism in patients experiencing dietary manipulation, specifically TPN. In other words, if the PACU nurse is caring for a patient on TPN and there are unexplained problems in recovery, the TPN should be considered as a contributing factor.

In a particular patient receiving total parenteral nutrition, several host factors (Fig. 15–5) may be in a state of dynamic change and interac-

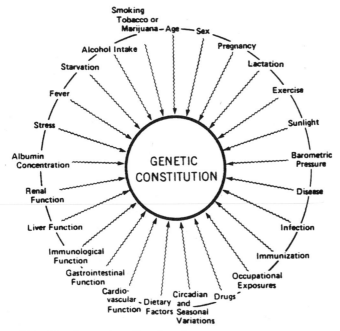

Figure 15–5. Host factors that affect drug disposition. *(Courtesy of Vesell. On the significance of host factors that affect drug disposition. Clinical Pharmacology and Therapeutics 31:2, Jan., 1982.)*

TABLE 15–14. CANCER CHEMOTHERAPY AND PRINCIPLES OF NURSING INTERVENTION

Agents	Indications for Use	Method of Administration	Side Effects/Toxic Effects	Nursing Interventions
Polyfunctional Alkylating Agents				
Methylbis (B-Chloroethyl) Amine HCL (HN₂, Mustargen) Mechlorethamine nitrogen mustard	Chronic leukemias, Cancers of the lung, breast, ovary, Hodgkin's disease, lymphosarcoma, reticulum cell sarcoma	IV	Nausea, vomiting, local phlebitis, marrow depression alopecia, jaundice, vertigo, tinnitus, decreased hearing, weakness, diarrhea, decreased sperm, skin eruptions, convulsions	Provide an emesis basin at bedside and empty after each use. Allay anxiety and stay with patient. Instruct patient to take deep breaths while nauseated. Give antiemetic drug as ordered, bland diet. Give mouth care to make patient feel refreshed. Note color, amount of vomitus and record. Avoid spillage on skin or infiltration since it can cause severe damage, use sodium thiosulfate to decrease reactions. Kaopectate, antispasmodics or Lomotil may be given for diarrhea. Wear gloves.
Busulfan (Myeleran)	Chronic granulocytic leukemia, polycythemia vera, primary thrombocytosis	PO	Pulmonary fibrosis, marrow depression, gynecomastia, hyperpigmentation of skin, amenorrhea, nausea, vomiting, testicular atrophy, bone marrow depression, systemic infection can occur, pseudomonas, candidiasis	Check results of lab tests, report abnormalities of CBC platelets. Initiate reverse isolation.

Drug	Uses	Route	Side Effects	Nursing Care
Chlorambucil (Leukeran)	Lymphosarcoma, Hodgkin's disease, cancers of breast, testis and ovary, chronic lymphocytic leukemia, lymphoma	PO	Nausea, vomiting, moderate depression of peripheral blood count, marrow depression, hepatic toxicity, bleeding, megaloblastic anemia	Same as above plus observe any bleeding. Check color of urine.
Cyclophosphamide (Endoxan, Cytoxan CTX)	Acute lymphocytic leukemia, chronic lymphocytic leukemia, cancer of the breast, ovary, lung, colon; Burkitt's sarcoma; Ewing's sarcoma, lymphosarcoma, Hodgkin's disease, multiple myeloma, neuroblastoma, reticulum cell sarcoma, Wilm's tumor; rhabdomyosarcoma	IV	Same as above, alopecia, hemorrhagic cystitis, anaphylactic reaction, liver dysfunction, stomatitis, mucositis, delayed wound healing, loss of virility, amenorrhea, dermatitis, darkened skin pigment	Same as above plus allow patient to verbalize feelings about self-image. Suggest use of wig or hairpiece. Provide physical comfort and emotional support. Ensure adequate hydration to prevent irritation of kidneys and bladder that cause hemorrhagic cystitis. For stomatitis give mouth care using lemon swabs rather than toothbrushes. Give soft, bland foods; do not give commercially prepared mouthwashes since they can irritate; instead give H_2O and H_2O_2 (1:1 proportion) then rinse with water; in case of severe pain, Xylocaine or Chloroseptic mouthwash may be given before meals.

(Continued)

TABLE 15–14. (Continued)

Agents	Indications for Use	Method of Administration	Side Effects/Toxic Effects	Nursing Interventions
Melphalan (Alkeran, Compound CB 3025, L-Sarcolysin, L-PAM, L-Phenylalanine mustard)	Multiple myeloma, cancer of breast, ovary or testis	PO	Nausea, vomiting, marrow depression, stomatitis	Stay with patient. Allay anxiety. Provide emesis basin and clean after each use. Give antiemetic as ordered. Note amount, color of vomitus and record. Check lab work and report findings if abnormal. Give after meals to prevent nausea.
Triethylenethiophosphoramide (ThioTEPA, TSPA)	Breast cancer, bladder cancer, cancer of ovary, Hodgkin's disease, retinoblastoma, lung cancer, lymphoma, control of effusions	IV, PO	Marrow depression, local pain, nausea, vomiting, dizziness, headache, anemia, GI perforation, potential allergic reaction	Check lab work. Report abnormal findings. Initiate reverse isolation. Protect patient from infection; use with caution if kidneys are impaired.
Triethylene melamine (TEM)	Breast cancer, lymphosarcoma, Hodgkin's disease, ovarian cancer, retinoblastoma	PO	Severe marrow depression, anorexia	Same measures as above. In addition, give sodium bicarb to promote absorption and activity of drug. Give before meals, acids inactivate the drug.
Antimetabolites				
Methotrexate (Amethopterin) MTX	Acute lymphocytic leukemia; breast cancer; choriocarcinoma; head and neck cancer; and testicular cancer; CNS leukemia; ostogenic sarcoma	PO, IV, intrathecal	Impaired kidney function, chills, fever, nausea, vomiting, pruritis, urticaria, drowsiness, visual blurring, headaches, photosensitivity, gastrointesti-	Provide mouth care. Protect from infection. Check vital signs at least qid. Give plenty of fluids, watch for bleeding. Since drug is excreted through

Drug	Route	Uses	Side Effects	Nursing Considerations
			nal ulceration; stomatitis; bone marrow depression; diarrhea; alopecia; fibrosis of lung, cystitis, diabetes, liver atrophy and necrosis	the kidneys, it should not be given in the presence of impaired renal function; keep antidote for drug on hand, i.e., leukovorin (folinic acid). Caution: not given to those with liver dysfunction; check liver function test results. Note: effect of MTX is decreased by salicylates, sulfonamides, and aminobenzoic acid; do not give with tetracyclines, vitamins, vaccines or chloramphenicol, Dilantin).
Cytosine arabinoside (Ara-C, Cytarabine, Cytosar)	IV	Lymphocytic and acute granulocytic leukemia	Marrow depression; megaloblastosis; leukopenia; thrombocytopenia; nausea, hepatic toxicity; esophagitis, thrombophlebitis	Check vital signs; report any rise in temperature. Care for nausea and vomiting as previously stated. Reduce exposure to infection; reverse isolation; drug crosses blood–brain barrier.
5-Fluorouracil (5-FU)	IV	Bladder cancer, ovarian cancer, breast cancer, cancer of stomach and colon, lung cancer cancer of uterus, liver, skin, oropharynx and prostate	Stomatitis, GI injury, marrow depression; nausea, diarrhea, alopecia, dermatitis, nail changes; cerebellar dysfunction	Meticulous mouth care. Avoid foods that cause curds. Give plenty of fluids. Check lab work and vital signs. Give Kaopectate as ordered; stomatitis indicates impending bone marrow depression.

(Continued)

TABLE 15–14. *(Continued)*

Agents	Indications for Use	Method of Administration	Side Effects/Toxic Effects	Nursing Interventions
6-Mercaptopurine (6-MP, Purinethol)	Acute granulocytic and lymphocytic leukemia, chronic granulocytic leukemia	PO	Marrow depression, nausea, vomiting (rare), hepatic toxicity, stomatitis, mouth ulcers	Check lab work and report abnormalities. Encourage verbalization of feelings.
6-Thioguanine (6-TG, Thioguan)	Acute myelogenous leukemia, chronic granulocytic leukemia		Photosensitivity, bone marrow depression, hepatic dysfunction, nausea, vomiting, skin rash, stomatitis, jaundice	Same as above. Avoid alcohol. Observe for rash and jaundice and report immediately to doctor.
Floxuridine (FUDR, Fluorodeuxyuridine)	Cancer of colon; gall-bladder, bile duct; liver metastasis	IV	Nausea, vomiting, diarrhea, stomatitis, alopecia, bone marrow depression	Give antiemetics; mouth care as previously stated, note any loose, watery stools and report; check WBC levels.
Antibiotics				
Actinomycin D (Dactinomycin, Cosmegen, Meractinomycin)	Choriocarcinoma, rhabdomyosarcoma, Ewing's sarcoma, Wilm's tumor, testicular cancer, oat cell cancer of lung	IV	Stomatitis, GI disturbances, alopecia, marrow depression, local phlebitis, tissue necrosis, nausea, vomiting, diarrhea, dermatitis, acne, abdominal pain, fatigue, malaise, lethargy, proctitis	Avoid skin infiltration (very toxic). Note: Not given if child has chicken pox since it would cause CNS chicken pox and resultant death. If given post-radiotherapy, it may reactivate radiation site.
Adriamycin (ADRIA, Doxorubicin)	Ewing's sarcoma, acute granulocytic and lymphocytic leukemia, cancer of	IV	Alopecia; GI disturbances; bone marrow depression; cardiac toxicity (at cumu-	Same as above, check any irregular and increased pulse rate and abnormal

Drug	Uses	Route	Side Effects/Toxicity	Nursing Considerations
	breast, bladder, thyroid; lung; Hodgkin's disease; multiple myeloma, neuroblastoma, osteogenic sarcoma, reticulum cell sarcoma		lative doses over 600 mg/m² can cause congestive heart failure with immediate toxicity: abdominal pain, nausea and vomiting within 4–6 hours, mouth ulcers); thrombophlebitis at injection site	rhythm. Observe for signs of cardiac decompensation (edema of legs, dyspnea, weakness). Dose is limited to 550 mg/m². Drug is red and causes red urine (do not confuse with hematuria).
Bleomycin (Blenoxane)	Head and neck cancer, lymphosarcoma, reticulum cell sarcoma, testicular cancer, Hodgkin's disease, epidermoid cancer lymphoma, urinary tract cancer, soft tissue sarcoma	IV	Phlebitis, fever, chills, pneumonia, mucocutaneous ulcerations, alopecia, pulmonary fibrosis, rarely stomatitis and myelosuppression; may have pain and hemorrhage from tumor site due to rapid destruction of tumor tissue	Check vital signs every 4 hours. Report any fever, chills. Give antipyretic drugs as ordered. Maintain proper room temperature and humidity. Avoid exposure to those with respiratory symptoms. Give mouth care. Note any difficult breathing. Dose limit is 400 mg total. Test dose is given before first dose.
Daunomycin (Rubidomycin, Daunorubicin)	Acute granulocytic and lymphocytic leukemia, neuroblastoma	IV	Nausea, vomiting, phlebitis, necrosis, marrow depression, alopecia, stomatitis, cardiac toxicity at cumulative doses over 25 mg/kg; mouth ulcer; diarrhea; fever with skin rash; CHF; PVCs; ST changes	Protect from infection. Check vital signs. Note pulse rhythm and rate. Drug is red and causes red color of urine. Dose is limited to 600 mg/m.

(Continued)

TABLE 15–14. (Continued)

Agents	Indications for Use	Method of Administration	Side Effects/Toxic Effects	Nursing Interventions
Mithramycin (Mithracin)	Testicular cancer, malignant hypercalcemia, trophoblastic tumors	IV	Anorexia, nausea, drowsiness, azotemia, thrombocytopenia, marrow depression, hypocalcemia, hypercalcemia, hepatic toxicity, hypokalemia, epistaxis, hematemesis, vomiting, diarrhea, stomatitis, change in renal and liver function with increased BUN and SGOT, headache	Note any complaint of tingling of extremities and muscle spasms. Serve foods attractively. Give nutritive fluids. Watch any bleeding and report immediately to physician, toxic to skin if infiltrated. Instruct patient not to drive or operate machinery after dose.
Mitomycin C (Mutamycin)	Cancer of colon, pancreas, cervix, breast, lung, head and neck cancers; gastric carcinoma, malignant melanoma	IV	Bone marrow depression, nausea, vomiting, severe skin reaction if given subcutaneously, stomatitis, severe malaise, fever, alopecia, pruritus, renal damage, paresthesias	Have vitamin B_6 on hand to counteract severe skin reaction; give stat after extravasation.
Steroid Hormones				
Androgen Testosterone propionate (Oreton) Halotestin, Teslac, Delatestryl, Drolban, Methosarb Cupusterone	Breast cancer postmenopausal or postcastration	PO IM	Fluid retention; masculinization, hirsutism, dyspepsia, increased libido, deepening of voice, hot flashes	Watch for edema. Weigh daily. Monitor blood pressure.
Estrogens Diethylstilbestrol (DES, Stilbestrol)	Breast cancer (palliative only), prostatic cancer (palliative therapy for advanced disease)	PO	Diarrhea, breast tenderness, headache, rash, paresthesias, anxiety, insomnia, changes in libido, changes in calcium and phosphorus metabolism, muscle weakness, polyuria, polydypsia	Note urinary output; push fluids, limit calcium intake via dairy products. Encourage ambulation to keep calcium in bones.

Drug	Indication	Route	Side effects	Nursing considerations
Estradiol cypionate (Depo-Estradiol)	Prostatic cancer	IM		
Chlorotrianesene (TACE)	Prostatic cancer	PO		
Estradiol valerate (Delestrogen)	Prostatic cancer	IM		
Estrone (Theelin)	Prostatic cancer	IM	Possible nausea, vomiting, sodium retention	Assess for occurrence of possible side effects.
Polyestradiol phosphate (Estradurin)	Prostatic cancer	IM		
Estrogenic substances conjugated (Premarin), esterified (Evex, Amnestrogen, Menest)	Breast and prostatic carcinomas	PO		
Progestin	Renal and breast cancer		When used with estrogens may cause nausea and vomiting, anorexia, abdominal cramps, thromboembolitic disorders, depression, backache, breast tenderness, hypercalcemia, fluid retention, libido changes	
Megestrol acetate (Megace)	Endometrial cancer	PO		
Prednisone (Deltasone, Merticorten, Orasone, Paracort, Delta-Dome, Servisone)	Acute leukemia (as combination chemotherapy; COAP)	PO	Stomatitis, gastric ulcers, alopecia, increased pigmentation, acne, urticaria, nail changes	Give with antacids and continue for at least 1 week after discontinuation of drug.
Hydrocortisone sodium succinate (Solu-cortef)	Acute and chronic lymphocytic leukemia, breast cancer, lymphosarcoma	IV	Potassium loss, sodium and fluid retention, gastric bleeding	Give foods high in potassium such as bananas, oranges, prunes, dates. Monitor blood pressure, weight and electrolytes

(Continued)

TABLE 15–14. (Continued)

Agents	Indications for Use	Method of Administration	Side Effects/Toxic Effects	Nursing Interventions
Dexamethasone (Decadron)	Same as above	PO	Immunosuppression, fluid retention, hypotension, hypertension, diabetes	Protect from infection. Watch for edema. Weigh daily. Check BP every 4 hours. Clinitest and Acetest urine after each voiding.
Methylprednisolone sodium succinate (Solu-Medrol)	Acute and chronic lymphocytic leukemia, breast cancer, miscellaneous tumors	IM IV	Depression, headache, hypertension, increased intraocular pressure, ulcer, menstrual abnormalities, atrophy at IM injection, muscle weakness, withdrawal symptoms, hypotension, dyspnea, fatigue, fever, hypokalemia, hypernatremia	Avoid sudden withdrawal of drug. Check BP, weight, serum electrolytes. Teach patient signs of early adrenal insufficiency: fatigue, muscular weakness, joint pain, fever, anorexia. Watch for depression or psychotic episodes.
Miscellaneous Drugs				
BCNU (1.3 bis (B-Chloroethyl)–1-nitrosurea, Carmustine)	Brain tumor, breast cancer, cancer of the lung and colon, myeloma, melanoma, lymphomas, gastric cancer, renal cancer	IV	Facial flushing, nausea, vomiting 6 hours after dose, renal toxicity, marrow depression, burning pain along vein, diarrhea, mild hepatotoxicity, anorexia	Observe amount and color of urine. Maintain I & O. Protect from infection. Give analgesics as prescribed. Crosses the blood–brain barrier, avoid skin contact (causes brown spots).
Hydroxyurea (hydrea)	Brain tumor, chronic granulocytic leukemia, melanoma	PO	Marrow depression; anorexia, diarrhea, megaloblastic anemia, nausea, vomiting, skin rash, rarely alopecia, oral and GI ulceration	Protect from infection. Note any complaints of tiredness and report to physician. Watch for pallor. Serve frequent small feedings that are attrac-

Drug	Uses	Route	Side effects	Nursing considerations
				tively presented. Note amount and frequency of defecation. Synergistic action with radiotherapy and may cause erythema. Note: Give with caution if liver or kidney is impaired. Crosses the blood–brain barrier.
Mitotane (O, p' DDD, lysodren, Ortho-para-DDD)	Adrenocortical cancer after excision	PO	Nausea, vomiting, anorexia, GI toxicity, diarrhea, CNS depression, dizziness, altered steroid metabolism, tremors, bone marrow depression	Instruct patient to be careful if concentration and coordination is needed. Steroid replacement may be necessary.
Streptozotocin (probably acts by alkylation)	Pancreatic insulinoma, carcinoid tumor, Hodgkin's disease, lung	IV	Nausea, vomiting, renal tubule defects, abdominal cramps, stomatitis, may cause hypoglycemia nephrotoxicity, diabetogenic	Inform patient of burning sensation on administration. Test urine for glycosuria (urinalysis).
Neocarzinostatin antibiotic (investigational drug)	Advanced bladder cancer, carcinoma of pancreas, stomach, ovaries, uterus, liver and kidneys, malignant melanoma, acute leukemia	IV	Nausea and vomiting, anorexia, diarrhea, anaphylactic reaction, elevation of liver enzymes, acute renal failure, skin rash, stomatitis, headache, chills	Give antiemetics as ordered, watch urinary output and report any oliguria. Mouth care as previously mentioned. Avoid sudden changes in room temperature. Report any chills or signs of anaphylaxis.

(Continued)

TABLE 15–14. (Continued)

Agents	Indications for Use	Method of Administration	Side Effects/Toxic Effects	Nursing Interventions
CCNU [1-(2-chloroethyl) 3-cyclohexyl-nitrosourea; Lomustine]; investigational drug (alkylating agent)	Hodgkin's disease, primary/ secondary CNS tumors, gastric, renal, bronchogenic carcinomas	PO	Nausea and vomiting, gastric irritation, hepatotoxicity, bone marrow depression	Give antiemetics. Give fluids on empty stomach. Crosses blood–brain barrier. NPO for 4–6° post-drug intake.
Methyl-CCNU [1-(2-chloroethyl)-3-(4-methylcyclohexy); 1-nitrosoureal]; MeCCNU; Semustine, Lomustine) investigational drug (more useful than BCNU in cancer of gastrointestinal tract)	Primary/secondary CNS tumors; cancer of stomach, colon, lung, pancreas; squamous cell carcinoma; malignant melanoma	PO	Nausea and vomiting, gastric irritation, anorexia, bone marrow depression, leukopenia, thrombocytopenia, renal and hepatotoxicity	Give on empty stomach 4 hours after meal. Give antiemetics and fluids. Avoid sources of infection.
Hexamethylmelamine (probably acts as an antimetabolite); investigational drug	Cancer of lung and ovary	PO	Nausea, vomiting, diarrhea, peripheral neuropathy after repeated doses, bone marrow depression, alopecia, motor weakness, incoordination	Give antiemetics. Note, record, and report watery stools. Drug may have to be stopped. Infection/ bleeding caution.
Imidazole carboxamide dimethyltriazino (DIC, DTIC, BIC, Imidazole Carboxamide, TIC Mustard, Imidazole Mustard); investigational drug	Hodgkin's disease, malignant melanoma	IV	Nausea, vomiting 1–2 hours after IV dose (lessens with further doses) flu-like syndrome with myalgia, headache and malaise up to 10 days, mild hepatotoxicity, bone marrow depression (rare)	Protect from light. Inform patient of possible burning sensation on injection, metallic taste, give antiemetics.
Cycloleucine (1-amino cyclopentane carbosylic-acid); investigational drug	Sarcomas	IV push or scalp vein needle	Nausea, vomiting, mild bone marrow depression, CNS toxicity, vertigo,	Give antiemetics. Protect from infection. Observe for early signs of CNS

Drug	Uses	Route	Side Effects	Nursing Considerations
Procarbazine (Matulane, Natulane, methylhydrazine, ibenzmethyzin)	Hodgkin's disease, myeloma, ovarian and oat cell cancer, non-Hodgkin's lymphomas	PO, IV	slurred speech, ataxia, weakness, diplopia, disorientation, immunosuppression Sedative effect, nausea, vomiting, bone marrow depression, myalgia, CNS irritability, psychosis (rare), orthostatic hypotension, inhibition of monoamine oxidase, mental depression, convulsion	toxicity (drug may have to be stopped). Synergistic action with phenothiazine and barbiturates, narcotic intolerance to alcohol. Note any facial edema. Instruct patient to avoid eating cheese, yogurt, bananas; do not drink chianti wine; avoid antihistamines, narcotics, sedatives, and alcohol. Drug crosses the blood–brain barrier. Give antiemetics. Watch for evidence of infection or bleeding and report stat.
BCG (Bacille-Calmette-Guerin); substrains: 1. Pasteur 2. Connaught 3. Tice 4. Glaxo nonspecific immunostimulant	Acute and chronic leukemia, lymphoma, malignant melanoma lung cancer	Intralesional, intradermal, IV, heaf gun, scarification, multipuncture	After injection, local inflammation (red papule) occurs in 7–10 days, then necrosis, eschar, and healing unless secondary infection sets in; flu-like syndrome with fever, myalgia, nausea, vomiting, lymphadenopathy near tumor sites, anaphylactic reaction	Avoid autoinoculation, keep site clean, dry, and exposed to air; give aspirin for flu-like syndrome; give antiemetics.
Cis-Platinum (II) diammine dichloride; inorganic metallic salt	Testicular and ovarian cancers, epidermoid tumors, head and neck cancer	IV	Nausea, vomiting, renal toxicity, deafness, diarrhea, bone marrow depression	Give antiemetics. Observe urinary output. Safeguard against infection.

(Continued)

TABLE 15-14. (Continued)

Agents	Indications for Use	Method of Administration	Side Effects/Toxic Effects	Nursing Interventions
Plant Extracts				
Vinblastine (Velban)	Breast cancer, choriocarcinoma, Hodgkin's disease, lymphosarcoma, reticulum cell sarcoma, testicular cancer	IV	Stomatitis, bone marrow depression, paresthesia, headache, vomiting, alopecia, constipation, diarrhea, abdominal pain, depression, loss of deep tendon reflexes, vesiculation of mouth, ileus, pain in tumor site, urinary retention	Apply previously mentioned care for nausea, vomiting, alopecia and bone marrow depression. Reassure patient when anxious about paresthesia. Avoid infiltration (very toxic). Caution: if splashed in the eye it can cause corneal ulceration, thus be careful in handling drug and wash hands after use; drug has cumulative toxicity.
Vincristine sulfate (Oncovin)	Acute lymphatic leukemia, breast cancer, Ewing's sarcoma, Hodgkin's disease, lymphosarcoma, reticulum cell sarcoma, Wilm's tumor; rhabdomyosarcoma, testicular cancer; choriocarcinoma	IV	Paresthesias, areflexia, muscular weakness, hoarseness, paralytic ileus, mental depression, constipation, mild bone marrow depression, impotence, visual disturbance, seizures, loss of deep tendon reflexes, upper colon impaction	Reassure patient. Assist in self-care. Watch for abdominal distention. Show interest in patient. Encourage involvement in some activities. Give plenty of fluids and fruits. Check lab results. Prophylactic stool softeners should be given; dosage limited by neurotoxicity; prevent skin infiltration—very toxic. Note: Use with caution in patients with preexisting neuropathies.

Enzyme

L-Asparaginase (Elspar)	Acute lymphocytic leukemia	IV	Fever, allergic reactions, hyperglycemia, hepatic toxicity, nausea, vomiting, renal toxicity, reversible encephalopathy, hypoalbuminemia, blood dyscrasias, malaise, hyper/hypolipidemia, decreased clotting factor, pancreatitis	Check vital signs. Give antipyretics as ordered. Check lab work. Report any abnormalities. Note urinary output—amount, and color. Test urine for glucose at least once a day. Avoid shaking vial—it harms enzymes.

Note: Due to the continued aggressive search for additional agents that can be used therapeutically in the treatment of cancer, this table cannot include everything that is being subjected to research and investigation.

(Courtesy of Baldonado AA & Stahl DA: Cancer Nursing—A Holistic Multidisciplinary Approach (2nd ed.). Flushing, N.Y.: Medical Exam Pub. Co., 1982, pp. 45–60.)

tion. The function of critical organs directly involved in drug disposition—including the heart, kidney, and liver—may be rapidly fluctuating. Effective blood concentrations of many drugs can differ from day to day, due not only to addition of new drugs and withdrawal of others, but also to changes in cardiovascular, hepatic, and renal function, hormonal status, and diet. In turn, these changes in drug blood concentration can alter, in often unpredictable ways, rates of drug elimination through effects on hepatic drug-metabolizing enzymes. Presence of infection, fever, and intercurrent disease offers additional opportunities for perturbation of a patient's normal rate of drug elimination. So many interrelated host factors converge simultaneously and change dynamically in surgical patients receiving total parenteral nutrition that it is often difficult to predict how a particular patient would respond to a particular drug.

Studies suggest that anesthesiologists should consider that the doses of many drugs given to surgical patients may need to be changed on commencement of total parenteral nutrition. Drugs eliminated primarily by hepatic metabolism especially require dosage adjustment. The extent of this dosage adjustment is not determined easily because numerous dynamically changing, interrelated host factors affect it.

Earlier experiments illustrate how various dietary manipulations dramatically alter hepatic drug metabolism. Use of laboratory animals permitted clearer elucidation of the mechanisms of these dietary effects than was possible in human subjects, since the activities of hepatic drug-metabolizing enzymes could be assayed directly in laboratory animals. In several species, the specific composition of the diet was demonstrated to influence the biologic fate of drugs and therefore their intensity and duration of action (Campbell, 1974, & 1977). Reduction in dietary protein decreased rates of metabolism of some drugs, whereas a high protein diet increased these rates (Kato, 1968; Kiejnen, 1971). Overnight starvation of rats markedly altered the activities of certain hepatic drug-metabolizing enzymes (Kato & Gillette, 1965), but in obese human subjects starvation produced no changes in antipyrine metabolism (Reidenberg, 1975). In mice, a diet high in carbohydrates diminished hepatic metabolism of drugs in vitro and in vivo (Strother & associates, 1971).

In 1951 Lanson and associates first demonstrated an effect of carbohydrate on drug disposition. On awakening from pentobarbital anesthesia, dogs would return to sleep if they received 10 ml of a 50 percent dextrose solution.

Once again a discussion of TPN is included here to alert the PACU nurse to the possibility that rates of drug elmination may change rapidly in surgical patients receiving total parenteral nutrition, probably because several host factors shown in Figure 15–5 may be fluctuating simultaneously and interacting dynamically.

Anesthetic and Nursing Responsibilities

For patients receiving hyperalimentation, hypertonic glucose calories are concentrated in normal daily fluid requirements in solutions containing protein hydrolyzates or synthetic amino acids. To diminish the likelihood of essential fatty acid deficiency, Intralipid, a soybean emulsion, can be added to the solution. The major complications of hyperalimentation are sepsis and metabolic abnormalities. The central lines used for TPN require an absolute aseptic technique and should not be used as an intravenous route for drug administration.

Major metabolic complications of TPN relate to deficiencies and hyperosmolar states that develop. Complications of hypertonic dextrose can develop if the patient has insufficient insulin (diabetes mellitus) to metabolize the sugar, or if insulin resistance is present, as in uremia, burns, or sepsis (Law, 1977).

Gradual decrease in the infusion rate of TPN prevents the development of hypoglycemia that can occur on abrupt discontinuance. Thus, the infusion rate of TPN should be decreased the night prior to anesthesia and surgery. The main reason for slowing or discontinuing TPN prior to anesthesia is to avoid intraoperative hyperosmolarity secondary to rapid infusion of the solution (Sheldon & Way, 1977). Hypophosphatemia is a particularly serious complication that results from administering phosphate-free or phosphate-depleted hyperalimentation solution. The low serum phosphate causes shifts of the oxygen dissociation curve to the left, and thus low 2, 3 diphosphoglycerate and ATP require increased cardiac output for the same oxygen delivery. Hypophosphatemia, when less than 1.0 mg/dl, may cause a hemolytic anemia, cardiac failure, tachypnea, neurologic symptoms, seizures, and death. In addition, trace metal deficiencies associated with long-term TPN include copper (refractory anemia), zinc (impaired wound healing), and magnesium deficiency. Based on the above considerations, some physicians slow TPN beginning the night prior to surgery, substituting 5 or 10 percent dextrose solution preoperatively; measure serum glucose, phosphate, and potassium concentrations preoperatively, and if abnormal, restore them to within normal limits; and maintain strict asepsis (Sheldon & Way, 1977).

THE OBESE PATIENT

The focus here is on the severely obese patient undergoing elective surgery. Obesity is defined using an anthropometric measurement, body mass index (BMI): weight (kg)/height^2 (m^2). Definitions of this index are: nonobese, < 25; overweight, 26–29; and obese > 30 (Bray & associates, 1976). Although variously defined, severely or morbidly obese patients manifest a weight two times ideal weight for height. M. S. Vaughan (1982) proposes that nursing care guidelines for this unique subset of the population must concentrate on the consequences of the obese state itself.

Transport from Operating to PACU

Immediately after the supine patient is transferred, the flexed knee position is instituted for the patient and the head of the bed elevated. Not only does this maneuver prevent postoperative patient migration to the foot of the bed, but more importantly, semirecumbent or lateral semirecumbent posture aids oxygenation. Special attention to guard the upper extremities during transport will avoid injury and inadvertent disconnection of intraarterial and venous lines. With the patient safely in bed (not a PACU cart), the drawsheet can be used to tuck arms and hands inside the confines of the bed for safe transport to the PACU.

Positioning and Oxygenation

Positioning can be a most beneficial element of postoperative nursing care. Vaughan and Wise (1975) found that semirecumbent rather than supine posturing was a valuable therapeutic adjunct to improve arterial oxygenation even in young, nonsmoking, obese but otherwise healthy women. Further studies document that the lateral ducubitus position (left or right) compared favorably with semi-erect upright position when oxygenation was measured in morbidly obese subjects (Vaughan, 1975). Thus, prudent nursing intervention to avoid the routine supine posture in postoperative severely obese individuals is documented by clinical research.

Supplementary oxygen (O_2) coupled with semirecumbent posturing is also advocated. In 1962, Nunn and Payne emphasized that arterial hypoxemia was the usual occurrence after any major operative procedure. Subsequently Palmer and colleagues (1965) studied nonobese subjects who underwent upper abdominal operations and found that profound lung volume disturbances (reduced functional residual capacity) occurred and lead to hypoxemia. More recently, data have been presented to delineate the frequency, extent, and duration of hypoxemia in obese subjects following jejunoileal bypass operations (Vaughan, 1974; Vaughan & associates, 1974). These patients experienced a greater degree of postoperative hypoxemia because, when compared with nonobese subjects matched preoperatively for age, a significant reduction in arterial oxygen tension (PaO_2) occurred in the nonoperated state. With the subsequent fall in PaO_2 incident to surgery, the oxygen levels that resulted in some patients were dangerously reduced. Especially on postoperative days one and two, severe decreases in PaO_2 were demonstrated in some patients. Without supplemental oxygen, tissue hypoxia could occur. With reduction in arterial oxygen tension, normal compensatory mechanisms become operative to increase cardiac output and maximize tissue oxygen delivery (Alexander & associates, 1962; Backman & associates, 1973). This additional requirement for an increase in cardiac output may be curtailed in patients with obesity-related diseases (such as hypertensive cardiovascular disease and advanced atherosclerosis secondary to diabetes mellitus). If any increased metabolic need for oxygen is added to this reduction in arterial oxygen tension, the potential for respiratory decompensation increases. Thus, preoperative physical status may have profound effects on developing hypoxemia.

Incisional Site

Postoperative hypoxemia, as previously implied, is influenced by the patient's operative site (peripheral versus abdominal). Further, in obese subjects with vertical operative incisions as opposed to transverse incisions, prolonged hypoxemia even to the third or fourth postoperative day has been demonstrated (Vaughan, 1975). Thus, a basic element of nursing care must incorporate continuous administration of supplemental O_2 during daily postoperative nurse–patient activities. A vertical incision signals the probability of supplemental O_2 therapy validated by arterial blood gas analysis.

Arterial Lines and Blood Gas Sampling

M.S. Vaughan (1982) warns us of the importance of proper anaerobic samplings of arterial blood for analysis. This caveat is crucial, because it is impossible to predict falls in arterial oxygen tension commensurate with the obese state. Therefore, arterial blood sampling errors may have potentially severe clinical consequences. For example, allowing small air bubbles to remain in the arterial sample will factitiously elevate the patient's reduced PaO_2. A false sense of security resulting in discontinuance of supplemental oxygen could result. Conversely, improper care to ice the arterial sample can lead to O_2 utilization by leukocytes within the sample. Subsequent measurement of a spuriously low PaO_2 could inappropriately initiate airway control and controlled mechanical ventilation.

To optimize intraoperative and postoperative blood-gas and pressure monitoring, many markedly obese patients have an arterial line placed preoperatively. Nursing care includes proper restraint and positioning of the extremity, observation for arterial disconnection, and knowledge of appropriate actions if disconnection does occur. An appropriate response would suggest immediate application of firm pressure on any portion of the artery proximal to the tip of the cannula. In addition, arterial lines are usually kept patent by continuous flushing with dilute heparinized saline (2 units/ml) utilizing an infusion pump. Using fluids without dextrose controls rouleaux of erythrocytes and subsequent clot formation. The nursing care principle of slow flushing of the intraarterial line with a small volume of fluid (usually 2 cc each time) was documented by Lowenstein and associates (1971). These investigators demonstrated, using retrograde angiography, that embolization of the cerebral circulation in the adult can occur using volumes as small as 3 ml.

Hypothermia and Shivering

Recent information relative to the obese postoperative adult in the PACU supports the contention that hypothermia (core body temperature < 36.0° C) or shivering can occur (Vaughan, 1980). Clinical data do not support the myth that severely obese individuals enter the PACU with minimal temperature imbalance compared with nonobese counterparts. Despite preconceived notions to the contrary, being severely obese does not guarantee PACU normothermia (36.0–38.0° C), nor does return to optimum body temperature occur at an accelerated rate. Nursing implications include monitoring of core body temperature at intervals throughout the PACU stay and as indicated thereafter.

Early Ambulation

A further adjunct to postoperative therapy beyond the PACU includes a regimen of early ambulation. Prolonged postoperative immobilization facilitates the development of phlebothrombosis (Postlethwait & Johnson, 1972). Pulmonary emboli secondary to peripheral venous occlusion occur frequently in obese patients following intraabdominal operation (Henderson, 1927; Pell & D'Alonso, 1961; Snell, 1927). Kakkar and associates (1970), using radioactive fibrinogen, confirmed a positive association between obesity and phlebothrombosis (the incidence was nonobese, 22.9 percent; obese, 47.9 percent). These and other findings suggest that treatment with heparin should be considered for markedly obese patients presenting for operative procedures greater than an hour in duration (Kakkar, 1975; Gallus & associates, 1976).

Fluid Management

Both volume and composition of electrolyte and colloid administration demand careful management in obese patients. Paul and colleagues (1976) demonstrated in 11 nonanesthetized obese subjects that change of posture from sitting to supine was associated with a 31 percent increase in mean pulmonary artery pressure and a 44 percent increase in pulmonary artery wedge pressure. Nevertheless, extracellular fluid losses do occur preoperatively, intraoperatively, and postoperatively. When the operative procedure involves colonic anastamoses, mechanical bowel preparation, such as clear liquid diet, cathartics, and enemas, is begun 48 hours prior to operation. Isotonic extracellular fluid (ECF) depletion results. Often such depletion can produce a deficit of 2 to 3 liters (Jenkins & Giesecke, 1974).

Balanced crystalloid solution is necessary. Use of a Foley catheter to assess urine output is a valuable aid during intraabdominal operations in severely obese subjects. Optimum fluid management during intraabdominal surgery in these patients should include monitoring of hourly urine output. Occasionally, central venous pressure monitoring is needed as well to facilitate evaluation of fluid volume status. Finally, obese subjects with coexistent severe cardiac dysfunction (as in open-heart surgery) benefit from Swan-Ganz catheter monitoring intraoperatively and postoperatively to guide fluid balance.

Table 15–15 summarizes postoperative nursing care considerations for the PACU and until hospital discharge.

THE SUBSTANCE ABUSER

Drug abuse may be defined as the self-administration of a substance for a purpose that deviates from accepted medical or social use (Jenkins, 1972; Isbell, 1971). Prolonged drug abuse leads to tolerance, psychologic and/or physical dependence, and in some instances life-threatening withdrawal symptoms when the substance is not continuously available.

An important consideration in the management of a patient who is known to abuse a drug or drugs includes an appreciation of the potential interactions of these substances with medications administered during the perioperative period. There may be cross-tolerance to the pharmacologic effects of drugs used during anesthesia. As a result, it can be difficult to predict analgesic or anesthetic requirements, or to achieve desired responses. Likewise, additive or even synergistic depressant drug interactions can occur. Finally, it is important to recognize signs of drug withdrawal in the perioperative period. Acute drug withdrawal should not be attempted at this time.

Narcotics

The patient addicted to narcotics or receiving methadone should have his narcotic requirement maintained during the perioperative period. These patients should receive a generous preoperative medication that includes their usual narcotic or methadone. Methadone 2.5 mg is equivalent to 10 mg of morphine (McGoldrik, 1980). There is no advantage in trying to maintain anesthesia with a narcotic. A volatile anesthetic is ideal—remembering, however, that these patients are likely to have

TABLE 15–15. POSTOPERATIVE NURSING MANAGEMENT FOR THE OBESE PATIENT

Immediate Care Considerations	Follow-up Care Considerations
Positioning	Cough and breathing exercises
Humidified oxygen	Intake and output
Vital signs	Early ambulation
Patency of drains	Skin care
Monitoring devices	
Radial artery line	
Arterial blood samples	
Pain management	
Reorientation to environment	

underlying liver disease. Intraoperative hypotension most likely reflects an inadequate intravascular fluid volume. Chronic pulmonary disease is often present, and a large alveolar-to-arterial difference for oxygen is likely. Postoperatively, a patient who has been on methadone will be tolerant to the analgesic effects of this drug and other narcotics. For reasons that are not clear, satisfactory postoperative analgesia is often achieved with average doses of meperidine, administered in addition to the usual daily intake of methadone or other narcotics (McGoldrick, 1980).

A rehabilitated addict should not receive a narcotic in the preoperative or intraoperative period. Anesthesia with a volatile drug is ideal. Postoperatively, analgesia should be provided with the smallest dose of narcotic possible, or with a continuous regional anesthetic technique.

Withdrawal from narcotics is generally not life threatening, although abrupt discontinuance has been associated with cardiovascular collapse. Seizures do not occur in response to withdrawal. Clonidine may serve a beneficial role in withdrawal, as this drug has been shown to prevent the signs and symptoms of acute withdrawal from methadone maintenance (Gold & associates, 1980). It is thought that clonidine acts by replacing opiate-mediated inhibition (absent during withdrawal) with alpha-2-mediated inhibition of sympathetic nervous system activity in the brain.

Barbiturates

Although barbiturate addiction is characterized by tolerance and by psychologic and physical dependence, the only suggestion of barbiturate abuse preoperatively may be excessive apprehension. This apprehension most likely reflects the patient's fear of not being able to obtain the drug. Intraoperatively, chronic abuse of barbiturates typically manifests as cross-tolerance to the sedative effects of anesthetic drugs.

In contrast to narcotics, withdrawal from barbiturates is potentially life-threatening. Signs of withdrawal, characterized by anxiety, tremors, and hallucinations, appear 24 to 48 hours after discontinuance of the drug. Acute withdrawal may culminate in grand mal seizures and death.

Amphetamines

Central nervous system stimulation that occurs during acute administration of amphetamines is most likely related to the release of catecholamines in the brain. Intraoperatively, a patient who is acutely intoxicated from ingestion of amphetamines may manifest hypertension, tachycardia, increased body temperature, and elevated requirements for volatile anesthetics. It would seem wise to monitor body temperature during the perioperative period. Furthermore, direct-acting vasopressors and drugs that sensitize the heart to catecholamines must be used with caution in these patients.

The response to cocaine abuse is similar to that seen with amphetamines.

Alcohol

The tolerance of alcoholics to alcohol is paralleled by similar resistance (cross-tolerance) to other central nervous system depressant drugs such as the barbiturates and volatile anesthetics. Indeed, there is evidence that chronic alcohol abuse increases anesthetic requirements (MAC) for Halothane (Han, 1969) and isoflurane (Johnston & associates, 1975). The most likely explanation is cellular tolerance.

Monitoring of intraoperative arterial blood gases, pH, and urine output, plus provision of exogenous glucose, are important principles of management of the alcoholic patient.

REFERENCES

Aldrete JA: Clinical implications of magnesium therapy. In SM Shnider & F Maya (Eds.), The Anesthesiologist, Mother, and Newborn. Baltimore: Williams & Wilkins, 1974, pp. 128–135.

Alexander JK, Dennis EW, Smith WG, et al.: Blood volume, cardiac output and distribution of systemic blood flow in extreme obesity. Cardiovasc Res Cent Bull 1:39–42, 1962.

Appel GB & Neu HC: The nephrotoxicity of antimicrobial agents. New England Journal of Medicine 296:663, 1977.

Backman L, Freyschuss V, Hollbug D, et al.: Cardiovascular function in extreme obesity. Acta Medica Scandinavica 193:437–446, 1973.

Baldonado AA & Stahl DA: Cancer Nursing—A Holistic Multidisciplinary Approach (2nd ed.). Flushing, N.Y.: Medical Exam Pub. Co., 1982.

Biebuyck JF: Total parenteral nutrition in the perioperative period—A time for caution? Anesthesiology 54:5, 360–362, May, 1981.

Biebuyck JF, Lund P, & Krebs HA: The protective effect of oleate on metabolic changes produced by halothane in rat liver. Biochemical Journal 128:721–723, 1972.

Brunner LS & Suddarth DS: Textbook of Medical-Surgical Nursing. Philadelphia: Lippincott, 1975.

Cahill CJ & Cahill JR: Starvation in man. New England Journal of Medicine 282:668–675, 1970.

Cooperman LH & Price HL: Pulmonary edema in the operative and postoperative period: A review of 40 cases. Annals of Surgery 172:883, 1970.

Dripps R, Eckenhoff J, Van Dam L: Introduction to Anesthesia (6th ed.). Philadelphia: Saunders, 1982.

Foldes FF: Factors which alter the effects of muscle relaxants. Anesthesiology 20:469, 1959.

Gallus AS, Hirsh J, O'Brien SE, et al.: Prevention of venous thrombosis with small, subcutaneous doses of heparin. Journal of the American Medical Association 235: 1980–1982, 1976.

Ghoneim MM & Long JP: Interaction between magnesium and other neuromuscular blocking agents. Anesthesiology 32:23, 1970.

Giesecke AG, Morris RE, Dalton MD, et al.: On magnesium muscle relaxants, toxemic patients, and cats. Anesthesia and Analgesia 47:689, 1968.

Gold MS, Pottash AC, Sweeney DR, et al.: Opiate withdrawal using clonidine: A safe, effective and rapid nonopiate treatment. Journal of the American Medical Association 243:343–346, 1980.

Goodman AG, Goodman LS, Gilman A: The Pharmacological Basis of Therapeutics (6th ed.). New York: Macmillan, 1980.

Han YH: Why do chronic alcoholics require more anesthesia? Anesthesiology 30:341–342, 1969.

Hawkins RA & Biebuyck JF: Ketone bodies are selectively used by individual brain regions. Science 205:325–327, 1979.

Henderson EF: Fatal pulmonary embolism: A statistical review. Archives of Surgery 15:34–37, 1927.

Isbell H: Clinical aspects of the various forms of nonmedical use of drugs. Part 2. Anesthesia and Analgesia 50:897–905, 1971.

Israel JS & DeKornfeld TJ: Recovery Room Care. Springfield, Ill.: Chas. C Thomas, 1982.

Jenkins LC: Anesthetic problems due to drug abuse and dependence. Canadian Anaesthetists Society Journal 19:461–477, 1972.

Jenkins MT & Giesecke AH Jr: Balanced salt solutions in clinical anesthesia. In SG Hershey (Ed.), ASA Refresher Courses in Anesthesiology (vol. 2). Philadelphia: Lippincott, 1974, pp. 107–116.

Johnston RE, Kulp RA, Smith TC: Effects of acute and chronic ethanol administration on isoflurane requirement in mice. Anesthesia and Analgesia 54:277–281, 1975.

Kakkar VV, Howe CT, Nicolaides AN, et al.: Deep vein thrombosis of the leg: Is there a "high risk" group? American Journal of Surgery 120:527–532, 1970.

Kakkar VV: Prevention of fatal postoperative thromboembolism by low dose heparin: An international multicenter trial. Lancet 2:45–51, 1975.

Ko KC & Paradise RR: The effect of halothane on the contractility of atria from starved rats. Anesthesiology 34:557–561, 1971.

Kuechel SW: Anesthesia and the Geriatric Patient. New York: Grune & Stratton, 1983.

Law DH: Current concepts in nutrition: Total parenteral nutrition. New England Journal of Medicine 297:1104, 1977.

Lowenstein E, Little JW, Hing ML: Prevention of cerebral embolization from flushing radial-artery cannulae. New England Journal of Medicine 285:1414–1415, 1971.

Luczun ME: Postanesthesia Nursing—A Comprehensive Guide. Rockville, Md.: Aspen, 1984.

Lueck J, Brewer JI, et al.: Observation of an organism found in patients with gestational tiophoblastic disease and in patients with toxemia of pregnancy. American Journal of Obstetrics and Gynecology 145(1):15–38, 1983.

McGoldrick KE: Anesthetic implications of drug abuse. Anes Rev 7:12–17, 1980.

Nunn JF & Payne JP: Hypoxemia after general anesthesia. Lancet 11:531, 1962.

Owen OE, Morgan AP, Kemp HG, et al.: Brain metabolism during fasting. Journal of Clinical Investigation 46:1589–1595, 1967.

Palmer KNV, Gardiner AJS, McGregor MH: Hypoxemia after partial gastrectomy. Thorax 20:73–75, 1965.

Paul DR, Hoyt JL, Boutras AR: Cardiovascular and respiratory changes in response to change of posture in the very obese. Anesthesiology 45:73–78, 1976.

Pell S & D'Alonso CA: Three-year study of myocardial infarction in a large employed population. Journal of the American Medical Association 175:463–470, 1961.

Pontoppidan H & Beecher HK: Progressive loss of protective reflexes in the airway with the advance of age. Journal of the American Medical Association 174:2209–2213, 1960.

Pontoppidan H, Geffin B, Lowenstein E: Acute respiratory failure in the adult. New England Journal of Medicine 277:690–698, 1972.

Postlethwait RW & Johnson WD: Complications following surgery for duodenal ulcer in obese patients. Archives of Surgery 105:438–440, 1972.

Roizen MF: Preoperative evaluation of patients with diseases that require special preoperative evaluation and intraoperative management. In RD Miller (Ed.), Anesthesia (vol. 1). New York: Churchill Livingstone, 1981, p. 59.

Sheldon GF & Way L: Total parenteral nutrition: The state of the art. Western Journal of Medicine 127:398, 1977.

Shnider S & Levinson G: Obstetric anesthesia. In RD Miller (Ed.), Anesthesia (vol. 2). New York: Churchill Livingstone, 1981, pp. 1133–1168.

Snell AM: The relation of obesity to fatal postoperative pulmonary embolism. Archives of Surgery 15:237–239, 1927.

Snyder SW, Wheeler AS, James FM: The use of nitroglycerin to control severe hypertension of pregnancy during cesarean section. Anesthesiology 51:563, 1979.

Speroff L: Toxemia of pregnancy: Mechanism and therapeutic management. American Journal of Cardiology 32:582, 1973.

Strauss RG, Keefer JR, Burke T, et al.: Hemodynamic monitoring of cardiogenic pulmonary edema complicating toxemia of pregnancy. Obstetrics and Gynecology 55:170, 1980.

Vaughan MS: Nursing treatment of hypothermia in adult recovery room postsurgical patients. Dissertation, University of Arizona, 1980.

Vaughan MS: Nursing care of the severely obese patient. In BR Brown (Ed.), Anesthesia and the Obese Patient. Philadelphia: Davis, 1982.

Vaughan RW: Anesthetic considerations in jejunoileal small bowel bypass for morbid obesity. Anesthesia and Analgesia 53:421–429, 1974.

Vaughan RW: Anesthetic management of the morbidly obese patient. In BR Brown (Ed.), Anesthesia and the Obese Patient. Philadelphia: Davis, 1982.

Vaughan RW, Engelhardt RC, Wise L: Postoperative hypoxemia in obese patients. Annals of Surgery 180:877–882, 1974.

Vaughan RW & Wise L: Choice of abdominal operative incision in the obese patient: A study using blood gas measurements. Annals of Surgery 181:829–835, 1975.

Vaughan RW & Wise L: Postoperative arterial blood gas measurement: Effect of position on gas exchange. Annals of Surgery 182:705–709, 1975.

Vesell: On the significance of host factors that affect drug disposition. Clinical Pharmacology & Therapeutics 31(1):2, 1982.

Walts LF, Miller J, Davidson MB, Brown J: Perioperative management of diabetes mellitus. Anesthesiology 55:104–109, Aug., 1981.

Walts LF: Managing diabetes during surgery. AORN Journal, 37(5):928–941, April, 1983.

Whelchel JD: Renal failure patients in the recovery room. Current Review for Recovery Room Nurses 2(12):1980.

PART IV

Professional Trends and Issues

Chapter 16

Coming Trends in Postanesthesia Nursing

Kay E. Fraulini

The present chapter discusses two trends that the author believes will significantly affect the future of postanesthesia nursing: specialization and computerization.

NURSE SPECIALIZATION

The clinical nurse-specialist has been defined by Baker and Kramer (1970) as a nurse prepared at the master's level who is responsible for or engaged in giving care to selected groups of patients. The goal of this specialist is the improvement of patient care, and the nurse-specialist's function may include direct patient care, the planning of patient care, patient and staff education, and consultation. In Pearson's view, the clinical specialist is a motivator; a knowledgeable person who supports and encourages personnel as they move toward independent thought.

The clinical nurse-specialist is role model, change agent, teacher, and consultant—someone with expert clinical competence and the ability to guide and evaluate nursing practice. Nurse-specialists who wish to pursue educational and administrative roles need a sound base in advanced clinical nursing through master's degree studies. Further, students wishing to prepare for a role in nursing education should have the opportunity to study the theories of teaching, learning, and the philosophy and mission of the institutions in which they expect to function. Similarly, preparation for administration should include organizational and management theories and political strategies related to health care systems (ANA, 1978).

Master's Degree Programs in Nursing

The nurse-specialist is one who functions within a specified and clearly designated field, drawing upon scientific knowledge and extensive experience. The specialist functions within defined practice boundaries using related theory and research.

Increased emphasis upon nursing theory and research for leadership roles is critical to the quality of nursing practice and education. The testing of theory and the utilization of research designs relevant to the improvement of nursing care are thus integral parts of master's programs in nursing. Examples of research studies appropriate in programs leading to the master's degree include medium-scale research problems or questions, replication of earlier clinical nursing studies, initiation of pilot projects to test hypotheses, testing of tools for research designs, participation in an ongoing investigation with a nurse-researcher, and development of group projects with faculty, students, and other health care providers so that students can contribute to a larger study of nursing and health care. Creation of a climate that encourages nursing and health research is vital to maintain the enthusiasm and excitement that are part of any scholarly setting (ANA, 1978).

The Clinical Nurse-Specialist in the PACU

As some organizations have discovered, there is a place in the PACU for the clinical nurse-specialist (CNS). Appendix 16–1 gives a job description of a CNS specific to the PACU developed at the University of California, San Francisco. UCSF has a clinical and administrative ladder similar to the levels of practice described in Chapter 2.

The clinical nurse-specialist brings highly desirable skills, training, and experience to the PACU. However, as it has with so much else the PACU has lagged behind other areas in recruiting, hiring, and developing clinical nurse-specialists. There are several reasons for this:

1. Nursing administrators have a very important part to play in the evolution of the clinical nurse-specialist role. To abdicate leadership responsibility after establishing and filling the CNS position is to endanger the achievement of the goal of improved patient care. The organization must plan for the introduction of the new role, offer guidelines for utilization of the role, and give clear-cut clues to appropriate behavior of other workers in relating to the role. Although time consuming and expensive, these activities are

necessary if the full benefit of the clinical nurse-specialist is to be felt (Baker & Kramer, 1970).

2. One of the functions of the CNS is change agent. Change is always difficult in a conservative profession. It has to be accepted that adjustment to new concepts and practices might be slow and sometimes painful. The introduction of any new role into an established organization requires staff involvement and administrative support. Practical questions raised by other workers in regard to the threat of a new role are: "Who is this person? What effect will the CNS have on my job? How do I relate to this nurse?" These are questions that need to be answered to some degree of satisfaction in order to avoid confusion. The introduction of a role in the process of unfolding presents even more demands. Not only is there the threat posed by the impact of the new role on existing roles, but there is also the concurrent fear and threat of unknown possibilities—what the new role may become.

3. Patients are another factor. In a study by Hardy (1975), patients were asked to evaluate nursing care following implementation of the clinical nurse-specialist role. Although patients evaluated nursing care very favorably, their failure to see nurses as personnel who should carry out many patient care activities and be involved in patient rehabilitation raises serious question as to why patients should support continuing or advanced education for nurses. Although it is not totally clear how patients perceive nurses, it has been suggested that nurses are perceived by the public as being skilled technicians rather than skilled professionals. If this is so, perhaps there is little reason for the public to feel the need to support the educational or research activities of nurses.

Yet is is the belief of the profession that if nursing is to have a significant impact in meeting the health needs of this nation, it must prepare scholarly practitioners who are able to translate their advanced preparation into practice (Rotkovich, 1976). It seems reasonable to expect that much of nursing literature in the next decade will be written by specialists as they attempt to apply the scientific method to clinical practice.

The Practitioner-Teacher

One of the structural issues that greatly saps the power and influence of nurses is the separation of education and service. In response to this, the practitioner-teacher role was developed and extensively implemented at Rush-Presbyterian–St. Luke's Medical Center in Chicago.

The Practitioner-Teacher: Implementing the Model. The idea of one nurse serving in both a service and educational position has been part of the nursing profession since the early days of collegiate education (Morton,

1973). The merging of service and education did not, however, develop as one would like. Instead, nursing split into two distinct areas of performance: (1) service, or the group stereotyped as task-oriented and resistant to change; and (2) education, or the group stereotyped as not working with reality but having an Ivory Tower Syndrome. In recent years, members of the nursing profession have begun to test various ways to decrease the split that developed between education and service. One such form of unification was given the title of dual role or joint appointment. In these types of roles, the identified extent of practitioner involvement tends to rest on the degree of flexibility and negotiation capacities of the respective service and educational institutions. Institutional backing and political aptitude, therefore, become major factors in performing a dual role.

A second type of role depicting unification is that of practitioner-teacher. In contrast to the dual role of joint appointment, the individual practitioner-teacher carries the major responsibility for flexibility and negotiation. All nursing service and education at Rush-Presbyterian is under one administration, which facilitates the practitioner-teacher assuming responsibility for negotiating within that system for the fullest expression of her or his professional role.

Both the joint appointment and practitioner-teacher approaches allow expression of the professional role and can result in improved nursing care. Sime and associates (1970) identified five reasons to close the gap between service and education. The reasons illustrate the need for increased effort in the area of unification.

1. The scarcity of experts in every area of nursing requires simultaneous utilization of skills.
2. Advances in nursing knowledge will come only when evolving theory can be seen as relevant to practice and can be applied to solving present-day nursing care problems.
3. Schools of nursing and service would complement one another for laboratories and nursing service for manpower.
4. Clinical specialists with master's degrees want jobs that combine the intellectual stimulation of the academic environment with the challenge of devising and providing quality nursing care.
5. Monies would be more available for salaries.

The practitioner-teacher position has capacities for full expression of the professional role: clinical practice, education, administration, and research (see Appendix 16–2).

The experience of putting into operation the practitioner-teacher model at Rush-Presbyterian has repeatedly revealed the need for strong administrative support of this role. On the other hand, the practitioner-teacher must maintain responsibility for developing skills in clinical practice, education, administration, and research.

Another key advantage of being part of the care endeavor is the defining of research problems. The nature and quality of the focus on the issues to be investigated is of a different order when they come from the real world of practice rather than the speculation of the classroom. In addition, the practitioner-teacher is in a highly advantageous position to disseminate research findings so that they become available to all nurses practicing in the organization. A cybernetic means for improving the quality of care comes out of this arrangement. The monitoring of care becomes scientific and manageable, and better safeguards are provided to patients. The practitioner-teacher role is the prime means of gluing the nursing efforts into a highly organized and sophisticated design (Christman, 1979).

There is a desperate need for research in the perioperative period. It is no longer acceptable to base practice on tradition, heresay, and inference. The clinical nurse-specialist, the practitioner-teacher, and the doctorally prepared nurse-researcher must (with the support of nursing and hospital administration) focus their efforts on building a scientific base for the practice of perioperative nursing.

These issues of nurse specialization are issues common to the profession as a whole and are linked to our survival. The full professional role for any clinical profession includes the four major components of service, education, consultation, and research. Society accords the rights and privileges of professional status in proportion to the extent that the full role is used to benefit society.

Mandate for the Future

Nurse-specialists, both clinical and administrative, must be sought out and used to their full capabilities in the PACU and during the perianesthetic period. This may be the only way for nurses to secure a place in the future of perianesthetic care. Clearly, there is a mandate for nursing and hospital administrators to support master's and doctorally prepared nurses in this critical care setting.

A growing handful of nurse-specialists practice in PACUs across the nation. It is exciting to see what they have already accomplished—the books and papers that are being written, the research underway, the growing peer relationships with anesthesiologists and other M.D.s, the contribution to nursing education, and so on. The potential for professional growth and the strengthening of autonomy is almost unlimited. Some changes that could be made by the influence of nurse-specialists on the future practice of perianesthetic nursing are described in the next few sections.

Research. More and more nursing practice will be based on scientific data generated by nurses and colleagues in the other disciplines. The nurse-specialist will increasingly demand quantitative answers to questions regarding patient care and personnel management. As an example, studies that have already contributed data include those on preoperative teaching (especially related to postoperative ventilatory function), temperature (hypothermia), predictive indices of postoperative morbidity, positioning as it affects various physiologic parameters, drug administration and circadian rhythm, and the development and validation of new postanesthetic assessment tools. The list is much longer, and the nurse-specialist must consider the communication of these research findings a primary responsibility. PACU nurses should understand that much research pertinent to their practice is being done. Nurses must think professionally, searching the research journals, attending scientific meetings, and so on. After critiquing the studies, the nurse-specialist and staff can make decisions relative to implementation of the findings.

Some very interesting findings will be gained from future nursing studies that look at postanesthetic complications. Many PACUs are currently collecting data on critical incidents. However, the PACU nurse knows little about the patient's later postanesthetic progress. It is suspected that many patients develop problems after leaving the PACU, and that in a large percentage of these cases the PACU nurse had a nagging hunch that the patient would benefit from continued intensive monitoring. It is possible that if we quantitate this we may have overwhelming indications for a Phase 2 recovery or Intermediate Care Unit. Walts, in writing about the diabetic patient, has proposed a postanesthetic endocrine area where the anesthesiologist could continue to monitor blood glucose; there are many other patients who would benefit from such vigilance.

We need to ask what exactly we accomplish in the PACU. Is it, in the literal sense, recovery from anesthesia? No. We know, for example, that the half-life of almost every drug administered far exceeds the average PACU stay. The patient therefore leaves the PACU with the lingering effects of numerous drugs and agents. What we have accomplished, with the general anesthetic patient at least, is return of consciousness. Perhaps the Swedes are right in calling the area "Uppvakningsavdelning," the "wake-up room." Once again, nursing studies that measure recovery of the various body systems from anesthesia must be undertaken in the future.

Some studies undertaken by physicians should lend themselves to future nursing study. Thompson and associates (1983), for example, have looked at music as a complement to anesthesia. They devised a compact, durable, clean, and personalized music system in order to provide music to surgical patients. When music was offered as an option in the PACU, 79 percent of patients expressed a desire to listen. Comments have shown that patients are enthusiastic over this method of passing time and relieving anxiety. Especially appreciative patients include those with sensory deprivation from bandaged eyes and patients immobilized from regional anesthesia. Ambulatory surgical patients found it a pleasant preoccupation while waiting for medications to wear off before hospital discharge. This would seem to be highly desirable and deserves further evaluation.

Consultation. The nurse-specialist should be able to function as a consultant in the PACU, operating room, surgical floors, intensive care units, outpatient facilities such as pain clinics, and so on. She or he can be consultant to the anesthesiologist. The nurse-specialist should be able to consult with other hospital PACUs (those that do not have benefit of nurse-specialists).

As beginning steps, the nurse-specialist and staff nurses could offer to publish a column in a departmental newsletter. This column could address topics of concern related to anesthesia and perioperative care. Other nurses could become aware of the PACU nurse's expertise.

Through professional organizations, PACU nurses can network to establish themselves as a resource in perianesthetic care.

Knowledge of broad concepts such as pain, hypothermia, preoperative and postoperative care, and resuscitation could make the PACU nurse-specialist a consultant to the general public.

Certain recurring problems would lend themselves to input from the PACU nurse-consultant:

1. Staffing and scheduling.
2. Patient classification systems.
3. Quality assurance.
4. Standards of care (available from ASPAN)—specifically, implementation and evaluation.
5. Clinical problems:
    Who should extubate the patient?
    Criteria for extubation.
    Standing orders.
    Who should discharge the patient?
    What type of pain medication?
    How should we collect physiologic data and how can we use it most effectively?
    Temperature monitoring.
    Care planning.
    Postanesthetic care beyond the PACU

Administration. Chapters 3 and 4 provide excellent examples of how the nurse-specialist can use the administration component in her or his PACU professional role.

Clinical Practice. It is acknowledged in nursing literature that the CNS position emerged in answer to the increasing lack of clinically skilled nurses at the bedside. This shortage resulted from the upward managerial movement of experienced nurses within the profession. These experienced nurses were advanced professionally but were thereby removed from administering direct patient care. The CNS role was envisioned as a reversal of this trend. Thus the provision of direct care to patients has been a major component of the definition of the nurse-specialist since its origin (Kohnke, 1977).

The CNS is responsible for delivering high-quality patient care and providing more advanced services and skills not yet available from the general nursing staff. Regarding the nursing staff, the CNS involved in direct care not only learns of but experiences the obstacles and constraints under which the staff must function, and can then better identify the need for reality-based nursing care methods and tools and can help to develop them.

The specialist's direct involvement may also improve and facilitate the health team's interdisciplinary effort, resulting in a heightened perception by other professionals of the validity of the nurse's role. With regard to physicians, the specialist can demonstrate clinical competence and establish collaborative, collegial relationships (Felder, 1983). From these relationships—begun at the bedside where both are caring for the patient—additional research and publications will be generated.

Education. The role descriptions given in the Appendixes provide clear direction for the CNS. Teaching responsibilities include the staff, nursing students, patients, and families. The CNS must be instrumental in bringing students to the PACU, designing learning experiences, and evaluating these experiences. She or he should actively recruit graduate nursing students to the area and serve as a preceptor.

COMPUTERIZATION

The past several decades have witnessed the growth of computers in health care institutions. It is predicted that in the next decade nursing will be the professional group that will demand and receive data-processing support. The profession and the technology have evolved to a point where this is now feasible.

Computer Support for Nursing Practice

Automated methods for recording nursing observations exist and are now commercially available from computer vendors.

Two general approaches to the automated recording of nursing observations were developed. The first approach was to create a computer-readable form consisting of statements arranged in groups adequate for describing most patient care or behavior in the most frequently used terms. More recently the reduced cost of computing equipment has resulted in abandoning the batch-processing mode in favor of on-line processing. A computerized library of frequently used phrases is arranged in subject categories; the nurse then chooses the phrase or combination of phrases that best describes the patient's condition. For example, by selecting a primary subject such as "sleeping habits," a screen "menu" of standard descriptions would appear, allowing the nurse to select additional comments such as "slept through breakfast—voluntarily" or "woke early at _____ A.M." When completed, the nursing station printer immediately prints a standard, easy-to-read, complete narrative that could then be attached to the patient's chart.

The second general approach has been to develop a "branching questionnaire." This approach utilizes a terminal with a display screen. The terminal is activated by a conventional typewriter keyboard. The terminal displays a list of choices, and the user selects a choice by pressing the corresponding number on the keyboard or touching the terminal with a light-sensitive input device called a light pen. The terminal then displays a further list of choices appropriate to the original selection. Thus, the nurse is led through a series of questions that can be "customized" for each patient. For example, a question might be "Skin intact? Yes, No." If yes, no further questions in that set would be necessary. If no then other choices might appear, such as a choice between "wounds" or "pressure sores." The option of free-form input is usually available via the terminal's keyboard. At the user's signal of completion of the entry, the computer processes the information and provides a narrative printout for the patient's chart.

Numerous advantages have been claimed for these approaches to the automated method of recording nursing observations:

- Increased numbers of observations as a result of forced recall.
- Increased accuracy and reliability of observations.
- Greater legibility and thus accuracy of the notes, which results in faster reading and therefore increased use.
- Less time spent writing notes.
- Ready statistical analyses and easier nursing audit because of the use of standard terminology.
- Use as a teaching tool by providing a guide for observations.

These advantages directly relate to nursing practice. Better observations—that is, increased number, accuracy, and reliability of observations—facilitate better assessment, planning, and evaluating of nursing care. Less time spent in writing the notes provides more time for assessment, planing, implementing, and evaluating care—that is, for the nursing process. Increased use and accuracy of interpretation of the notes furthers consistency and continuity of the plan for nursing care. Statistical analysis facilitates research that would ultimately lead to refinements in the nursing process and to improvement in patient care.

Planning Patient Care

The following is a summary of the advantages of automated care plans over the traditional methods of using nursing care plans:

- Time is saved by eliminating the necessity for daily handwriting of patient assignments and by decreasing the amount of verbal explanation required.
- Accountability is increased because personnel have printouts of care plans of each of their patients.
- Errors and omissions are decreased.
- Consistency of care from shift to shift and day to day is increased; patient care is more complete and comprehensive.
- Judgments for nursing care become the specific responsibility of the professional nurse, who now has tools available to assist in making nursing judgments.

Patient Monitoring

Originally, the major area of development of automated patient monitoring was coronary care. In coronary care units and pacemaker clinics, computers were inititally used to monitor electrocardiograms, analyze the information, and reduce the volumes of data formerly produced to manageable proportions—generally to some type of graph. The computers were also programmed to recognize deviations from accepted norms and to alert attending personnel to the deviation by an indication such as an alarm or light.

In addition to monitoring arrhythmias, computers are used today in acute care areas such as emergency, intensive care, coronary care, and neonatal intensive care for hemodynamic and vital sign monitoring, calculation of physiologic indices such as peripheral vascular resistance and cardiac output, and environmental regulations of isolettes. Sophisticated computerized ICU monitoring systems for management of patient data are now in use around the world. In the United States, Spain, and Canada, as well as other countries, ICU computer systems are used to monitor patient heart rates, arterial blood pressure, temperature, respiratory rate, central venous pressure, intracranial pressure, and pulmonary artery pressures.

These automated approaches to patient monitoring free the nurse from the technician role of watching machinery and permit the nurse to focus attention on the patient, the family, and the nursing process. It is now widely accepted that computerized cardiac monitoring of patients dramatically increases the early detection of arrhythmias and contributes to decreased mortality of CCU patients. Additionally, such systems have been shown to facilitate data retrieval for comparison of the patient's current conditions with conditions at an earlier time (Beckman & associates, 1981). Finally, Beckman and coworkers (1981) have identified an increase in consultation among members of the health care team in relation to the interpretation of the information generated by these computerized physiological monitoring systems.

Integrated Patient Data Bases

As hospital information systems moved beyond the developmental stage and were marketed and installed on a wide scale, they provided nurses with access to a great deal of information about their practice and increased time to analyze and consider this information. Simultaneously, the level of educational preparation of nurses began to rise. During the 1960s and 1970s the profession saw the proliferation of master's and doctoral programs that produced a core of nurses with much greater appreciation for, as well as sophistication and skill at, data analysis and research. Ball and Hannah (1984) believe that the consequence of this concurrent evolution of both technology and the nursing profession is about to coincide and facilitate advances in nursing practice of astronomical proportions. We are just beginning to initiate the cycle whereby information availability promotes greater understanding of nursing decision-making and diagnosis, which in turn facilitates higher-level functioning of nurses, which in turn generates additional information and further stimulates the cycle (Fig. 16–1).

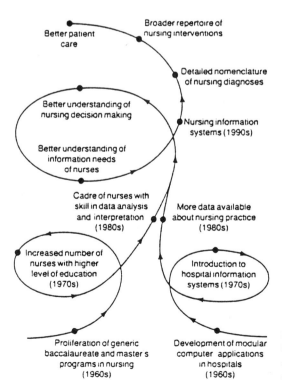

Figure 16–1. The nursing information cycle. *(Courtesy of Ball MJ & Hannah KJ: Using Computers in Nursing. Reston, Va.: Reston, 1984.)*

However, one more technological advance is necessary. The development of relational data base management systems for use in patient care is imperative for nursing to fully exploit technology. As McHugh and Shultz (1982) suggest:

> Hospital nursing departments have followed the . . . frozen-asset path for their data resources. Information contained in existing modular and turnkey systems cannot be easily merged with other computer stored information.

Experienced users of computers in business have largely abandoned the traditional modular approach to computer file handling that is currently being marketed to the health care industry. Data-based management systems have long been available (Fry & Sibley, 1976) to reduce data redundancy, provide quality data, maintain data integrity, protect data security, interface relatively easily with technological advances, and facilitate access to a single integrated collection of data for numerous applications of multiple user groups.

Application to the PACU
The foregoing points have application to nursing in the PACU. Undeniably, the practice of anesthesiology continues to affect the practice of PACU nursing. As an example, computerized anesthesia records are being developed and plans are for PACU records to follow. The authors suggest that the system that generates this record is designed for flexibility, allows full editing of any data, whether entered manually or automatically, and that the plotter prints the record with accuracy and clarity heretofore unattainable (Rosen & Rosenzweig, 1985).

Presently, the computer is also being used for operating room scheduling, workload monitoring, physiologic monitoring, and the processing and distribution of supplies. The onus of computer literacy is on the PACU nurse, and the challenge of level-III (Table 16–1) proficiency will hopefully entice some. What can we do to prepare ourselves?

Preparing Nurses to Use Computers
Farsighted individuals have long recognized the benefits of the use of computers in health care delivery and advocated the widespread dissemination of this technology. Health care professionals, including nurses, have created an extensive body of literature documenting experiences in the fields of health care computing and medical informatics. The current need is for the formal development of curricula that address educational training in medical informatics for health care practitioners at all levels. Anderson and associates (1974) clearly identified the necessity for more and better education of both practitioners and students of the health care disciplines about medical informatics. Many experts have consistently

TABLE 16–1. LEVELS OF COMPUTER PROFICIENCY

Roles of Nurses in Medical Informatics	Levels of Educational Preparation in Medical and Nursing Informatics
Consumer Role Users of automated medical information systems.	*Level I* General knowledge of computers and data processing.
Provider Role Participate in designing and selecting systems to be implemented. Articulate to computer program designers and systems engineers the needs of nurses and patients relative to automated medical information systems. Teach and interpret the jargon and basic tenets of nursing to information specialists. Teach nursing students and practitioners to use automated medical information systems.	*Level II* Maintain nursing orientation and focus, but communicate and participate with data processing professionals in developing solutions for computing problems related to nursing.
Participate as consultants to companies developing computer systems for use in health care or as project directors of studies on the effects of implementing such systems on health care delivery and nursing practice.	*Level III* Major commitment to computing and data processing, training in both nursing and computer science, primarily involved in developing and initiating new computer systems.

(Courtesy of Ball MJ & Hannah KJ. Using Computers in Nursing. Reston, Va.: Reston, 1984.)

identified the lack of education of users and systems engineers as a major problem in the failure of attempts to implement automated health care systems. Unfortunately, as Ronald (1979) points out, little progress has been made toward meeting this need:

> The development of automated systems in nursing has progressed very slowly . . . [and] the success of many computerized information systems has been extremely limited. Two basic reasons for this are the lack of technical literacy on the part of health professionals combined with the lack of knowledge of the health care field by computer scientists.

Continuing Education

The need of practicing nurses for information about the use of computers in nursing can be accomplished by providing continuing education workshops. These have been sponsored by universities, community colleges, hospitals, and professional associations. The objectives for such workshops are consistent with achieving level I preparation (Table 16–1) and are aimed at developing basic computer literacy among a cadre of practicing nurses. Increasingly, PACU nurses must demand this as part of their orientation or continuing education.

REFERENCES

American Nurses Association: Statement on graduate education in nursing. Kansas City, Mo., 1978, pp. 1–7.

Anderson J, Gremy F, & Pages JC: Education in Informatics for Health Personnel. Amsterdam: North-Holland, 1974.

Baker C & Kramer M: To define or not to define: The role of the clinical nurse specialist. Nursing Forum, 9:45–55, 1970.

Ball MJ & Hannah KJ: Using Computers in Nursing. Reston, Va.: Reston, 1984.

Beckmann E, Cammack BF, & Harris B: Observation on computers in an intensive care unit. Heart & Lung 10(6):1055–1057, 1981.

Christman L: The nurse clinical specialist. In Riehl J & McVay JW (Eds.): The Clinical Nurse Specialist: Interpretations. New York: Appleton-Century-Crofts, 1973.

Christman, L. The practitioner-teacher. Nurse Educator, 8–11 March–April, 1979.

Felder LA: Direct patient care and independent practice. In Hamric AB & Spross J: The Clinical Nurse Specialist in Theory and Practice. New York: Grune & Stratton, 1983, pp. 59–60.

Fry & Sibley: Evaluation of data-base management systems. ACM Computing Surveys 8(1), 1976.

Hamric AB & Spross J: The Clinical Nurse Specialist in Theory and Practice. New York: Grune & Stratton, 1983.

Hardy ME: Implementation of unit management: Patient's perception of the quality of general hospital care and nursing care. In Batey M (Ed.): Communication Nursing Research: Critical Issues in Access To Data. Boulder, Co.: Wiche, 1975, 325:8.

Kohnke M (Ed.). The Case for Consultation in Nursing: Designs for Professional Practice. New York: Wiley, 1977.

Luczun MF: Postanesthesia Nursing—A Comprehensive Guide. Rockville, Md.: Aspen, 1984.

McHugh M & Schultz S: Computer technology in hospital nursing departments: Future applications and implications. In Blum BI (Ed.), Proceedings of the sixth annual symposium on computer application in medical care, Institute of Electrical and Electronics Engineers, Los Angeles, 1982, pp. 557–561.

Morton BF: Nursing service and education in a comprehensive health care center. Journal of Nursing Administration, May–June, 1973.

Riehl J & McVay JW (Ed.): The Clinical Nurse Specialist: Interpretations. New York: Appleton-Century-Crofts, 1973.

Ronald JS: Computers and undergraduate nursing education. Journal of Nursing Education 18(9):4–9, 1979.

Rosen AS & Rosenzweig W: Computerized anesthesia record. Anesthesiology 62(1):100–101, Jan., 1985.

Rotkovich, R. (Ed.). The Role of the Clinical Nursing Specialist. New York: Wiley, 1976.

Sime E, Sparrow A, Harriman V: Faculty-supervisor: A dual position. Nursing Outlook 18:3, March, 1970.

University of California, San Francisco: Job description, Clinical Nurse V, San Francisco.

Walts LF: Managing diabetes during surgery. AORN Journal 37(5):828–841, April, 1983.

APPENDIX 16–1

Job Description of Clinical Nurse V (PACU)

REQUIREMENTS

1. Current licensure as R.N. in the State of California; diploma or associate degree with 5 years of recent clinical critical care experience; or baccalaureate degree in nursing with 3 years of recent clinical critical care experience; or a master's degree in nursing with 2 years of recent clinical care experience.
2. Clinical experience includes demonstrated advanced skill and expertise in critical care nursing.
3. A minimum of 1 year recent experience in administration and/or education.

General Description: The Clinical Nurse V has in-depth knowledge of critical care and postanesthesia nursing and, under general direction, applies theories and concepts derived from the biologic, natural, and behavioral sciences and areas related to her nursing specialty; and in addition may perform the duties prior to her job as Clinical Nurse V. Responsibility and Accountability: Responsible for nursing care behaviors described in Clinical Nurse V job description and accountable to the Administrative Level IV.

BEHAVIORS

I. Nursing Process

A. Assessment
1. Utilizes a patient-centered approach to assess specific needs of the PACU patient population.

2. Uses knowledge of a variety of conceptual models in order to consider alternatives that explain and predict present or potential patient and/or staff problems.
3. Selects and adapts models for meeting the needs of the PACU staff and patient population.
4. Uses specialized clinical knowledge to assess the needs of the PACU staff and population.
5. Uses a wide repertoire of assessment tools to determine the data base for the PACU staff and patient population.
6. Modifies and adapts assessment tools to meet the needs of the PACU staff and patient population.
7. Develops assessment tools to meet the emerging needs of a changing staff and patient population.
8. Assesses the social system of the work setting to identify directions for change in the delivery of nursing care service for the PACU patient population.
9. Assesses the needs for the numbers and levels of personnel required to provide quality nursing care for a particular patient population in collaboration with the Clinical Nurse IV, and makes recommendations to Administrative IV.
10. Demonstrates advanced understanding of physiologic monitoring and physiologic alterations and treatments occurring in the immediate postoperative period.
11. Assesses learning needs of PACU staff and modes of delivering appropriate information and learning experiences; such as orientation, continuing education.

B. Planning
1. Plans the selection of a specific patient population for direct care in order to:
   a. classify the common nursing needs that define the relationship between cause and effect of nursing intervention.
   b. test nonstandardized nursing interventions with unpredictable outcomes and bring them into the realm of predictability.
   c. determine methods of orienting patients to the nursing care plan developed to meet specific needs.
2. Collaborate with other unit personnel and departments to provide support services that facilitate the delivery of patient care.
3. Participate in groups to plan strategies for affecting changes in health care system.
4. Plan educational programs and experiences, such as orientation programs and continuing education programs, to meet learning needs of PACU staff.

C. Implementation
1. Identifies methods of problem identification in order to assess her own practice and serve as a positive role model for staff.
2. Gives direct care to patients to:
    a. explore areas of patient problems.
    b. identify learning needs of staff.
3. Collaborates with Clinical Nurse IV to develop, implement, and evaluate models of practice for PACU patient population.
4. Collaborates with Administrative IV and submits specifications for the numbers and levels of personnel needed to care for the PACU patient population.
5. Participates in efforts to affect changes in health care delivery and in legislation that affects nursing practice.
6. Serves as a chairman of the Quality Assurance Committee for the PACU and makes recommendations for change to Administrative IV.
7. Participates in and monitors programs designed to produce effective and efficient use of supplies and equipment.
8. Implements clinical programs designed to provide ancillary support services that facilitate the delivery of patient care.
9. Implements education programs for PACU staff—e.g., orientation and continuing education.

D. Evaluation
1. Develops, with Administrative IV, evaluation mechanisms to be used by clients to evaluate the quality of nursing care received.
2. Develops, with Administrative IV, criteria to establish evaluation protocols.
3. Evaluates the environment in which care is given and makes recommendations for change.
4. Evaluates the long-term consequences of nursing interventions.
5. Submits annual report that evaluates the program of care within the PACU, forecasts directions for change, and reflects self-evaluation.
6. Establishes future goals based on evaluation of yearly activities.
7. Submits to Administrative IV the outcome of the nursing audits with suggested action.
8. Evaluates the effectiveness of auxiliary services designed to facilitate the delivery of patient care.
9. Evaluates educational programs and experiences and makes

appropriate revisions based on needs of changing patient and employee populations.

II. Teaching

   A. Patient and Family
1. Initiates the development of written criteria for teaching standards for specific groups of patients.
2. Collaborates with Clinical Nurse III to formulate written objectives based on the learning needs of the PACU patient population.
3. Evaluates and revises teaching standards based on the needs of a changing patient population.

   B. Staff
1. Develops written criteria for a planned unit level orientation program for staff.
2. Collaborates with Clinical Nurse IV to formulate written objectives and contracts based on learning needs of the specific new employee.
3. Collaborates with Clinical Nurse III and IV to adapt the planned unit level orientation to the identified learning needs of the specific new employee.
4. Evaluates and revises the planned unit orientation program based on the needs of a changing client and staff population.
5. Collaborates with the Clinical Nurse III and IV to plan appropriate learning experiences for all levels of staff.
6. Collaborates with Administrative IV to provide situations in which knowledge is articulated and disseminated to staff.

   C. Program
1. Develops theoretical framework that guides decisions about patient and staff teaching programs.
2. Establishes teaching/learning priorities for patients and staff.
3. Develops learning resource materials to facilitate the teaching process for both patients and staff.
4. Actively contributes to the growth and development of the Clinical Nurse III:
   a. orients and assists Clinical Nurse III to role function.
   b. counsels and supports Clinical Nurse III to role function.
   c. participates in peer review for Clinical Nurse III.
5. Collaborates with Administrative IV and Clinical Nurse IVs and Vs to develop and implement intradepartmental teaching programs for patients and staff.

      6. Participates in the evaluation of the total educational program with PACU staff and Administrative Levels IV.

D. Students
    1. Secures a nonsalaried clinical appointment to faculty of the School of Nursing if and when appropriate.
    2. Participates in curriculum development of the School of Nursing when appropriate.
    3. Serves as a preceptor for students at a variety of learning levels.
    4. Identifies ongoing learning programs available to the PACU and invites students and faculty to participate.
    5. Participates in evaluation of student clinical experience and individual evaluation with the Clinical Nurse III and provides feedback for clinical faculty of record.

E. Communications
    1. Participates in designing communication systems to facilitate the exchange of information between PACU and OR as well as other departments.
    2. Promotes an effective communication network in the PACU.
    3. Initiates planned change and evaluates the outcomes to improve quality of patient care through conscious, deliberate, and collaborative effort.
    4. Communicates rationale, progress, and evaluation of change before implementation.
    5. Designs the methodology used in the change process.
    6. Establishes and maintains a communication system with other departments and agencies that are used as resources for patient care needs—e.g., Respiration, ECG, X-ray, CSR, Pharmacy.
    7. Provides consultation to Clinical Nurse III for conflict resolution.
    8. Communicates final decisions regarding standards of nursing practice to all levels of personnel.

III. Evaluation

A. Uses systematic methods of scientific inquiry to investigate patient care and nursing problems.
    1. Audits patient charts and care plans and submits audit results to Administrative IV.
    2. Observes practice.

3. Reviews guidelines for practice and helps develop new tools or revise existing ones.
4. Supports and encourages spirit of inquiry in others.

B. Works toward the modification or removal of agency and other restraints on improving the quality of patient care and nursing practice.

C. Recommends appointment of candidates for Clinical III, IV positions.

D. Evaluates the clinical competency of personnel and makes formal recommendations for retention and promotion.

E. Evaluates own personal performance based on attainment of immediate and long-term goals which are congruent with agency objectives.

F. Begins to develop framework for joint practice review.

IV. Research

A. Actively participates in clinical research.
1. Investigates methods of delivering care.
2. Studies response to illness in order to plan and implement preventive and rehabilitative measures.
3. Assists staff in interpreting and implementing research findings.
4. Uses research findings to modify theory as it relates to clinical practice.

B. Communicates research findings.

(Courtesy of the University of California, San Francisco.)

Job Description of Practitioner-Teacher

GENERAL DESCRIPTION

Practitioner-teachers are faculty members who actively effect quality patient care in the clinical and classroom settings through an integrated role as clinician, educator, consultant, and researcher. The practitioner-teacher (P.T.) role is highly individualized; each P.T. contracts with the departmental chairperson a balance of the components of the role, which may vary on a quarterly basis.

CLINICAL

1. Functions as a clinical practitioner in area(s) of expertise.
2. Assists in planning and implementing health education programs for patients and families with the primary nurse.
3. Collaborates with the health care team to assess, plan, direct, and evaluate the treatment approach.
4. Serves as a resource person to the nursing personnel in the evaluation of nursing care.
5. Serves as a consultant in patient care situations/settings.

ADMINISTRATION

1. Participates in the operational management of the Department, College of Nursing and Division of Nursing.
2. Participates in unit and departmental decision making.
3. Participates in the management of a unit as negotiated with the head nurse/unit leader and departmental leadership.

EDUCATION

1. Directs the learning of students in the clinical setting.
2. Facilitates the learning of students in the classroom setting.

3. Interprets the Rush University programs to patients, staff, and others.
4. Participates in unit and department educational efforts.
5. Participates in the development and implementation of continuing education.

RESEARCH

1. Applies research findings in one's own practice and teaching.
2. Interprets research project findings to nursing staff and students.
3. Collaborates with members of related disciplines in research activities.
4. Assists with the development and implementation of nursing and health related studies.
5. Plans, implements, and publishes studies and projects as negotiated.

QUALIFICATIONS

A professional nurse with the minimum of a clinical master's degree in nursing from an accredited school of nursing, who holds current licensure in the State of Illinois.

(Courtesy of Rush-Presbyterian–St. Luke's Medical Center, Chicago.)

Chapter 17

Legal Considerations in Postanesthesia Nursing

Nancy J. Brent

The practice of nursing has become increasingly complex as medical and scientific advances in the health care field have proliferated. These advances have helped to improve the quality of patient care provided by nurses and other health professionals. In addition, the advances have also created the need for the health professional to continually update his or her skills and knowledge in order to provide nonnegligent care to the consumer of health care. The PACU nurse is not exempt from this requirement. An important part of the knowledge base needed for the PACU nurse is a working understanding of the legal issues and concerns inherent in this specialty area. This chapter presents an overview of the concept of professional negligence or professional malpractice. Specific issues for the PACU nurse will be covered, including the scope of practice concerns, the documentation in medical records, and the importance of liability insurance. The nurse-anesthetist's role is also highlighted. Cases involving PACU nurses and nurse-anesthetists are included where possible.[1]

---

[1] This chapter is designed to provide accurate and authoritative information concerning the subject matter presented. It is prepared with the understanding that the author is not engaged in rendering legal or other professional service. If legal advice or other expert assistance is required, the services of a competent professional person should be sought. (Adopted from a Declaration of Principles jointly adopted by a Committee of the American Bar Association and a Committee of Publishers and Associations.)

PROFESSIONAL NEGLIGENCE OR MALPRACTICE

Negligence is included in the law of torts. A "tort" is a wrongful civil act or injury. Torts do not include actions based on contract; rather, the law of torts is concerned with compensating an individual—usually with money—for injury to person, property, or both. (Prosser, 1971, 2.) Before this compensation can occur, however, the allegations of injury must be proven. In relation to an allegation of negligence, certain requisite elements must be proven in order for an injured party to prevail. The four essential elements vital to a cause of action in negligence are:

1. The existence of a duty, established or recognized by law, requiring a person to conform to that duty in order to avoid unreasonable and forseeable risks of harm to another.
2. Failure of the person to uphold or conform his or her behavior to the duty.
3. The failure to conform to the duty must be the "legal cause" or "proximate cause" of injury to the victim.
4. Actual damages recognized by law must be suffered by the victim. (Prosser, 1971, p. 143; Second Restatement of Torts, 1965, ¶ 281.)

In short, then, negligence can be defined as "conduct which falls below the standard established by law for the protection of others against unreasonable risk of harm" (Gifis, 1975), and may involve acts of omission as well as acts of commission. (Second Restatement of Torts, 1965, ¶ 284.) An individual's conduct in a particular situation in which negligence is alleged is compared with the behavior of the ordinary, reasonable, and prudent person in the same or similar circumstances. (Prosser, 1971, 149–165).

It is important to note that every person is responsible for his or her own behavior. As a result, it is generally very difficult to defend oneself against alleged negligent behavior by attempting to reassign one's duty of care to another.

The discussion of negligence thus far has focused on negligence in general. However, it also has applicability to professional negligence or malpractice. Professional negligence concerns itself with the duty(ies) of professionals—including nurses—and whether or not that duty of care is upheld in a certain situation. Although the four elements necessary for a cause of action in negligence presented earlier must also be satisfied when a cause of action in professional negligence is at issue, the standard of conduct by which the professional's behavior will be measured varies slightly. Thus, when professional negligence is alleged, the standard of conduct will be measured by that degree of knowledge and skill customarily used by the (specific) professional in the same or similar circumstances in the same or similar community. Jury instructions may vary from state to state, but the main idea is always the same: that the conduct in a particular situation will be looked at by comparing it to an objective professional standard. If the professional has additional skills and expertise, then the law will hold that professional to a standard of other specialists in the same or similar circumstances in the same or similar community (Prosser, 1971, 149–163).

The laws of torts and negligence also apply to employers, and the employers of nurses are no exception. Under the doctrine of *respondeat superior* or "let the master speak," the employer of a nurse or other health professional can also be held indirectly liable for the negligent actions of an employee if the negligent act occurred during that employee's employment and the employee was acting within the scope of his or her employment (Prosser, 1971, 458–468). Similarly, under the theory of corporate or institutional liability the employer can be held directly liable for its own negligence when it breaches its duty of care to patients in a particular situation. This theory gained support in Darling v. Charleston Community Hospital decided in 1965.[2] These two theories of liability, then, allow an injured patient to select who to include in a negligence action: the employer alone (the hospital or institution), the employer and the employee (the hospital and the nurse), or the employee alone (the nurse).

It is important for PACU nurses to understand how these concepts apply to their practice by exploring several cases that utilize them.

Postanesthesia nursing is a speciality area where the potential for injury to the patient is high. Two major areas of concern for the PACU nurse include failing to perform nursing procedures correctly and following incorrect or inappropriate orders (Rabinow, 1985). In Goldsby v. Evangelical Deaconess Hospital,[3] the failure to follow correct nursing procedures is tragically illustrated. In this case, the patient was admitted to the PACU after an open reduction and internal fixation of a mandibular fracture was performed. The jaws were wired. The patient was extubated in the operating room but a patent airway was present. The patient was received in the PACU in good condition with orders stating how the patient should be positioned and that wire-cutters should be at his bedside at all times.

The PACU nurses then asked a circulating nurse to care for the patient while they attended an in-service program. The circulating nurse, inexperienced in postanesthesia nursing, followed standard PACU procedures and checked the patient 15 minutes after he had arrived in the unit. Unfortunately, however, the patient had suffered an obstructed airway, had suffocated, and could not be resuscitated.

The patient's family filed suit against the anesthesiologist, the oral

---

[2]   211 N.E.2d 53 (1965).
[3]   74-004-754 N.M. (1978).

surgeon, and the hospital. The anesthesiologist and the oral surgeon were dismissed from the suit, but the hospital—as the employer of the nurse involved in the care of the deceased patient—was found liable. At trial, it was discovered that in addition to the negligent care given by the nurse involved, the patient was not positioned as specified by the anesthesiologist's order; nor were the wire-cutters at the patient's bedside.

Likewise, in Laidlow v. Lion Gate Hospital,[4] two nurses in the PACU were observing two patients, an adult and an infant. Five of the operating rooms were scheduled for surgeries on that day. At about 10:25 A.M., one of the nurses—with full knowledge of her supervisor—took a coffee break. Shortly after she left, a third patient was sent to the PACU, and one of the nurses on duty began providing care to her. Soon thereafter, a fourth and fifth patient were admitted to the PACU, and the nurse had to provide care to both of them as well.

The fifth patient was quite restless and his anesthetist ordered an injection of Demoral "stat." The nurse on duty prepared the injection and gave it. As she was completing the injection, the phone rang and the nurse answered it. Upon returning to check the third patient—the one she had been caring for prior to the admission of the fourth and fifth patients—she noticed that the patient was not breathing. The nurse called for assistance from a doctor who was in the PACU at the time making a phone call, and care was provided to the patient. She did survive, but extensive permanent brain damage resulted due to an insufficient supply of oxygen while under the influence of anesthesia in the PACU.

A suit was filed against the hospital as the nurse's employer, alleging negligence on the part of the one nurse in failing to provide the necessary observation of the patient and leaving the patient unattended and unobserved for a long period of time. The charge nurse was also alleged to be negligent under a negligent supervision theory for agreeing to the requested coffee break. Likewise, the nurse who left for the coffee break was also sued for negligence for leaving the PACU when she did.

The court entered a verdict in favor of the injured patient and against the hospital. Testimony and evidence at the trial clearly indicated that two registered nurses were to be on duty in the PACU and relief for coffee breaks was to be arranged prior to patients arriving in the PACU or by obtaining a substitute nurse to provide care if patients had already arrived. Decisions concerning relief were the responsibility of the nursing supervisor, according to the evidence.

The trial court, in deciding the case as it did, said:

> The function of this room [the PACU] is to provide highly specialized care, frequent and careful observation of patients who are under the

---

[4]   70 W.W.R. 727 (1969).

influence of anesthesia. Respiratory arrest is not an uncommon occurrence in the . . . recovery room. . . . The nurses in this room are there for the purpose of promptly recognizing any respiratory problem, cardiovascular problem, or hemmorrhaging. They are expected to take corrective action and/or summon help promptly. . . .

The patient in this room requires the greatest attention because it is fraught with the greatest potential dangers to the patient. This hazard carries with it . . . a high degree of duty owed by the hospital to the patient. . . . There should be no relaxing of vigilance if one is to comply with the standard of care required in this room. . . . (Canadian Nurse, 1970; Hershey, 1970).

The second type of error in the PACU involves following an incorrect order or procedure. This may include not questioning an order for medication or other care that appears incorrect. Clearly, this is a nursing responsibility that has been documented time and time again (Creighton, 1981; Rhodes & Miller, 1984). Other legal risks concerning negligence that PACU nurses should be aware of include, but are not limited to, potential liability for equipment failures, injury to patients when using equipment to provide postsurgical care, medication administration (for example, wrong dose, wrong route, wrong patient), blood transfusion (for example, patient reactions, wrong blood) change in patient condition during transfer from the PACU to the unit (Rabinow, 1985), communicating changes in patient condition to the appropriate health care provider, and intervening to provide care when the patient's condition warrants it (Creighton, 1981; Rhodes & Miller, 1984). Clearly, this potential liability extends not only to PACU nurses but also includes potential liability for negligent supervision or delegation of tasks to others.

The PACU nurse can help to avoid potential liability for negligence by practicing this area of nursing in a preventive manner. Adequate staffing in the PACU is vital. Equally important, however, is competent staffing to perform the care that must be done. Well-developed nursing policies and procedures can help PACU nurses prepare themselves to gain the skills they need in this area of practice. Good documentation of the care given can reflect that standards of care were upheld. Continuing education and constant updating of skills can also aide the PACU nurse in keeping abreast of new information necessary to provide competent, nonnegligent care.

DOCUMENTATION

The medical record is an important document that is used in many ways. In addition to serving as a communication between health professionals providing care to the patient and with risk-management, quality-assurance, third-party reimbursement, hospital-accreditation, and other personnel, the medical record is a legal document that can be used to prove or disprove professional negligence. Because of this possible use, accurate, complete, and timely nursing (and other) entries in the record can be the best defense against a professional negligence suit (Roach, 1985).

This principle is also applicable to the PACU and the nursing entries must be done with this preventive approach in mind. First and foremost, for example, it is vital that the nursing entries be legible. An illegible entry can create difficulties for other health professionals who must read and determine the care already given in order to provide additional care. When negligence is alleged, an illegible entry can be welcome ammunition for an injured patient's attorney.

All nursing entries should be dated and timed pursuant to hospital policy. They should likewise contain objective, factual information concerning the patient and the care provided. Entries reflecting the nurse's opinions and subjective remarks may create more problems than they solve during a lawsuit, especially for the nurse (Roach, 1980).

No erasures should ever be present in the patient's record. If an error in the record occurs, a single line drawn through the error—with the date, nurse's initials, and any other documentation required by the hospital's policies (for example, "error in charting")—should be recorded. Under no circumstances should errors be obliterated, since a question as to what was obliterated can be raised by the patient's attorney and thus raise doubt and suspicion in the minds of the jurors should the case go to trial.

Especially important for the PACU nurse to keep in mind is that no abbreviation should be used in the patient's medical record unless it is capable of being interpreted in only one way. The abbreviation CP, for example, could be interpreted as meaning capillary pressure, constant pressure, cor pulmonale, close pressure (spinal tap), or creatine phosphate, to name a few (Documenting Patient Care Responsibly, 1983). The PACU nurse should use abbreviations with only one meaning. This can be done by developing a hospital policy for the PACU and the rest of the hospital that allows only certain abbreviations with specified meanings to be used in the patient's record.

Nursing entries should always be made in ink, whether they be in narrative form or on a flow sheet or other PACU form. Ink is permanent and it copies well, should a duplicate of the medical record be necessary. Under no circumstances should pencil be utilized for patient care documentation.

In addition to documenting the care and medications given by the PACU nurse, the nurse should also be certain to include the patient's reaction to that care and medication. If, for example, a change in the patient's position due to difficulty in breathing was instituted by the nurse, the nurse should document improvement in the patient's breathing, if present. If not, then any additional interventions necessary should be instituted and those interventions and subsequent patient responses documented.

Along a similar vein, many PACU nurses provide care based on written, standing orders and protocols. When doing so, the nurse should not only document the care provided and the patient's response, but also should document the clinical signs and symptoms observed that she or he utilized in exercising nursing judgment to carry out those orders. In addition to conforming with good nursing practice, PACU nurses who document in this way also protect themselves against any allegations of practicing medicine without a license, a topic discussed at greater length later in this chapter.

The PACU nurse must also be certain that no blank spaces are present in the entries or on any flow sheets or other PACU forms. Blank spaces can again be a welcome piece of information for an injured patient's attorney should there be a question as to whether or not the blank space or ommitted information contributed in some way to the patient's injury. Therefore, a single line should be drawn for any entry which is not completely used by the PACU nurse. If information is requested that is not pertinent to a particular patient's care, then a notation such as "n/a" or a notation contained in the institution's policy and procedure manual concerning documentation should be utilized.

The PACU nurse is often the one who accompanies the patient from the PACU to the medical, surgical, or other postoperative unit. If this is the case, the PACU nurse should document the patient's condition prior to transfer, during transfer, and upon arrival to the unit. If the PACU nurse does not accompany the patient from the PACU, well-documented data concerning the patient's condition prior to transfer are vital.

Although not a complete list of all the documentation guidelines important for the PACU nurse to follow, those discussed can help the nurse document the good patient care given and, at the same time, provide a ready defense against any allegation of malpractice should one arise.

SCOPE OF PRACTICE ISSUES

PACU nurses, like colleagues in other areas of nursing that require expanded role functions, must be concerned with practicing in conformity with the state's nurse practice act. State nurse practice acts, among other things, define professional nursing as including permissible acts, functions, and roles of the professional nurse. Likewise, other practice acts—such as the pharmacy act and the medical practice act—define those respective professions. When the nurse functions in an expanded role, the question often arises if the nurse is truly practicing nursing with a license or one of the other professions without a license. Most often, this question arises in relation to the medical practice act, expecially since nurses are now performing many functions once traditionally within the purview of the physician.

One case which challenged two nurses' expanded role functions was a 1983 Missouri case, Sermchief v. Gonzales.[5] In this case, two nurse-practitioners were charged with practicing medicine without a license by the Missouri State Board of Registration for the Healing Arts after the board investigated them. The nurse practitioners were licensed R.N.s in the State of Missouri and had postgraduate special training in obstetrics and gynecology. Five physicians who had developed individualized, specific written protocols and standing orders for each of the nurse-practitioners were also charged by the board with aiding and abetting the unauthorized practice of medicine. The services provided by the nurse-practitioners pursuant to those written protocols and standing orders included, but were not limited to, history taking; breast and pelvic examinations; dispensing certain medications; community education; performing lab tests of pap smears, blood serology, and gonorrhea cultures; and providing oral contraceptives, IUDs, and condoms.

It is important to note that no allegations were made that any of the nurse's actions caused any injury to the patients they cared for.

Once a formal complaint was filed by the board after its investigation, the nurse-practitioners and the physicians filed a declaratory judgment action and injunction petition in the Missouri circuit court asking the court to hold that the nurse-practitioners were practicing nursing pursuant to the nurse practice act and not medicine, and to enjoin the board from taking any further action, civil or criminal, against them or the physicians until the court made its decision. The trial court held against the nurses and physicians, who then appealed directly to the Missouri Supreme Court.

The Missouri Supreme Court reversed the trial court's decision, holding that the Missouri nurse practice act's language clearly contemplated nurses functioning in expanded roles.[6] In addition, the court noted that there had been wide legislative and public support for that definition. Finally, the court clearly held that a nurse is making a *nursing diagnosis*,

---

[5]   600 S.W.2d 683 (Mo. en banc 1983).

[6]   The definition of nursing in Missouri at the time the case was before the court was: "the performance for compensation of any act which requires substantial specialized education, judgment and skill based on the biological, physical, social and nursing sciences, including but not limited to: (a) responsibility for the teaching of health care and prevention of illness . . . ; (b) assessment, nursing diagnosis, nursing care and counsel of persons who are ill, injured or experiencing alterations in normal health processes; or (c) the administration of medications and treatments as prescribed by a person licensed in this state to prescribe . . . ; or (d) the coordination and assistance in the delivery of a plan of health care with all members of the health team; or (e) the teaching and supervision of other persons in the performance of any of the foregoing." (RSMo Supp. §334.155, 1982)

not a medical one, when following physician-based standing orders and protocols when providing treatment, as the nurses did in this case.

Although not involving PACU nurses, the Sermchief case has implications for nurses in the PACU. Because the PACU nurse often initiates treatment, the importance of written protocols and standing orders cannot be stressed enough in order to avoid the possibility of similar charges against those nurses (Regan, 1970). Likewise, as the Sermchief case discussed, the "hallmark of the professional is knowing the limit of one's professional knowledge" (Regan, 1970). The PACU nurse, then, must know when she or he can no longer handle a particular patient situation, and obtain the appropriate health professional to initiate and prescribe further care. Last but by no means least, PACU nurses must be familiar with their state's definition of professional nursing. In addition, membership and active participation in the many professional associations is vital in order to contribute to those organization's development of the role and functions of professional nursing in general and PACU nursing in particular. Political activism, including the exercise of the privilege of voting, is also necessary to ensure that the respective nurse practice acts truly reflect an accurate and up-to-date definition of professional nursing, which provides a solid legal base for expanded role areas.

LIABILITY INSURANCE

Because most nurses, including PACU nurses, are associated with an institution as an employee, they often do not investigate the value of having their own professional liability insurance. For the most part, this is based on the decision to rely on the professional liability insurance policy their employer has which covers them as employees. In making that decision, however, few nurses are truly informed consumers concerning that reliance. Whether nurses decide to rely solely on their employer for professional liability coverage or decide to purchase their own policy, certain areas should be investigated before making that decision.

To begin with, the nurse should know the definition of professional nursing as it is defined in the policy, as well as any exclusions. For example, most professional liability policies do cover allegations of negligence but do not cover alleged intentional torts such as assault and battery. Likewise, the limits of coverage of the policy should be known.

The obligations of the nurse under the policy should be understood by the insured nurse. Most policies, for example, require that the insured person cooperate fully with the company when a suit has been filed or is being contemplated, and require the insured person to notify the company as soon as possible when those situations arise.

Insured nurses should also know what rights they have under the policy. Can they, for example, have input into the final decision as to whether or not a suit is settled or goes to trial, or is this decision made solely by the company?

Perhaps the most important information the professional nurse should know about a policy is if it is a claims-made or an occurrence policy. Generally, a claims-made policy covers a suit that is filed *only* while the policy is in effect, whereas an occurrence policy will cover any occurrence while the policy is in effect even if the suit is filed *after* the policy is no longer in existence. Occurrence policies provide better protection for the insured nurse, but they are clearly more expensive.

Whatever type of policy and whatever coverage is selected by the professional nurse, carrying her or his own professional liability insurance is vital. Despite employee status, PACU nurses are responsible and accountable for their own negligent acts. To rely on another, then, to carry liability insurance for those acts is contradictory. Likewise, it may be that in certain situations, the PACU nurse's position may not be the same as that of the employer's. If so, relying on the employer's liability insurance may be quite uncomfortable and not legally wise. Additionally, if the nurse is sued individually rather than as an employee, the employer's liability insurance will not be applicable. Finally, should the nurse need to utilize the private liability insurance, a defense attorney is provided for by the policy.

It must be noted that if a PACU nurse functions as an independent contractor or in some type of private practice arrangement, professional liability insurance is vital.

In summary, PACU nurses should carry their own malpractice insurance. Indeed, the premiums are a small price to pay for the peace of mind obtained should a negligence suit be filed against the nurse.

NURSE-ANESTHETISTS

No text on PACU nursing would be complete without acknowledging the nurse-anesthetist. This specialty began in the late 19th century in Erie, Pennsylvania when Sister Mary Bernard, a student nurse at St. Vincent's Hospital, began administering anesthesia (Mannino, 1982). Since that time, nurses have continued to provide anesthesia to patients. The development of the American Association of Nurse Anesthetists and its councils on practice, certification, recertification, and accreditation clearly underscores the acceptance of this specialty area of nursing (Mannino, 1982). Recent statistics indicate that over 50 percent of the anesthesia given in the United States is administered by nurse anesthetists (Biggins, 1971).

Like their professional colleagues, nurse-anesthetists must be concerned with professional liability suits and challenges that they are practicing outside the scope of the state's nurse practice act.[7] Although the latter question was settled in 1936 when a California case held that nurse-anesthetists were practicing nursing and not medicine,[8] many legal challenges to the nurse-anesthetist's practice, and to the quality of that practice, continue.

In addition to legal challenges, nurse-anesthetists must also be concerned with carefully documenting the medications used for anesthesia. One case illustrating this legal duty is Hogan v. Mississippi Board of Nursing.[9] In that case, Patricia Hogan, a certified registered nurse-anesthetist at Lawrence County Hospital in Mississippi, was fired by her employer and charged by the Mississippi Board of Nursing with 17 violations of the state's nurse practice act after a 1981 audit revealed that substantial amounts of Demerol signed out by Hogan could not be accounted for.

The Mississippi Board found Hogan guilty of misappropriation of the missing Demerol, and revoked her license to practice as a registered nurse. Hogan appealed that decision to the Mississippi Supreme Court, arguing that the Nursing Board found only that she had failed to reasonably account for the missing Demerol and had not proven she had misappropriated it by clear and convincing evidence. The court agreed with Hogan's argument, and held that her license should not have been revoked, that her license must be restored, and that her costs for the appeal should be paid by the board. Despite the holding in her favor, the court discussed the lax policies in force in the hospital dealing with narcotics and their dispensation.

It is important to note that although Hogan won her suit, she did not gain back her position at the hospital.

Nurse-anesthetists must also be concerned with the legal duty to be truthful during a lawsuit, despite the results. In Sides v. Duke Hospital,[10] a nurse-anesthetist sued after she was fired from her job because she refused to falsely or incompletely testify in a medical malpractice trial against two physician anesthesiologists and other defendants. The injury that was the subject of the malpractice case was permanent brain damage allegedly caused by the negligent administration of anesthesia by one of the anesthesiologists.

Prior to Side's deposition in the malpractice case, she was told by the attorneys for Duke Univesity Medical Center and the other defendants that she should not tell all she had seen of the patient's treatment, and

---

[7] This is especially so in states in which the Nurse Practice Act does not specifically define nurse-anesthetists. Some states have practice acts that do include a definition of nurse-anesthetists, including Massachusetts, New Mexico, Nevada, South Carolina, and Florida.

[8] Chalmers-Francis v. Nelson, 6 Cal 2d 402 (1936).

[9] 457 So. 2d 931 (1984).

[10] 328 S.E. 2d 818 (1985).

that if she did, she would "be in trouble." Despite these threats, Sides testified truthfully and fully at her deposition and at trial. The jury entered a verdict of $1.75 million in favor of the estate of the injured patient. Shortly after the verdict, Sides was discharged from her job, and she sued alleging wrongful discharge and wrongful interference with her employment contract.

The court, in holding in favor of Sides, discussed at length the at-will employment doctrine, employment by contract, and other legal theories. The court held her firing from the Medical Center should not have occurred, regardless of whether that employment was protected by a contract that was breached by her employers or by the doctrine that at-will employees cannot be discharged for an unlawful reason or purpose that contravenes public policy. Furthermore, the court clearly stated the physicians in the case were motivated by their "malicious and wrongful desire to retaliate against the nurse anesthetist because of her truthful testimony against them in [a] malpractice action."

Nurse-anesthetists must be vigilant to ensure that quality anesthesia care is being provided, that their scope of practice is within the nurse practice act of the state, that documentation of anesthetics given is honest, and complete, and that above all, honesty—despite its ramifications—must always be the principle followed.

SUMMARY

As has been seen, the practice of PACU nursing is not without its legal pitfalls. Yet knowledge of those pitfalls is a good way to avoid being trapped by them. Continued interest in the legal developments in postanesthesia nursing, and nursing in general, can help those pitfalls to disappear.

REFERENCES

Biggens D, et al.: Survey of anesthesia service—1971. American Association of Nurse Anesthetists Journal 39:5, 1971.
Canadian Nurse. Negligence in the recovery room. Canadian Nurse 66:26, July, 1970.
Creighton H: Law Every Nurse Should Know (4th ed.). Philadelphia: Saunders, 1981.
Documenting Patient Care Responsibly. Springhouse, Pa.: Intermed Communications, 1983.
Gifis S: Law Dictionary. New York: Barron's, 1975.
Hershey N: Prudence and the coffee break. American Journal of Nursing 70:2389, Nov., 1970.

Mannino MJ: The Nurse Anesthetist and the Law. New York: Grune & Stratton, 1982.

Prosser W: Handbook on the Law of Torts (4th ed.). St. Paul: West, 1971.

Rabinow J: Avoiding legal risks in the O.R. Nursing Life 5:6, 1985.

Regan W: Clinical problems. Regan Report on Nursing Law 10: 4, 1970.

Rhodes A & Miller R: Nursing and the Law (4th ed.). Rockville, Md.: Aspen, 1984, chap. 7.

Roach WH, et al.: Responsible intervention: A legal duty to act. Journal of Nursing Administration 7:23–24, 1980.

Reach WH, et al.: Medical Records and the Law. Rockville, Md.: Aspen, 1985.

Second Restatement of Torts. 1965.

Index

Italicized *t* and *f* indicate tables and figures, respectively.